Texts in developmental psychology

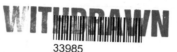

33985

Series Editor
Peter Smith

D0276367

TEXTS IN DEVELOPMENTAL PSYCHOLOGY SERIES

Published titles:
FRIENDS AND ENEMIES
Barry Schneider

CHILDREN'S INTERACTIONS IN SCHOOL
Peter Blatchford and Anthony Pellegrini

Forthcoming titles:
AGEING AND DEVELOPMENT
Peter Coleman

CHILDREN'S LITERACY DEVELOPMENT
Catherine McBride-Chang

Attachment and development

Susan Goldberg BA MS PhD
Psychiatry Research Unit, Hospital for Sick Children, Toronto

Hodder Arnold

A MEMBER OF THE HODDER HEADLINE GROUP

Class no.
155.418 Gol
Accession no.
33985
Date catalogued
10.09.09

First published in Great Britain in 2000
This impression reprinted in 2007 by
Hodder Arnold, an imprint of Hodder Education
and a member of the Hodder Headline Group,
an Hachette Livre UK Company,
338 Euston Road, London NW1 3BH

www.hoddereducation.co.uk

© 2000 Susan Goldberg

All rights reserved. No part of this publication may be reproduced or transmitted in
any form or by any means, electronically or mechanically, including photocopying,
recording or any information storage or retrieval system, without either prior
permission in writing from the publisher or a licence permitting restricted copying.
In the United Kingdom such licences are issued by the Copyright Licensing Agency:
Saffron House, 6-10 Kirby Street, London EC1N 8TS.

The advice and information in this book are believed to be true and accurate at the
date of going to press, but neither the authors nor the publisher can accept any legal
responsibility or liability for any errors or omissions.

British Library Cataloguing in Publication Data
A catalogue entry for this book is available from the British Library

Library of Congress Cataloging-in-Publication Data
A catalog record for this book is available from the Library of Congress

ISBN 978 0 340 73171 0

8 9 10

Typeset by J&L Composition Ltd, Fiely, North Yorkshire
Printed and bound in India by Replika Press Pvt. Ltd.

What do you think about this book? Or any other Hodder Arnold title?
Please visit our website at www.hoddereducation.co.uk

Contents

Preface

Writing this book was not my idea. I was approached by the editors of the series and asked whether I would be interested in contributing to it with a volume on a topic of my own choosing. At first I demurred, not on the grounds that I had nothing to say, nor because I find writing onerous (it is one of my favourite activities), but because I could not imagine adding the task of writing a textbook to my ongoing responsibilities. By the time I was pressed to reconsider, the idea of attempting a broad, integrated and critical view of attachment theory and research had become appealing. In 1998, attachment dominated the study of parent–child relationships and their effects on development, and had produced numerous edited volumes on specific aspects of attachment, as well as one textbook. Moreover, this work had provoked several vehement controversies. It seemed that a critical review of attachment theory and research was now overdue.

I undertook this task as one who has worked in the field of parent–child relationships for many years, both before and after attachment came on the scene. In fact, I was one of the original sceptics. When I moved to the Hospital for Sick Children in Toronto in 1981, I joined a team studying development of preterm infants and assessing infant attachment at 1 year. No one had yet learned to score the videotapes of these assessments, and I volunteered to do so. Training was minimal at that time. I spent two half days with Everett Waters, correctly classified 10 videotapes that included only episodes with the mother, and was sent on my way! Somewhere in the process, I became intrigued and joined the world of attachment researchers. However, I remained someone primarily asking other questions who found attachment theory and methodology useful in the process, rather than an attachment researcher *per se*. In writing this volume, I do so both as an 'insider' and as an 'outsider,' and I hope that this perspective enables the reader to understand and appreciate attachment work while simultaneously grasping its limits and limitations.

Two significant events in the world of attachment marked the last months of this endeavour. To my great chagrin, the long-awaited *Handbook of Attachment* became available just as I was putting the finishing touches to this manuscript. Of course, it is a book I should have read from cover to cover before attempting my own, but such are the ways of the publishing world. Chapters of the *Handbook* cited in this book are either ones that were made available to me as preprints, or ones which I raced through the moment my copy arrived. I hope that these limited references will alert those who are serious about pursuing attachment work to this valuable resource.

The second was a less happy event, namely the death of Mary Ainsworth in March 1999. I wish she had been able to read this book. Her approval of its contents would have meant a great deal to me. Because she was so instrumental in initiating the research traditions on which this book is based, thinking of her reminds me of the debt I owe to those cited in the text and the many pages of references. Some are friends and colleagues, some acquaintances, and some only faceless names attached to books and journal articles. However, some have had a more direct impact on this work.

First there are the many colleagues, students and fellows with whom I shared working days, conferences, symposia, runs, dinners and/or friendships. These have all been opportunities for me to beg, borrow and steal ideas shamelessly, but often they were pressed upon me! In many cases I no longer know exactly whose ideas they are, but some of the most likely culprits are Canadian colleagues from Ontario and Quebec, especially David Pederson and Greg Moran, with whom I pondered, discussed and argued about the mysteries of attachment through the years of Home County Attachment Workshops. Joan Grusec, Jennifer Jenkins and I taught a graduate seminar on attachment and subsequently used that experience to write a 'thought paper' that has infiltrated Chapter 15. Parts of Chapters 5 and 9 were published in French as a single book chapter.

Although writing is often a solitary task, I felt supported by the many colleagues who responded generously to questions about their work, engaged in e-mail dialogues, and sent reprints and preprints. I cannot list them all, as to do so would surely exceed my space allotment, and I would be bound to omit someone. You know who you are and I am grateful for your help. The list of those who intended to help but who never got round to it is shorter and easier to compile, but it would be graceless to include it. (You know who you are as well!) I do want to thank publicly those who read drafts of chapters and saved me from embarrassing errors. George Tarabulsy read parts of Chapters 5 and 9 in their previous incarnation. Deborah Finkel read the genetics section of Chapter 5, Leslie Atkinson read Chapter 10, Emma Adam and Megan Gunnar read Chapter 12, and Robert Maunder read Chapter 14. Undoubtedly, some embarrassments remain. They are my responsibility and I shall undoubtedly hear about them from diligent readers.

Finally, I owe a significant debt to the Hospital for Sick Children, not only for being my intellectual home for close to 20 years, but for granting me the sabbatical leave during which this book was written.

Susan Goldberg
Toronto, July 1999

Part I

Introduction

1 Origins of attachment theory

In our time, the view that parent–child relationships play a central role in a child's psychological development has been widely accepted. Periodically there are valiant efforts to dislodge this belief from its prominent position – such as the *Nurture Assumption* (Harris, 1998) and *Altering Fate* (Lewis, 1997) – but they appear to have had little effect on the prevailing ideology. These convictions are so strong that it is hard to believe that, until recently, it has proved difficult to amass convincing empirical evidence to document the importance of parent–child relationships in development. Attachment theory and the research that it generated played an important role in producing this evidence. Clearly the human infant is not equipped to survive without adult caregivers who provide food, warmth, and protection from illness and injury. Yet our intuitive concepts go beyond the confines of physical care and include the notion that individual differences in later functioning – indeed, the core of personality – are shaped by the experiences we have with a small number of early caregivers. The emergence of attachment theory, as articulated by John Bowlby, and the discovery by Mary Ainsworth of a way to assess individual differences in attachment behaviour patterns, laid the groundwork for intensive, ongoing, fruitful attempts to examine the psychological effects of early relationships. In this chapter, we shall trace the origins of these ideas and introduce the rest of the volume. Bretherton (1992), Grossmann (1995) and Holmes (1993) provide excellent detailed historical accounts of attachment theory and research.

Empirical roots

One logical way to understand the effects of early care and relationships is to examine what happens in their absence. Thus some of the first attempts to study the psychological effects of early care focused on the development of children raised without the benefit of a consistent caregiver, namely those reared in orphanages. In the 1940s when orphanages were common in North America, there were many such studies and they indicated not only that these children were developmentally delayed, but also that their social and emotional behaviour was unusual. They did not seem to form close relationships, and were instead described as inappropriately friendly towards everyone, including strangers (e.g. Bender and Yarnell, 1941;

Goldfarb, 1943a; Skodak and Skeels, 1949; Spitz, 1945, 1946). When they were later adopted or reared in foster homes, improvements were noted in many domains, but some cognitive and affective defects persisted (e.g. Goldfarb, 1943a, 1943b, 1945).

These data were generally interpreted as the effects of 'maternal deprivation' (Bowlby, 1951; Goldfarb, 1955; Spitz, 1956), and this view was buttressed by the now classic experiment of Skodak and Skeels (Skeels, 1966; Skodak and Skeels, 1949). They found that orphanage children who were moved to an institution for mentally retarded adults were usually 'adopted' by a particular older resident who lavished individual attention and affection on them. These children were more likely to develop normally, leave the institution and become fully contributing members of society than those who remained in the orphanage. Now we are more aware that the privations of institutional care cannot be attributed to maternal deprivation alone. They include the absence of fathers, siblings and a family context. Nevertheless, at the time, these data played a major role in formulations concerning the mother–child relationship. They were also a catalyst for the demise of institutional care for young children and the increasing use of foster care placements as an alternative. Ironically, when current forms of foster-care break down and children experience repeated placements, the resulting psychological effects are highly consonant with earlier descriptions of institutionalized children (Karen, 1994, chapter 1).

Other attempts to understand the role of early care in development were being made through naturalistic observations of animal behaviour as well as laboratory studies where rearing conditions could be experimentally manipulated. For example, ethologists documented the phenomenon of imprinting in precocial birds (those in which infants are mobile at birth). The term 'imprinting' was introduced by Lorenz (1935) in his studies of behaviour in geese, and there was subsequently much debate as to how imprinting should be defined (e.g. Bateson, 1966; Sluckin, 1965). The general notion is that during a 'critical' or 'sensitive' period shortly after birth, exposure to a specific figure sets in motion a series of behavioural processes that result in later preferential behaviour (e.g. following, mating) towards that figure. Under normal rearing conditions, this figure is a biologically appropriate one (the mother or another species member), but experimental manipulations can lead to striking examples of imprinting on anomalous figures – for example, the famous photograph of Konrad Lorenz being followed by a line of goslings. Related behavioural phenomena were also observed in maternal behaviour. Among sheep and goats (Hersher et al., 1958), if the young are removed from the mother shortly after birth for a prolonged period, she will not accept them back into her care. Thus the initial experiences of the mother sheep or goat influence caregiving behaviour. Data such as these suggest that early contact between mother and infant has an important biological function which normally ensures or enhances caregiving and development.

In his Wisconsin Primate Laboratory, Harry Harlow and his colleagues began their studies of rhesus monkeys raised with various types of 'mother surrogates.' These studies originated in a very practical problem, namely how to rear monkeys under laboratory conditions. Wire frames covered with terry cloth to which monkeys could cling for comfort, and attached bottles containing food allowed the monkeys to grow and develop in a fashion that initially appeared normal, particularly when some exposure to peers was provided (Harlow and Harlow, 1962). Later studies (Harlow and Harlow, 1965) showed that this type of rearing resulted in abnormal social behaviours, namely inability to mingle with peers and have normal sexual relations and, if females were impregnated, grossly neglecting and/or abusive behaviour towards their infants.

Bowlby and the beginnings of attachment theory

This information on the effects of early experience in the absence of normal care was accumulating at the time when John Bowlby's clinical experience was drawing him towards intensive consideration of the nature of early mother–child relationships. Bowlby entered the field of child psychiatry after working as a volunteer at a school for maladjusted children, where he was struck by the impoverished family lives of some of his young charges. These observations convinced him that family life was important to emotional development and its problems, and that appropriate treatment for maladjustment required family involvement. However, this was not the custom of the time, and Bowlby's ideas engendered much conflict with his analytic supervisors, Melanie Klein and Joan Riviere. He also diverged increasingly from many of his psychoanalytic colleagues (who were preoccupied with internal phantasy) in believing that children's actual experiences form the basis of their notions about themselves, others and relationships. Perhaps it was his childhood experience of growing up between a slightly older brother (with whom he competed) and a younger brother of more limited talents (towards whom he felt protective) that spurred Bowlby on to challenge current doctrine and champion the needs of young children (Holmes, 1993). Perhaps it was the experience of being raised by relatively distant parents who valued individual achievements, but Bowlby was determined to produce evidence in support of his position. His first empirical paper (Bowlby, 1944) was based on case-notes from experiences at the London Child Guidance Clinic. In it he presented the histories of 44 juvenile thieves to show links between their affectionless behaviour and their childhood experiences of chaotic families marked by lack of a consistent caregiver.

After World War II, he became head of the Children's Department at the Tavistock Clinic, where he again found himself at odds with staff clinicians who dismissed family interactions as relatively unimportant. Consequently, he established his own research unit in order to focus on family experiences and mother–child separation in particular. Here he collaborated with John Robertson in collecting data on hospitalization and its effects on children. Parent visiting in hospital at the time was minimal, discouraged and tightly controlled. The feeling among hospital staff was that parental visits were 'upsetting' to children, and that these upsets made the children more diffi-cult to manage. Robertson found the grief and pain he observed in his young subjects so upsetting that he was moved to do something to help them (Holmes, 1995). As a result, Robertson (1953) produced *A Two-Year-Old Goes to Hospital*, a simple documentary film of the heart-wrenching experiences of one child. This film had a powerful impact and played a major role in initiating changes in hospital practices that supported and encouraged parental involvement in children's care in hospital.

Soon afterwards, Bowlby was asked by the World Health Organization (WHO) to prepare a report on the mental health of homeless children. The resulting monograph, *Maternal Care and Mental Health* (Bowlby, 1951) was published in a popular edition, *Child Care and the Growth of Maternal Love* (Bowlby, 1953), and became an instant best-seller. Its major conclusion, based on the available empirical evidence, was that in order to develop normally, it is necessary for the infant/young child to experience a 'warm, intimate, and continuous relationship with his mother (or permanent mother substitute)'. However, Bowlby felt that this statement required a theoretical explanation. His traditional theoretical orientation, namely psycho-analysis, was problematic, for despite his public success, he was a highly controversial figure and much criticized by psychoanalysts. Soon he found himself seeking out friendlier colleagues in other disciplines, especially ethology, and engaging them in ongoing seminars. His efforts at theoretical elucidation, culminating in the major three-volume work, *Attachment and Loss* (Bowlby, 1969, 1973, 1980), reflect these efforts to marry ethology, psychoanalysis and developmental research.

Enter Ainsworth

Mary Salter Ainsworth arrived at the Tavistock Clinic in 1950 when Bowlby's work on the WHO monograph had already started. She had completed her doctorate 10 years earlier at the University of Toronto as a student of William Blatz, with a thesis entitled 'An Evaluation of Adjust-ment on the Concept of Security' (Salter, 1940). Blatz's theory of security was anchored in the belief that the experience of security within the family forms the basis from which individuals branch out as they mature and develop new skills and interests. In fact, he used the term 'secure base' (now so fundamental to attachment theory) to describe the role that this early family experience plays in later exploration.

While she was at the Tavistock Clinic, one of Ainsworth's projects was to work on data from the hospitalization study. In 1953, she left for Uganda where her husband had a research position, intending to pursue the theme of mother–child separations. She was thoroughly familiar with Bowlby's developing thoughts on attachment, but was not convinced that his ideas about ethology were useful to her own work on the development of infant–mother relationships (Ainsworth and Marvin, 1995). Her plan was to conduct a study among the Ganda, who traditionally separated infants from their mothers as part of the weaning process. When she found that this practice was no longer common, she reoriented her work to study the development of infant–mother attachment, and it was the resulting obser-vations that shifted her thinking to be more consonant with that of Bowlby. This work was undertaken before Bowlby actually published the seminal papers in which he laid out attachment theory (Bowlby, 1958, 1959, 1960). When he wrote the first volume of the 'Attachment Trilogy' (Bowlby, 1969), it was one of only two existing empirical studies that informed his analysis of attachment in humans. The other, by Schaffer and Emerson (1964), was based on conducting interviews with 60 mothers of infants every 2 weeks over the first 12 months of the infant's life and then again when the infant was 18 months old. These interviews focused on the types of infant behaviours considered to be important for attachment (separation protest, clinging, following, reaching to be picked up), and the individuals towards whom infants directed these behaviours. Ainsworth was not the first to make direct observations of infant–mother interactions, but the Ganda study and the work in Baltimore that followed it were the first studies to be framed by the concepts most relevant to attachment.

When Ainsworth returned to North America, she initiated a study in Baltimore designed to explore further the ideas generated by her work in Uganda. In this study she followed 26 mother–infant pairs with intensive home observations every 3 weeks during the first year of life. Separations in the home environment in Baltimore proved to be much less distressing than those she had observed in Uganda. In an attempt to examine more stressful brief separations, mother–infant dyads were brought into the laboratory at the end of the first year for a series of structured separations and reunions. The format of the observation session was inspired by Bowlby's ideas, as well as Ainsworth's own elaborations, with particular emphasis on the concept of the caregiver providing a secure base for explor-ation (Ainsworth and Wittig, 1969). This structured sequence, which was called the 'strange situation,' enabled Ainsworth to detect three different patterns of infant attachment behaviour and to link them to the previous home observations (Ainsworth et al., 1978).

The idea that individual differences in a 25-minute structured laboratory observation could be a marker for behaviour in the home soon led to widespread use of the strange situation as an assessment of attachment, and rapidly accumulating data to validate its use. Indeed, it was the existence of this empirical tool that formed the basis for the rapidly proliferating research on attachment, attempts to develop parallel assessment tools for other age groups, and elaboration of theory concerning individual differences in attachment patterns, their origins and consequences.

An introduction to attachment theory

General functions and operation of the attachment system

Bowlby's original exposition argued that affectional ties between children and their caregivers have a biological basis that is best understood in an evolutionary context. Since human infants do not survive without adult care, our evolutionary history has selected 'prewired' dispositions on the part of both infants and adults to behave in ways that increase the likelihood of the infant's survival. Thus infants are biased to behave in ways that maintain and enhance proximity to caregivers and elicit their care and investment. Conditions that threaten health and survival (i.e. when the infant is tired, ill or faced by external dangers in the environment) serve as triggers to evoke their attachment behaviours. Similarly, adults are biased to engage in protective behaviour in response to infant signals of exhaustion, illness or perception of danger, and to monitor, prevent and/or alter potentially dangerous situations. This focus on protection and its central role in early infant–caregiver relationships was both innovative and unique. While other theories of the time emphasized the role of the caregiver in reducing physiological arousal (e.g. psychoanalytical theory) and teaching (e.g. learning theory), attachment theory focused on caregivers as protectors and providers of safety and the psychological concomitant of security.

Sometimes the concepts of attachment theory are confused with those of bonding (Klaus and Kennell, 1976). The latter was introduced to describe the emotional bonds that parents form with their children, and the processes by which this occurs. Although this is now thought to be a lifelong process, much of the initial emphasis was on the impact of events surrounding birth and delivery. In contrast, attachment theory has focused on the processes whereby infants and young children develop confidence in their parents' protection.

During the first year, the infant's repertoire of proximity-promoting behaviours (both orienting signals such as vocalizations and cries, and direct actions such as approaching and clinging) become organized into a goal-oriented behaviour system focused on a specific caregiver. This first attachment figure is usually the mother, but can be any individual who has been consistently responsive to the infant's signals. Eventually there may be several attachment figures, but early on Bowlby emphasized the concept of 'monotropy,' namely a bias to have a hierarchy of preferences, with one highly preferred primary attachment figure.

When the attachment behavioural system is in its goal state (i.e. there is adequate proximity and contact for the environmental conditions), attachment behaviours are not evident, but if threats to safety are perceived, attachment behaviours are activated. Bowlby envisioned the attachment system operating in the context of other behavioural systems (e.g. exploration, sociability) with its 'set goal' adjusted to fit the context. Thus the healthy 12-month-old in a safe environment may be comfortable enough to move some distance away from the attachment figure within the same room, but if the infant becomes tired, encounters an unfamiliar person or place, or the attachment figure moves out of their visual range, the goal is 'reset' for greater proximity and/or contact. The goals of the attachment system are also modified as the child develops, so that longer separations and greater distances are deemed to be 'safe.'

This concept of attachment includes social, emotional, cognitive and behavioural components. Attachment is a property of social relationships in which a weaker, less skilled individual relies on a more competent and powerful one for protection. Each participant experiences emotional ties to the other and forms an internal representation (which Bowlby called a 'working model') of the relationship and its participants, and the participants engage in behaviours that reflect and maintain the relationship. It is the nature of and relationships between components that change with development.

In particular, cognitive components and internal working models play an increasingly important role as the child matures into adulthood. Bowlby used the term 'working model' to indicate that these representations are influenced by experience and are subject to change as new experiences accumulate. However, the manner in which new information is added to or integrated in the model is shaped by its existing nature. Hence the effects of early experiences are carried forward in these models, even as they undergo change. Furthermore, Bowlby believed that some aspects of these internal working models, particularly those that are not accessible to consciousness, would be especially resistant to change. Each individual's working model of a particular relationship includes concepts of the self and the other, as well as expectations of the relationship. With development and experience, a general working model of relationships evolves which reflects an aggregation of experiences in different relationships. Presumably some relationships are more influential than others in shaping this model.

In contrast to the passive role given to the infant in many theories, the infant's active signalling is crucial to the process of forming and maintaining attachments from birth onwards. Likewise, although initially they are not very elaborate, infants do form internal working models. Because they are not encoded linguistically, aspects of working models that are laid down in infancy are relatively inaccessible to consciousness, and are thus (for Bowlby) included among the features of internal working models that are difficult (but not necessarily impossible) to change.

Rather than viewing early attachment as a stage to be outgrown and supplanted, attachment theory assumes that attachments can endure throughout the lifespan even as they undergo developmental transformations. A striking example of adult attachment to a parent is the comment made by a 40-year-old woman after her mother's death: 'I never realized, until she was gone, how much my own sense of confidence depended on knowing that if I ran into trouble I could always go to her for help and advice.' However, with developmental change and experience, new attachment figures may be added to the hierarchy and the relative preferences for attachment figures may also change. Thus, in adulthood, one may prefer a friend or other peer to a parent as a primary attachment figure.

Individual differences

Bowlby's focus on the universal facets of attachment, its evolutionary history, functions and course of development was soon supplanted by interest in individual differences. As was noted earlier, Ainsworth's observations of infant behaviour in the strange situation were the main catalyst for this shift. Bowlby was not uninterested in individual differences. The clinical work that led him to develop his theory presented him with striking individual differences. Even in the first volume of the trilogy, *Attachment* (Bowlby, 1969), which devotes 15 of 17 chapters to evolutionary origins and functions of attachment, individual differences in human attachment are featured in the last two chapters. However, data on individual differences in human attachment were scarce. As he wrote the second and third volumes of the trilogy, *Separation, Anxiety and Anger* (Bowlby, 1973) and *Loss, Sadness and Depression* (Bowlby, 1980), there was an increasing body of research on individual differences in attachment patterns to inform this work.

Ainsworth's typology identified three basic patterns in infancy, which she called 'secure,' 'avoidant,' and 'resistant' (or 'ambivalent') on the basis of distinctive organization of behaviour in the strange situation. Secure infants gave evidence of confidence in the mother's ability to provide comfort, avoidant infants seemed oddly unconcerned with the mother's presence or absence, and resistant infants seemed to be preoccupied with getting maternal attention/contact to the exclusion of other activities. In Ainsworth's Baltimore sample and several other early studies (Ainsworth *et al.*, 1978), these patterns of behaviour in the strange situation were linked to behaviour observed in the home. These links and subsequent demonstrations that behaviour in the strange situation was related to later features of social development established the validity of the strange situation as a tool for assessing the quality of early attachment relationships.

The first 10–15 years of research on the strange situation were devoted to collecting normative data and documenting the precursors and sequelae of these three patterns. Detailed descriptions of the three patterns will be presented in Chapter 2, and data from these studies will be discussed in detail in subsequent chapters. Typically, these studies report differences between secure and insecure infants in both previous experience and later functioning.

Attempts to study clinical populations (e.g. infants born prematurely, those who were maltreated, or offspring of depressed mothers) soon followed. Although there had always been a small number of infants who did not readily fit into one of Ainsworth's original patterns, work in these clinical populations produced significantly larger groups of 'unclassifiable' infants, as well as anomalous results such as the finding that the behaviour of a substantial number of maltreated infants fitted the description for the secure classification. These difficulties soon led Mary Main (who received her doctorate under Ainsworth's tutelage) and her students to review large numbers of unclassifiable and anomalous strange situations. The concrete result of this review was the introduction of a fourth classification, which was not a distinct pattern of organization but was characterized by lack of organization or breakdown in organized attachment behaviour. Main and Solomon (1986, 1990) termed these infants 'disorganized/disoriented' with respect to attachment, and evidence that this pattern occurred with a high frequency among maltreated infants and those with depressed mothers led to the notion that disorganized attachment is a very insecure pattern.

Beyond infancy

Bowlby considered attachment to be a feature of selected relationships throughout the lifespan. Most of the initial research focused on infancy, and theoretical developments reflected this interest, with a focus on how early attachments develop and a search for mechanisms that could account for the influence of attachment on subsequent development. However, the initial theory asserted that attachments themselves change and develop beyond infancy, and the need for assessment of attachment in other age groups eventually emerged. Attempts to develop such assessments led to parallel classification schemes for preschool children (Cassidy and Marvin with the MacArthur Working Group, 1987), 5 to 7-year-olds (Main and Cassidy, 1988), and adults (George *et al.*, 1984), with others well under way (e.g. Hillburn-Cobb, 1996). Such developments opened up the possibility of tracking attachment relationships over time, the study of stability and change in attachment patterns, and consideration of the mechanisms which serve to maintain and alter attachment patterns. These concerns are very much a part of attachment research and evolving attachment theory.

Clinical concerns: another look

The rapid proliferation of attachment research and its continuing expansion resulted in a massive body of data documenting links between the quality of early experience in the attachment relationship and subsequent development. Although there is much critical discussion in the field on interpretation, meaning and problems with the data, the net result is a body of evidence which provides a scientific basis that was previously lacking for evaluating assumptions underlying clinical work. By virtue of the sheer mass of studies (both completed and ongoing), attachment research and its underlying ideas have become familiar to many clinicians. In fact, 'attachment' has become the term that is commonly used to refer to infant–parent relationships (sometimes inappropriately) by many who have little idea of its theoretical underpinnings.

The expansion of attachment ideas into the clinical domain was enhanced by studies in which developmental researchers chose to study clinical populations (e.g. maltreated children) and necessarily engaged their clinical colleagues in these efforts. A further impetus came from the development of a method for assessing attachment in adults, namely the Adult Attachment Interview (George *et al.*, 1985), whose content was readily recognized by clinicians as being consonant with material elicited from clients during assessment and therapy. Edited volumes began to appear with such titles as *Clinical Implications of Attachment* (Belsky and Nezworski, 1988) and *Attachment and Psychopathology* (Atkinson and Zucker, 1997), testifying to the bridges being built between researchers and clinicians. Although these bridges are as yet incomplete, Bowlby (who died in 1990) was fortunate to be long-lived enough to see many of his formerly controversial views widely accepted even by some of the very psychoanalysts who had once been his antagonists. Similarly, Mary Ainsworth (who died in 1999 as this book was being completed) encountered much controversy and criticism in the early years of her attachment work, but lived to receive many enthusiastic accolades and awards. Together, Bowlby and Ainsworth exerted a powerful influence on our views of children and parent–child relationships, and inspired the scholarly endeavours that form the basis for this book.

The rest of this book

The remainder of this book is organized into three general sections. The remaining two chapters in Part I elaborate the discussion of the development of attachment in infancy (Chapter 2) and beyond (Chapter 3), and introduce the variety of methods that have been or are being developed to assess individual differences in attachment. Armed with an understanding of how attachment is assessed, we shall proceed in Part II of the book to consider those factors which influence the development of attachment patterns. In successive chapters, we shall consider the influence of the primary caregiver (Chapter 4), the infant (Chapter 5), the family (Chapter 6) and influences beyond the family (Chapter 7). A separate chapter is devoted to the influence of particularly adverse early experiences such as maltreatment or institutional care (Chapter 8). Part III is concerned with the influences of attachment on different aspects of development, namely emotion regulation (Chapter 9), information-processing (Chapter 10), social competence (Chapter 11) and physiology (Chapter 12). The role of attachment in these developmental phenomena is indicative of the broader implications of attachment for general health and well-being, which form the subject matter of Part IV. Here we discuss both mental health (Chapter 13) and physical health (Chapter 14). Part V (Chapter 15) is an attempt to evaluate critically the contributions of attachment theory and research.

Selection of material

One of the purposes of a textbook such as this is to introduce students to the primary sources on which it draws – in this case, empirical and theoretical papers on attachment. The literature in most domains is extensive, and it is impossible to review all of the studies that bear upon each issue. Therefore, instead of trying to review each area comprehensively when studies are numerous, individual studies are introduced primarily as examples. Wherever possible I shall refer to comprehensive reviews. These reviews not only provide a good overview of a topic area, but have inclusive bibliographies that will be useful to the student who wishes to pursue the topic.

Many of these reviews are described as 'meta-analyses' or 'statistical reviews.' I use these terms interchangeably. For those who have not previously encountered meta-analyses, these are endeavours which aggregate data from related studies and subject them to statistical analysis. The advantage of such statistical reviews is that they allow hypotheses to be evaluated for large numbers of subjects with much greater statistical power than can be achieved in individual studies. They can also provide answers to questions that cannot be asked of individual studies. For example, we can ask whether studies which used one measure of attachment differ significantly from those that used a different measure, or whether published studies differ from unpublished ones. The potential limitation of such meta-analyses is that they are dependent on the quality of the original studies and the soundness of the strategies used by the investigator to aggregate information.

A philosophy of science

Attachment theory is no longer a single theory. There are as many versions of attachment theory as there are attachment researchers. Although I make every effort to represent some of this diversity, in the end I am telling the story of attachment theory and research from my own particular perspective. The ground rules of science are designed to create a filter of objectivity through which we seek to understand the world, but they are imposed not upon a blank slate but on existing schemas. When I was an undergraduate, I had a philosophy professor who repeatedly asserted that what we call 'data' (that which is given) should more accurately be called 'capta' (that which is taken). We do not begin our study of attachment or any other phenomenon without preconceptions about where and how to look and what kinds of phenomena are salient. Although my goal is to provide a comprehensive overview of the attachment field, I too have been selective – in deciding both what topics to cover and which sources to review and reference.

Attachment theory and research have been controversial, and much of what is said in the following pages may be hotly contested. Where there has been open controversy, I try to give a fair presentation of the different perspectives. However, in the end I have a preferred 'story' and cannot be fully objective. I do not think I am unique in this respect. I believe that the best opportunity for objectivity is provided by explicit presentation and identification of the perspective from which the story is told. I find the concepts of attachment theory very appealing, yet it is clear that some predictions lack empirical support. I also believe that some of the most interesting predictions of attachment theory have not been adequately pursued, often because researchers have been stymied by practical problems in doing so. I encourage the student to recognize and critique the biases embedded in the text as a central part of the adventure on which we shall now embark.

Suggested reading

Ainsworth, M.D.S. and Marvin, R.S. (1995) On the shaping of attachment theory and research: an interview with Mary D.S. Ainsworth (Fall 1994). In Waters, E., Vaughn, B.E., Posada, G. and Kondo-Ikemura, K. (Eds), Caregiving, cultural and cognitive perspectives on secure-base behaviour and working models. *Monographs of the Society for Research in Child Development* **60**, 3–24.
Mary Ainsworth's backward glance and reflections on her work and its offshoots guided by a former member of her Baltimore research team, an eminent theorist and researcher in his own right.

Bretherton, I. (1992) The origins of attachment theory: John Bowlby and Mary Ainsworth. *Developmental Psychology* **28**, 759–75.
An historical account of the Bowlby–Ainsworth collaborations and their contributions.

Grossmann, K.E. (1995) The evolution and history of attachment research and theory. In Goldberg, S., Muir, R. and Kerr, J. (Eds) *Attachment theory: social, developmental, and clinical perspectives*. Hillsdale, NJ: The Analytic Press, 85–122.
The origins of attachment theory in the broad historical and cultural context.

Holmes, J. (1993) *John Bowlby and attachment theory*. London: Routledge.
The official biography of Bowlby and an analysis of his theories by a psychoanalyst with an elegant writing style.

2 Early development and assessment of attachment in infancy

The major impetus for the empirical study of attachment was the development of a convincing methodology for assessing infant attachment. Although, as we shall see, the emergence of the current dominant methodology was somewhat serendipitous, it arose in the context of naturalistic study of the development of infant–mother relationships and reflected a consensus that, regardless of the theoretical framework adopted, the formation of a special relationship with a primary caregiver is consolidated by the end of the infant's first year of life and is a major developmental milestone. We shall briefly review the early development of attachment before considering its assessment.

Development of attachment in infancy

There are now many accounts of the initial development of the primary infant–caregiver relationship. Whether based in attachment theory or not, there is general agreement that there is an initial phase (encompassing the first few weeks of life) during which there is little evidence of discriminative orientation or signalling to specific caregivers, a second phase (encompassing the remainder of the first 6–7 months) during which preferences begin to develop, followed by the clear emergence and consolidation of a special relationship. Bowlby and Ainsworth agreed on three developmental phases which occur during infancy and a fourth phase that is initiated in the preschool years. Ainsworth (1973) provided detailed descriptions of the infant phases, which she called 'preattachment,' 'attachment-in-the-making' and 'clear-cut attachment,' respectively.

Bowlby envisioned the human infant as having evolved with a bias towards forming social relationships. Thus from birth the neonate is equipped with a repertoire of behaviours designed to attract the attention of adult caregivers and to respond to the caregiver's reciprocal behaviours. In phase 1 (pre-attachment), behaviours such as crying, orienting, cuddling, grasping and clinging are initially either undirected, or directed towards any available adult. Furthermore, the features of human adults, particularly those that mark their interactions with infants, are particularly attractive to infants. For example, face-like stimuli elicit more attention from neonates than abstract patterns. Neonates are visually attentive to areas of high contrast and to motion. The human face, when animated in the exaggerated fashion typically used with babies, is thus a strong attractor. Similarly, infants are best able to hear sounds in the range of the human voice, particularly higher-pitched voices and are especially attentive to the kinds of changing pitch contours that are typically exaggerated in speech directed to infants.

Even during the neonatal period, infants rapidly learn to discriminate between different adults and their patterns of interacting. For example, breast-fed newborns recognize the odour of their own mothers as demonstrated by a head-turning preference towards the breast pad their mothers have used over that used by a stranger (McFarlane, 1975; Porter *et al.*, 1992). If a baby has had a consistent primary caregiver for several days in hospital care, a shift in this figure is reflected in changes in infant behaviour (Sander, 1975). These rapid learning phenomena probably reflect species-specific learning biases (Waters *et al.*, 1991).

In phase 2 (attachment-in-the-making), as infant vision and audition improve and patterns of interaction with one or more caregivers become established, infants discriminate between familiar and unfamiliar faces, voices and interaction styles and begin to develop expectations concerning the effects of their own behaviour and the reactions of caregivers. When social smiling first appears (after the first month), babies smile indiscriminately, but they gradually start to smile more at familiar figures and less and less at strangers. Nevertheless, studies of infant cognition suggest that early discrimination and preferences are rooted in concrete experiences and lack the concept of a specific person who continues to exist in the absence of direct sensory contact. In an innovative experiment, Bower (1975) used mirrors to expose infants to multiple images of their own socially responsive mothers. Prior to the age of 5 months, babies happily smiled, vocalized and generally played with these multiple images. Beginning at around 5 months and older, babies showed confusion and upset which suggested that they recognized the anomalous nature of this experience. It has been suggested that, during this phase, the mother functions for the infant primarily as the intersection of previously unco-ordinated sensorimotor schemes such as looking, grasping and sucking (Waters *et al.*, 1991).

Clearly, the formation of a special relationship requires the understanding that an enduring specific other exists apart from concrete interactive experiences. This understanding develops in the second half of the first year. Studies by Piaget and his followers used the technique of hiding objects and observing infant search patterns to show that the general notion of object permanence is consolidated by 8 to 9 months of age. At first, infants do not search at all for an object they are handling when it is withdrawn and hidden. Later, they search for an object where they have previously found it, even if they have just seen it hidden elsewhere. Some time around 8 to 9 months, they cease to make this error. Although there are further developments in object permanence, with the infant gaining ability to follow increasingly complex and delayed hiding strategies, the achievement of this first simple success is considered to mark the emergence of object permanence.

What about analogous concepts of people? When do infants achieve person permanence? Sylvia Bell (1970) was the first to examine person permanence in infants. She adopted methods used in earlier Piagetian studies which had each infant's mother hide behind screens in sequences that mirrored those used with objects. In general, she found that person permanence emerged slightly earlier than permanence for inanimate objects, particularly for infants who were developing secure attachments. Thus some time in the second half of the first year infants gain the cognitive concepts that are prerequisites for attachment.

The other major development at this time is the emergence of locomotion. Although the development of crawling, standing and walking is highly variable, most infants begin to crawl some time between 9 and 12 months. Until the infant acquires this ability to locomote on his or her own, the work of maintaining proximity occurs through caregiver responses to the signals of a stationary infant. Once the infant is mobile, he or she can assume more of the responsibility for contact by going to, following and seeking out the caregiver. Infant mobility is also accompanied by new dangers. The curious infant soon has access to new aspects of the physical world and is able to touch things that are hot or electrified, handle objects that are breakable, trip and fall over unexpected obstacles or ledges, and mouth small objects. The consolidation of the first attachment is contemporaneous with the need for a new way of organizing infant protection.

Assessing infant attachment: the strange situation

Assessing relationships is no easy task, and assessing relationships when one participant is an infant involves further complexities. Much of current attachment research and theorizing about individual differences was made possible by the fortuitous emergence of the strange situation as a paradigm for assessing infant attachment. This paradigm played a pivotal role in the development of attachment research. First, it provided one of the few standardized validated instruments for assessing infant–parent relationships. Secondly, it served as the basis for the development of other measures both in infancy and in later age periods. In the remainder of this chapter we shall examine the logic of the strange situation, the associated classification scheme and the strengths and limitations of alternative approaches to attachment assessment.

The first and most widely used assessment procedure for infants, namely the strange situation, made its first appearance as a laboratory-based addition to an ongoing intensive observational study of infant–mother interaction in homes in Baltimore, Maryland. The purpose of the laboratory visit was to study the effects of separation from the mother in an unfamiliar environment. The structure of the session was based on Bowlby's concept of the protective function of attachment and Ainsworth's developing ideas regarding the attachment figure as a secure base for exploration. Ainsworth's previous work, both in Uganda and in Baltimore, had involved naturalistic observations in the home. The strange situation incorporated numerous features of naturalistic observation. It was designed to resemble situations which an infant and mother might encounter in everyday life and, within the general structure, participants were free to behave as they would normally do.

The structure is a series of brief (3-minute) and increasingly stressful episodes interspersed with opportunities for recovery. The room is equipped with toys of interest to a 12 to 18-month-old child. Perception of stress should activate the infant's attachment behaviour, while new interesting toys should activate exploratory behaviour. In short, this is an opportunity to see how the child balances these two systems (exploration and attachment), and how the attachment figure is used as part of the strategy for coping with stress. If this strategy is successful, attachment behaviour will be reduced and the child will confidently explore the environment. The attachment figure can be any significant caregiver. The strange situation has been used with mothers, fathers, and alternative caregivers such as the metapelet on the Israeli kibbutz (e.g. Fox, 1977; Sagi *et al.*, 1985). However, Ainsworth's original study used mothers, and since most of the research to be discussed involved mothers, the description below features the mother as the attachment figure.

Table 2.1 (Ainsworth *et al.*, 1978) provides an outline of the strange situation. To understand its logic, it may be useful to imagine that you are a 12 to 18-month-old participating in the strange situation. You are able to crawl or perhaps walk, if a bit unsteadily, but you only have a few words, if any, to make your needs known to others. Three minutes is a very long time, and you have no way to measure time. Your mother brings you to a strange place. An unfamiliar person shows you a strange room with interesting toys and soon departs. Your mother shows you some of the toys and then sits down and begins to read a magazine (episode 1 and 2). What do you do? Are you interested in the toys, or are you looking around the room? Are you worried that your mother is preoccupied with reading? Do you try to get your mother's attention, and how does she respond? (She has been

Table 2.1 Episodes of the strange situation[a]

Episode	Participants	Duration	Description
1	Mother, baby, experimenter	<1 minute	Experimenter brings mother and baby to the room, gives instructions
2	Mother, baby	3 minutes	Mother sits in chair and reads, baby explores. M responds if approached but does not initiate
3	Mother, baby, stranger	3 minutes	Stranger enters, silent (1 minute), converses with mother (1 minute), approaches baby (1 minute)
4	Baby, stranger	3 minutes[b]	First separation: mother departs, stranger comforts baby if needed, otherwise sits in chair
5	Mother, baby	3 minutes	First reunion: mother returns, greets and/or comforts baby, returns to chair and reads
6	Baby	3 minutes[b]	Second separation: mother departs, saying 'bye-bye'
7	Baby, stranger	3 minutes[b]	Second separation continues: stranger enters, comforts baby if necessary, otherwise sits in chair
8	Mother, baby	3 minutes	Second reunion: mother returns, greets, comforts baby if needed, and is then free to interact as she chooses

[a] Adapted from Ainsworth et al. (1978) with permission.
[b] These episodes are shortened if the baby does not settle within 20–30 seconds.

instructed not to initiate activities, but to respond appropriately if approached.)

After a while, yet another unfamiliar person enters (episode 3). She sits quietly for a while, chats with your mother, and then attempts to play with you. What do you do? Does the appearance of this stranger worry you? Do you look at or go to your mother for reassurance? Do you respond to the stranger's initiative? Then there is a knock and your mother leaves the room (episode 4). What do you do? Are you upset? Do you worry about when or whether your mother will return? Do you think it is OK to be with this stranger? Are you crying? Do you go to the door and try to open it or call to your mother? Finally, your mother returns and calls you from the door (episode 5). What do you do? Do you rush over to greet her? Do you go back to play? Are you worried that she might leave again?

In fact, in a short while she does leave again (episode 6). What do you do? Do you understand what is going on? Are you able to continue playing or do you break down and cry? Do you go to the door and call? To make matters even worse, the next time the door opens, where you expected to see your mother, the strange person comes back and tries to comfort you (episode 7). What do you do? Are you willing to settle for this stranger? Are you even more worried about the return of your mother? At last your mother does come back (episode 8), calling to you from the doorway. What do you do? Do you go to her? Are you angry with her for leaving you? If so, do you try to tell her that? Are you relieved that she is back? Do you go back to play? Or do you want to stay even closer to your mother?

In this procedure, any separation episode (4, 6 or 7) is curtailed if the infant cries hard for more than 20 seconds. In the Baltimore sample and three other early studies, curtailments were necessary for 53 per cent of the infants. Later studies showed that even infants who do not cry experience substantial increases in heart rate indicative of distress (Donovan and Leavitt, 1985; Sroufe and Waters, 1977a).

Patterns of attachment

Ainsworth's original patterns

Nowadays the entire session is videotaped, and trained coders review the tapes. In the original studies, descriptions of behaviour were dictated into a tape recorder. This record was later transcribed into a narrative report, and behaviour was coded from these transcripts. Specific behaviours were coded in each episode, and there were systematic differences in infant behaviour from episode to episode (Ainsworth *et al.*, 1978). However, none of these specific behaviours in the laboratory were related to individual differences in infant or mother behaviours in the home. What did relate to home behaviour was the way in which the infant organized behaviour to use the attachment figure as part of his or her coping strategy. Although the original emphasis had been on separations, infant behaviours at reunion were particularly salient in these patterns of organization.

Attachment patterns (classifications) are established from global ratings made in each episode. These describe the infant's proximity-seeking, contact-maintaining, avoidance of the mother, resistance to comforting, search behaviour during separation, and distance interaction (looking and vocalizing) with the mother.

The infants that Ainsworth termed 'secure' used the mother as a secure base for exploration, as expected. That is, when the mother was present, they freely explored the environment, with occasional visual, verbal or physical contact. When she departed, their exploration was diminished. They might or might not cry, but when she returned, they greeted her positively, and if they were visibly upset, they went to her, were soon comforted and returned to exploring. The infants Ainsworth termed 'avoidant' explored with little reference to the mother, showed little distress at her departures, and visibly ignored or snubbed her when she returned. Sometimes they were more sociable and friendly to the stranger than to the mother. The infants Ainsworth termed 'resistant' or 'ambivalent' seemed to be preoccupied with the mother. They were reluctant to explore even in her presence, and were extremely distressed by her departures. At reunions they made strong efforts to make contact with her, but they also resisted her comforting efforts – for example, by squirming when picked up, rejecting toys she offered, or simply continuing their displays of distress. These behaviours had an either angry or passive emotional quality.

In order to avoid the effects of judgemental labels, Ainsworth gave letter names to the three groups, namely B, A and C for the secure, avoidant and resistant groups, respectively. However, through association with the descriptive labels, 'B' has come to have positive connotations, while 'A' and 'C' have come to have (often undeserved) negative connotations. Within each of these major patterns, Ainsworth noted subgroups – four in the secure group (B_{1-4}), two in the avoidant group (A_{1-2}) and two in the resistant group (C_{1-2}). Throughout most of this book we shall use the descriptive labels rather than letter names for attachment patterns, except when distinguishing subgroups.

In the secure group, B_1 and B_2 babies were somewhat like avoidant babies in that they showed minimal upset and displayed less contact-seeking during reunions than B_3 and B_4 babies. However, they were distinguished from the avoidant group by their positive responses to the mother. B_3 and B_4 babies were somewhat like resistant babies in being readily upset by separations and engaging in strong contact-seeking at reunions. B_4 babies were also relatively slow to settle. However, these babies differed from the resistant group in being unambivalent about their desire for contact, and in being less angry. Thus babies that show the secure pattern differ in the amount of distress they exhibit, but are similar in showing a positive response to the mother at reunions and in their ability to return to exploration in her presence.

In the avoidant group, A_1 babies were consistently avoidant whereas A_2 babies showed mixed behaviour, namely some tendency to greet or approach the mother mixed with a marked tendency to move away or look away at reunions. Thus the A_2 baby might start to approach the mother on her return, but then continue past her to the door or veer off towards the toys. The common feature in both avoidant groups is the inability to approach the mother directly after separations or to express overt pleasure at her return.

In the resistant group, C_1 babies were overtly angry, while C_2 babies were more passive and helpless, signalling to be picked up at reunions rather than actively approaching. The C_2 babies were also thought to be angry, but showed their anger through pouting and inappropriate helplessness rather than overt protests. Babies in both groups share an inability to engage in exploration and play after separations. Figure 2.1 shows the full range of attachment patterns along a continuum that reflects the threshold for activating attachment behaviour. Thus, at the far left, the threshold is relatively high (attachment behaviour is not easily elicited), and it decreases as one moves to the right, where the resistant (C) babies have an extremely low threshold for activating attachment behaviour (even objectively safe conditions activate attachment behaviour).

Each of the three patterns reflects a strategy for enlisting the caregiver in the service of alleviating stress. The secure infant explores freely and seeks contact with the attachment figure as necessary. The avoidant infant focuses on exploration, and monitors and maintains proximity to the attachment figure, but does not express attachment needs in order to avoid risking rejection. The resistant infant is preoccupied with the availability of an inconsistent caregiver, making repeated high-intensity demands to ensure that at least some of the latter elicit attention.

Links to home behaviour

These three main patterns were linked to behaviour at home (Ainsworth *et al.*, 1978). Although both infant and mother behaviours in the home

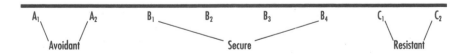

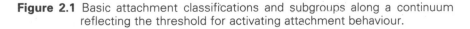

Figure 2.1 Basic attachment classifications and subgroups along a continuum reflecting the threshold for activating attachment behaviour.

differed from attachment patterns in the strange situation, links with maternal behaviour were emphasized because Ainsworth's hypothesis was that 'different experiences in interaction with the mother are largely responsible for the qualitative differences in infant–mother attachment' (Ainsworth *et al.*, 1978, p.298).

Mothers of securely attached infants were most sensitively responsive to infant signals, including cries. They were described as emotionally expressive and flexible in dealing with their babies. In the last quarter of the first year, they were more psychologically accessible to their infants than the mothers in other groups, accepting rather than rejecting, and co-operative rather than interfering.

Mothers of avoidant infants were described as 'rejecting' (Ainsworth *et al.*, 1978, p.300) – slow to respond to distress, and uncomfortable with close body contact. Their positive feelings about the baby were often overcome by anger and irritation. They were minimally expressive, relatively rigid in dealing with their infants, and often interfered unnecessarily with their infants' activities.

Mothers of resistant infants were inconsistently responsive. Like the mothers of avoidant infants, they were relatively insensitive to infant signals, but were less rejecting. They were more likely to be inept in physical contact with their infants, and they showed little spontaneous affection.

There have been numerous efforts to replicate these relationships between infant behaviour in the strange situation and prior maternal behaviour in the home, which have met with varying degrees of success. Although many research teams noted similar associations, few found effects as strong as those described by Ainsworth and her colleagues in the original studies (De Wolff and van IJzendoorn, 1997). There has also been ongoing controversy about the importance of infant contributions (especially infant temperament) in determining attachment patterns (e.g. Goldsmith and Alansky, 1987). The issues surrounding both maternal and infant contributions to patterns of attachment are discussed in detail in Chapters 4 and 5. However, the initial thrust of these studies was to show that infant behaviour in the strange situation is an indicator of prior home experiences and how the infant's attachment system operates.

Soon after Ainsworth and her colleagues developed the strange situation, it was being widely used by others, in some cases within the framework of attachment theory, and in others simply as a general measure of the infant–mother relationship. Ten years after the publication of *Patterns of Attachment*, it was possible for van IJzendoorn and Kroonenberg (1988) to provide a statistical summary of strange situation data from around 2000 infants from 8 countries. The distribution of the three main attachment patterns was remarkably similar to that of Ainsworth's Baltimore sample: (65 per cent secure, 21 per cent avoidant and 10–14 per cent resistant).

Disorganized attachment

In the course of these studies, investigators found a small number of infants whose behaviour could not be classified in the three-category scheme. Furthermore, as studies expanded to include populations with known parenting problems such as maltreatment (Crittenden, 1985) and parental depression (Radke-Yarrow *et al.*, 1985), not only were there children who could not be classified, but there were some for whom classifications seemed to be anomalous in view of known family information (Main and Solomon, 1986). Some children in these groups displayed both avoidance and resistance, a combination not previously seen. Both Crittenden (1985) and Radke-Yarrow and her colleagues (1985) added an A/C category to characterize such infants, and they found that this pattern occurred with high frequency in the most seriously disordered families.

Main and Solomon (1986) undertook the review of 55 videotapes of infants from community samples whose responses to separation and reunion in the strange situation failed to meet the criteria for any of the three known attachment patterns. What these infants had in common was not new patterns of behaviour, but rather sequences of odd behaviour which lacked an obvious goal or explanation. These unusual behaviours made more sense if they were interpreted as signs that the infant had confused expectations or was fearful of the caregiver. These infants were described as 'disorganized/ disoriented ' with respect to attachment. A subsequent review of additional 'unclassifiable' cases resulted in detailed criteria for identifying disorganized/ disoriented attachment (Main and Solomon, 1990).

In contrast to secure, avoidant and resistant infants who exhibit organized strategies for relating to the caregiver when distressed, those who are disorganized with respect to attachment are unable to maintain a consistent strategy. They either lack a strategy or their preferred strategy fails, giving rise to the unusual behaviours that Main and Solomon (1986, 1990) described. Thus an infant who avoids the caregiver while crying hard may prefer an avoidant strategy, but it fails to relieve his or her distress. Similarly, an infant who repeatedly approaches his or her mother but stops short and shifts from one foot to the other looking down at the toys may have an underlying secure strategy but be unable to implement it successfully.

Because disorganization is not a pattern in and of itself, there is no clear description of disorganization. Rather, there are seven categories of behaviour that are considered in scoring disorganization: (1) sequential or (2) simultaneous displays of contradictory behaviour (e.g. strong proximity-seeking followed by strong avoidance, avoiding the parent while extremely distressed); (3) undirected, misdirected, incomplete and interrupted movements and expressions (e.g. attempting to follow the stranger out of the room); (4) stereotypies, asymmetrical movements and anomalous postures (e.g. huddling prone on the floor for more than 20 seconds when the infant is clearly not tired); (5) freezing, stilling and slowed movements and expressions (e.g. no movement and a dazed expression); (6) direct indices of apprehension of the parent (e.g. fearful expression on being picked up); (7) direct indices of disorganization or disorientation (e.g. flinging hands about or in front of the face in response to the parent's return).

If an infant is thought to fit the disorganized category best, an effort is also made to determine the underlying strategy (secure, avoidant or resistant). Thus an infant may be classified as disorganized–secure, disorganized–avoidant or disorganized–resistant. If there does not appear to be an underlying strategy, the alternative may be 'unclassifiable,' followed by a guess (e.g. disorganized–unclassifiable–avoidant). The unclassifiable category (U) may also be used for infants who show no signs of disorganization but who do not fit the description for any of the other choices.

The antecedents and sequelae of disorganized infant attachment have yet to be explored fully, but initial research suggests an association with particularly inadequate care – disorganization occurs with high frequency in samples of maltreated infants and those with depressed mothers (Lyons-Ruth, 1996). In low-risk samples, disorganized infant attachment is associated with the parent's experience of attachment-related loss or trauma that has not been resolved (Main and Hesse, 1990). Current thinking is that disorganized attachment reflects the infant's inability to resolve the dilemma created by a caregiver (who should be a haven of safety and allay fear) who engages in behaviour that is frightening to the infant (Main and Hesse, 1990). Overt maltreatment is one form of frightening caregiver behaviour, but subtle and brief behaviours can also be frightening (e.g. suddenly looming over the infant without giving a clear signal that a game is intended, exaggerated startles in response to the infant's fall, or periods of being dazed and unresponsive). These more subtle behaviours have been found to occur more often in mothers with experiences of unresolved attachment losses or traumas and in mothers of disorganized infants (Lyons-Ruth et al., 1999; Schuengel et al. 1999).

Strengths of the strange situation

The strange situation was designed to observe secure base behaviour, and it is generally agreed that it provides a good basis for doing so (Goldberg et al., 1999; Waters et al., 1995). It represents a unique combination of experimental and clinical methods, as the procedure itself is well standardized but allows controlled opportunities for natural interactions. Human observers employ well-trained intuitions to make clinical judgements. However, unlike clinical judgements in everyday practice, the judgements made in strange-situation classifications are well described and can be highly reliable when they are made by trained coders.

When making classifications, the observer focuses on the infant, considering caregiver behaviour primarily as the context for infant behaviour. For example, ignoring the mother on reunions gets a higher score for avoidance if the mother makes repeated active efforts to gain the infant's attention than if the mother goes to her chair and quietly reads. The caregiver's behaviour is also constrained by instructions in most episodes. The advantage of relying on infant behaviour is that, whereas the mother can make inferences about the purpose of the observation and may try to please the experimenter or be a 'good mother,' infant behaviour is free of such biases and is more transparent. The classifications that are made are based on inferences about the infant's expectations when the caregiver is briefly unavailable.

Since the strange situation was first developed, a considerable body of research has been amassed showing that Ainsworth's attachment patterns are not only linked to prior home behaviour but are also associated with a range of later developmental outcomes throughout the lifespan (to be reviewed in Chapters 4, 5 and 9 to 13 inclusive). Although this body of work has its limitations, it stands as a substantial mass of research validating the use of the strange situation as an indicator of the quality of infant–mother relationships. The evidence supporting the use of the strange situation with other caregivers is not consistent (see Chapters 6 and 7). However, the heuristic value of the strange situation procedure as a catalyst to developmental research is unparalleled in the study of social development.

Limitations of the strange situation

Of course, the strange situation and its classification scheme are not without problems (Waters and Deane, 1985). It was designed for 12 to 18-month-olds, and although it has been used with some success in older children (see Chapter 3), it is not well suited to assessing changes in the attachment system over a wide age range. Initially, researchers used the strange situation as a marker of early home experience and turned their attention to its prediction of later competence (e.g. Lieberman, 1977; Matas et al., 1978; Renken et al., 1989). While this work was invaluable and continues to generate important information, the development of attachment per se was neglected. Ainsworth herself expressed disappointment as the 'success' of the strange situation drew researchers away from the naturalistic observations that she considered to be crucial to the developmental enterprise (Ainsworth and Marvin, 1995).

Second, early attempts at reliability assessments (Ainsworth et al., 1978) revealed that the strange situation could not be readministered within a narrow age range. Infants remembered their previous experiences and were highly distressed and upset on repetition. It has been recommended that a period of 4–6 weeks elapse between repetitions of the strange situation.

Thus we cannot readily evaluate the test–retest reliability of this procedure for assessing attachment. Furthermore, it is labour-intensive (and hence costly), requiring a minimum of at least two people, video equipment for recording, and review by trained coders who must make ongoing reliability checks.

Third, the data yielded by the strange situation are categorical and thus qualitative rather than quantitative. The statistical methods that are most prominent in developmental research are based on quantitative procedures. Thus investigators using the strange situation are confronted with serious limitations in the types of data analysis that they can use. As a further complication, the distribution across categories is markedly uneven, which leads many researchers to combine avoidant and resistant cases to form a larger 'insecure' group, or to omit the resistant group (the smallest) altogether. This results in loss of important information and undermines one of the unique aspects of attachment theory, namely the differences between different types of insecurity.

Efforts to overcome these limitations include attempts to organize the classification system into a linear security scale (e.g. Crittenden, 1985; Cassidy, Marvin and the MacArthur Working Group, 1987; Schneider-Rosen, 1990) and use of global rating scales to create scores on dimensions (such as security and avoidance) underlying the classification scheme (Richters et al., 1988). None of these has been satisfactory enough to be widely adopted. One successful alternative to the strange situation is the Attachment Q-sort developed by Waters and Deane (1985) for infants and toddlers.

The Attachment Q-sort

Origins and procedures

Ainsworth was not alone in her concern that researchers would lose sight of primary attachment phenomena. After considering the limitations of the strange situation, Waters and Deane (1985) set out to develop an alternative method. Q-sort methodology had been previously used in both personality and developmental research. This technique requires a set of items selected as indicators of a construct (or constructs) that are sorted by observers or judges into several categories ranging from most characteristic to least characteristic of the target individual. The sorting is further constrained by requiring a normal distribution of items – the largest number in the middle category and increasingly smaller numbers in the more extreme categories. Several statistical techniques can be used to analyse the distribution of items.

The first Attachment Q-sort consisted of 100 items reflecting 7 clusters of behaviour – those characterizing the attachment system (e.g. does not stay closer to adult in unfamiliar environment), affectivity (e.g. predominant mood is happy), social interaction (e.g. laughs easily with observer), object manipulation (e.g. prefers animate toys), independence/dependency (e.g. is independent with adult), social perceptiveness (e.g. is aware of social environment) and endurance/resiliency (e.g. becomes bored quickly). Items are sorted into nine piles ranging from least to most characteristic of the target child.

The Q-sort has been used with both mothers and trained observers. When mothers are the sorters, they are first familiarized with the items and then observe their child for a set period of time (e.g. 1 week) before actually sorting the cards. Usually they are assisted by a trained researcher. For observers, one or more prolonged home visits (e.g. 2–4 hours each) are made before attempting to characterize a child's behaviour. Although Q-sorts can be scored in a variety of ways, the common procedure for the Attachment Q-sort is based on 'criterion sorts' made by 'expert judges.' To develop these, experienced attachment researchers sorted the items to correspond to the 'ideal' secure, dependent and sociable child as well as for social desirability. The item sorts of mothers or observers are compared to the criterion sorts by comparing the informant's card placements with those of the criterion group. Thus, a child can be scored from -1 to $+1$ for security, indicating the correlation between mother/observer card placements and the criterion sort for security.

Efforts to demonstrate links between strange situation classifications and Q-sort scores have been mixed, partially reflecting the evolving nature of the Q-sort instrument. For example, van Dam and van IJzendoorn (1988) found only modest correlations between Q-sort security scores from mother reports on an early version of the instrument and security in the strange situation. Later, Vaughn and Waters (1990) were more successful in finding that observer security scores were related to attachment classifications in the strange situation. As expected, secure infants scored higher on the security scale than insecurely attached peers. They also scored higher on sociability but not on dependency (Vaughn and Waters, 1990). Avoidant and resistant infants did not differ from each other on these scales. Furthermore, the ratings used to make attachment classifications (proximity-seeking, avoidance, resistance, etc.) each contributed significantly to predicting home security scores, but not to predicting sociability or dependency scores.

A recent meta-analysis (van IJzendoorn and Riksen-Walraven, in press) reviewed over 60 studies which used the Attachment Q-sort, and concluded that observer sorts showed moderate convergence with assessments based on the strange situation and strong links with maternal sensitivity measures. Thus observer Q-sorts were judged to be a reasonable alternative to the strange situation. Maternal Q-sorts showed less convergence with the strange situation, weaker relationships with maternal sensitivity and considerable overlap with temperament procedures, and were therefore considered to be less adequate measures of attachment.

Strengths of the Attachment Q-sort

The Attachment Q-sort is a tool for home observation that encouraged many attachment researchers to engage in detailed examination of the primary attachment phenomenon, namely secure base behaviour in the home. It has the advantage of having carefully defined criterion behaviours and allowing for quantitative analyses. Because it provides a quantitative measure, it can circumvent the problem of the uneven distribution of attachment patterns. Whereas investigators working with classifications may discard or combine infrequent classifications and thus 'lose' data, Q-sort methods allow the investigator to make full use of all cases providing data.

Limitations of the Attachment Q-sort

The Attachment Q-sort, like the strange situation, is a labour-intensive procedure. In studies where observers complete the sort, they have spent 4–10 hours on home observations in order to do so. In studies where mothers complete the sort, research staff invest considerable time in 'training' mothers in observation and sorting. It is possible that even with intensive training and assistance, mothers may not be reliable reporters for attachment assessments (van IJzendoorn and Riksen-Walraven, in press). In particular, the same limitations in objective perception that lead mothers to behave in ways that shape insecure attachment may contribute to sorting bias.

Although the Attachment Q-sort might eventually include criterion sorts for the prototypic avoidant and resistant infant, at present it does not do so. It is conceptually possible to develop a criterion sort for organization/disorganization, but this would be extremely difficult using current information, because there is no simple description of disorganized behaviour. Although one attempt has been made to derive classifications from the Q-sort (Howes and Hamilton, 1992a) the different forms of insecurity are not inferred from standard use of the Q-sort. Since much of current theorizing is focused on individual differences in attachment patterns, the Q-sort is of limited usefulness in such enterprises. In fact, there is a danger that the Q-sort forces thinking about attachment into a simple good (secure, 'B-ness') vs. bad (insecure 'not-B-ness') dichotomy and loses one of the unique features of current attachment theory, namely the notion that there are several variants of insecure attachment which may have different consequences. However, the original purpose of the Q-sort was not to replace the strange situation but rather to complement it.

Pederson–Moran home assessment

Origins and procedures

The most recent attempt to bring attachment researchers back to home observations was designed to maintain the classificatory approach that had been so successful for Ainsworth. Pederson and Moran (1995) were well versed in both the strange situation and Q-sort methods when they began their efforts to develop a classification system for home behaviour. In fact, they had developed a Q-sort of their own to measure maternal sensitivity during home observations. In their home-based attachment procedure, two trained observers conduct a 2–hour home visit. In the first study to use this procedure (Pederson and Moran, 1995), such visits were made when infants were 8 and 12 months of age. During each of these visits there were several scheduled activities, including assessment of infant development, an interview with the mother, and the mother's completion of the Attachment Q-sort. Thus during at least part of the visit the mother's attention had to be divided between a structured task (the interview or the Q-sort) and the needs of the infant. Both visitors took detailed notes during the visit.

After the visit each observer described the visit and the observations to an experienced attachment researcher who had no other knowledge of the mother–infant pair, This description was in the context of a very detailed semi-structured interview paying particular attention to attachment-relevant incidents and behaviours of both participants (e.g. infant comfort-seeking behaviour, mother's accessibility to the infant during the visit). The interviewer then summarized the impressions of the dyad, and the reporting observer confirmed or corrected them. Finally, the interviewer and the observer classified the relationship using descriptions modelled after Ainsworth's original ones for the strange situation.

Pederson and Moran (1996, 1998) used this procedure in several studies, documented good reliability of the classifications, and found home classifications to be related to those in the strange situation. For secure/insecure comparisons, home and laboratory comparisons were in agreement 84 per cent of the time. When the three-category scheme (secure, avoidant, resistant) was used, the level of agreement was excellent (> 75 per cent) for secure and avoidant classifications, but was weak for the resistant category (40 per cent). Home classifications also showed strong associations with measures of maternal behaviour expected to predict attachment. Thus there is preliminary evidence to support the validity of the home-classification procedures.

Evaluation of home classifications

Because the home-classification procedure is relatively new, it has not been widely used. It is not yet clear how readily these procedures can be transferred to other laboratories and maintain equally strong reliability and validity. It is clearly a labour-intensive procedure, but combines the advantages of direct observations of the primary phenomenon (interaction in the home) with those of Ainsworth's original classifications. At present, the disorganized classification is not included. Like any classification scheme, it limits the options for statistical analysis and is subject to some of the same problems as the strange-situation classifications (e.g. uneven distribution leading to aggregation or discarding of categories).

Overview of attachment assessments in infancy

In this chapter we considered three different procedures for assessing infant attachment. All of them were found to be labour-intensive. While this limits, for example, their clinical utility, this shared feature indicates that there may not be short cuts for assessing the quality of dyadic relationships, particularly with infants or young children who are unable to provide verbal reports. Because it came first, has been used extensively and represented a major breakthrough in attachment research, the strange situation continues to be regarded as the 'gold standard' measure against which others are compared. However, the emergence of other techniques, such as the Q-sort and home-classifications scheme, indicates that the realm of attachment assessments will continue to expand in the future.

Suggested reading

Ainsworth, M.D.S., Blehar, M.C., Waters, E. and Wall, S. (1978) *Patterns of attachment*. Hillsdale, NJ: Lawrence Erlbaum.
A summary report of several early studies with the strange situation and the standard reference for conducting and scoring the strange situation.

Waters, E. and Deane, K.E. (1985) Defining and assessing individual differences in attachment relationships: Q-methodology and the organization of behavior in infancy and early childhood. In Bretherton, I. and Waters, E. (Eds), Growing points of attachment theory and research. *Monographs of the Society for Research in Child Development*, 50, 41–65.
A description of the origins and development of the Attachment Q-sort.

Marvin, R.S. and Britner, P.A. (1999) Normative development: the ontogeny of attachment. In Cassidy, J. and Shaver, P.R. (Eds), *Handbook of attachment theory and research*. New York: Guilford Press, 44–67.
A detailed account of the early development of attachment and its theoretical context.

Pederson, D.R. and Moran, G. (1995) A categorical description of infant–mother relationships in the home and its relation to Q-sort measures of infant–mother interaction. In Waters, E., Vaughn, B., Posada, G. and Kondo-Ikemura, K. (Eds), Caregiving, cultural and cognitive perspectives on secure-base behavior and working models. *Monographs of the Society for Research in Child Development*, **60**, 111–33.
The first description and validation of a method for home classifications of attachment.

van IJzendoorn, M.H. and Riksen-Walraven, M.J.M.A. (in press) Is the Attachment Q-sort a valid measure of attachment security in young children? In Vaughn, B.E. and Waters, E. (Eds), *Patterns of secure base behavior: Q-sort perspectives on attachment and caregiving*. Hillsdale, NJ: Erlbaum.
A critical evaluation of the Attachment Q-sort using meta-analytic techniques.

3 Later development and assessment of attachment beyond infancy

What happens to attachment over time? How often do patterns of attachment change or stay the same over the course of development? What factors influence stability or instability? Do children develop attachment behavioural patterns that match those of their parents? Or do they develop complementary patterns? These are interesting and important developmental questions, but they cannot be answered without measures of attachment that extend across the lifespan. Bowlby envisioned attachment as a lifespan construct, but the success of the strange situation led, at first, to a narrow focus on infancy. Indeed, Bowlby's description of the development of attachment culminated in the emergence of what he called the 'goal-corrected partnership' in the preschool years. Most people would intuitively expect attachment to undergo further developmental changes in the school years and adolescence and, in fact, the need to develop ways of assessing attachment at later ages was soon evident. In this chapter we shall first consider changes in attachment beyond the infant period and then go on to review the corresponding development of assessment tools.

Continuing development of attachment

The preschool years are marked by burgeoning linguistic, cognitive and motor skills that enable the child to have more control and to move towards increasing autonomy. The fourth phase of attachment development noted by both Bowlby and Ainsworth, namely the 'goal-corrected' partnership, emerges during this period. The child becomes aware of attachment figures as individuals with distinct goals and needs of their own, and recognizes that meeting his or her own needs and desires must be negotiated within this context. The child gains knowledge about the social rules, is capable of verbal expression and can understand explanations regarding parental separations. Longer separations are more routine and less likely to be upsetting. Much of this change is captured in the notion of a transition to the increasing reliance on representational thought in organizing the attachment system.

The most detailed description of development in middle childhood reflects the thinking of Waters and his colleagues (Waters, *et al.*, 1991) concerning the way in which the secure-base concept can be elaborated to encompass the developmental accomplishments of this period. As the child gains skill in self-protection and moves increasingly outside the family context, there is again exposure to both new delights and new dangers. This is accompanied by the need for a new kind of parental protection which is qualitatively different to that required by infants, toddlers and preschoolers. The concept of identification, central to analytical theories of development, is invoked in a more contemporary form (Richters and Waters, 1990) to describe the child's orientation towards parent and family values. It is suggested that, in middle childhood, the child and parents gradually develop a 'supervision partnership.' Thus the goal of the attachment system becomes the maintenance of supervision. Relevant behaviours for the child include accepting parental discipline, informing the parent of plans when leaving the home, reporting changes of plans, and reporting problems to the parent, whether these be physical, psychological or social. In middle childhood, the child also appreciates the care that he or she has received, as well as the parent's feelings and needs for help – for example, with household chores or care of siblings.

In adolescence, hormonal changes serve as a catalyst for a major shift in social relationships directed towards seeking and establishing exclusive pair bonds, most often with a member of the opposite sex. These relationships often include an attachment component. Although such attachments may occupy a higher position in the preference hierarchy than attachment to parents, they do not supplant them. Most commonly, these lasting pair bonds are associated with establishing new households in young adulthood, reproduction and the assumption of caregiving roles. The latter entail serving as an attachment figure for a young infant.

Strategies for developing assessments

Several different strategies have been used in developing new measures of attachment. The first of these built on the tradition of attachment research and capitalized on the impressive success of the strange situation by using it as the basis for parallel classification schemes for older children and adults. This approach assumes that patterns of infant attachment have analogues at other age periods, and that these patterns are relatively stable not only across age periods, but also across generations. The resulting assessments include observational procedures for preschoolers (Cassidy, Marvin and the MacArthur Working Group, 1987, 1992) and 5 to 7-year-olds (Main *et al.*, 1985) as well as an interview for adults (George *et al.*, 1985). Table 3.1 notes the measures that used this strategy.

A second approach does not begin with the strange situation but instead draws on the theory and developmental principles to elaborate salient features of attachment at different stages of the life cycle as the basis for assessment procedures. Here no assumptions are made about relationships with the strange situation. Undoubtedly, this is a conceptually more challenging task, but several programmatic efforts of this type are in progress for assessing attachment in preschoolers (e.g. Crittenden, 1992, 1995), adolescents (Hillburn-Cobb, 1996) and adults (e.g. West and Sheldon-Keller, 1994). Some of these are also listed in Table 3.1.

A large number of adult measures (questionnaires and interviews) originate from the tradition of social psychology research on adult relationships. Most of these focus on romantic relationships and translate the constructs used by Bowlby and Ainsworth into this context. The first questionnaire of this type simply presented descriptions of Ainsworth's three attachment patterns and asked adults to indicate which of these was most like themselves (Hazan and Shaver, 1987). Several subsequent questionnaires were elaborations to make the instrument more sensitive and improve its psychometric characteristics (e.g. Collins and Read, 1990). However, some also developed new approaches or interpretations of the traditional attachment constructs. For example, Bartholomew and her colleagues conceived of four adult attachment styles based on positive and negative evaluations of self and other (e.g. Bartholomew and Horowitz, 1991), and developed interviews and questionnaires to assess these four styles in different relationship contexts.

Infancy measures necessarily focus on behavioural observations. Adult measures concentrate on questionnaires and interviews that rely on language skills. As discussed in previous chapters, from infancy onwards, attachment emotions, cognitions and sensory motor behaviours are represented internally as 'working models.' Internal working models become progressively more elaborated and differentiated and, as Main and her colleagues suggested, it may be appropriate to 'move to the level of representation' in assessing attachment (Main *et al.*, 1985). Thus, beginning in the preschool period, there are narrative as well as observational methods of assessing attachment. At present none of these are well developed or widely used, and they will be considered only briefly here. We shall reconsider these measures in Chapter 10.

Because the instruments in use for this wide age span (preschool to adulthood) are so numerous, it is impossible to discuss each of them in the same detail that was given to procedures for infants. Instead, we shall focus first on observational measures for children, considering all age groups together. Secondly, we shall consider the Adult Attachment Interview in some detail as a prototype for narrative approaches. Then we shall briefly consider narrative measures for children and questionnaire measures for adults.

Table 3.1 Attachment terminology across the lifespan[a]

Age	Method	Classifications		
		Secure	*Insecure*	
Infancy	Observation Strange situation (reunions)	Secure (B)	Resistant or ambivalent (C)	Avoidant (A)	Disorganized (D)
Preschool	Observation Strange situation Other reunions	Secure or balanced (B)	Dependent or coercive (C)	Avoidant or defended (A)	Controlling (D) Insecure-other
5–7 years	Observation	Secure or balanced (B)	Dependent or coercive (C)	Avoidant or defended (A)	Controlling (D) Insecure-other
7–11 years		No standardized classification scheme available		
Adolescence	Observation Revealed differences Reunions	Balanced (B)	Preoccupied (C)	Limiting (A)	Disorganized (D)
		Adult questionnaires and measures have also been used with older adolescents		
Adult	Discourse Analysis Adult Attachment Interview	Autonomous (F)	Preoccupied (E)	Dismissing (Ds)	Unresolved regarding loss or trauma (U)

[a] This table does not include all of the numerous adult measures which vary in classification terminology.

Reproduced from Goldberg, Muir and Kerr (1995) with permission.

Observational measures for children

The Attachment Q-sort (Waters and Deane, 1985) was designed to extend beyond the infancy years and is used with toddlers and preschoolers without major changes in methodology. Although the strange situation was originally developed specifically for 12 to 18-month-olds, it too was soon being used with toddlers and preschoolers (e.g. Lyons-Ruth et al., 1987; Marvin and Greenberg, 1982). However, it was evident that the classification descriptions needed to reflect the more sophisticated cognitive, affective and behavioural repertoire of older children (Marvin, 1977). For preschoolers the brief separations of the strange situation may not reliably activate attachment behaviour, and differences in attachment behaviour patterns are likely to be much more subtle. For older children, this is even more the case. For this reason, behavioural assessments of older children have used longer separations (e.g. for the duration of an experimental testing situation of 30–60 minutes) and rely on detailed evaluation of affective expression, conversational exchange and subtle body language. In addition, in some cases the salience of attachment issues has been heightened by involving both the child and the parent in attachment-related activities during the separation. For example, Main, Kaplan and Cassidy (1985) asked children to draw a picture of their family, showed them a family photograph taken when they first arrived, and conducted the Separation-Anxiety Test (Klagsbrun and Bowlby, 1976). Meanwhile, the parent participated in an Adult Attachment Interview. Thus, when the reunions on which the classifications were based took place, the attachment system had already been 'primed.'

With adolescents, Hillburn-Cobb (1996) also used attachment-related activities for both the parent and the child during separations in a half day of tasks. In addition to reunion observations, the adolescent and the parent were observed during discussions that entailed potential conflict. For example, the pair watched a film about child–parent separation, responded to written questions and were then asked to discuss the responses on which they had disagreed. In another task, the child and parent were asked to discuss vignettes involving parent–child conflicts.

When these techniques are used, behavioural patterns emerge that parallel the three main infant patterns. The labels given to these patterns vary. For the purpose of clarity, Table 3.1 summarizes attachment patterns from infancy to adulthood in so far as they have been described. Note that measures for 7 to 12-year-olds have not been explored in sufficient detail to yield a general measure.

Secure attachment is characterized by positive relaxed reunion behaviour, namely comfortable, appropriate, occasionally prolonged eye contact, fluent discourse (which may be personal) and a shift in posture or position to orient towards the attachment figure. Like the secure infant who balances exploration and attachment needs, the secure older child integrates attention to play/exploration or a task with attention to the attachment figure. The child greets the parent but continues his or her ongoing activity and finds a way to include the parent. With younger children there may be casual relaxed physical contact. The affective expressions of the parent and child are well matched.

Avoidant attachment is marked by neutral affect and minimal but polite responses. This pattern is also described as 'defended' (Crittenden, 1992) or 'limiting' (Hillburn-Cobb, 1996). While the avoidant infant snubs or ignores the returning parent, the older child recognizes the violation of the social rules implicit in extreme avoidance, and follows the rules but ignores the relationship. The child is polite but gives the impression of being 'too busy' to respond to the attachment figure, glancing only briefly – usually when the likelihood of eye contact is minimal. The parent carries the responsibility for initiating interactions and may use inappropriately bright affect in an attempt to engage the child. Thus the parent may ask repeated questions with the child giving single word (yes/no) answers. Child initiatives, if they occur, are predominantly instrumental (e.g. seeking help with a task or toy).

The pattern analogous to infant-resistant attachment has been variously termed 'dependent' (Cassidy and Marvin, with the MacArthur Working Group, 1987, 1992), 'coercive' (Crittenden, 1992) or 'involving' (Hillburn-Cobb, 1996). Like the ambivalent/resistant pattern in infancy, it is characterized by preoccupation with the relationship at the expense of exploration/play or attention to the task in hand. Among younger children, it may be marked by overt upset and difficulty in settling. There may be brief avoidance, but it is sulky rather than neutral in affect. The child's activity is interrupted during exchanges with the parent, and the episode is ridden with parent–child conflict. Such conflicts may arise over the child's repeated 'testing' of the parent by engaging in inappropriate activities (e.g. wanting to leave the room) or disagreement over minor details in attempted play or discussion (e.g. 'Look at my truck!' 'No, it's a car,' 'No, it's a blue truck,' 'That's not blue, it's green'). Alternatively, the struggle may reflect inappropriately helpless or babyish behaviour on the part of the child. This use of feigned immaturity to engage the parent includes whispering, twisting and coy squirming by the child in response to queries from the parent and/or wheedling attempts to persuade the parent to do something. In some cases, especially with older children and adolescents, it takes the form of silliness, giggling and teasing. Among younger children, where there is physical contact, it is ambivalent (e.g. backing into or sidling over to the parent).

These three main patterns correspond to the three strategies for relying on an attachment figure at times of stress that Ainsworth described in infants. What would be analogous to disorganization beyond infancy? Here it is more difficult to speak generally of all age groups. In some children, particularly younger preschoolers, brief moments of frank behavioural disorganization (as described by Main and Solomon, 1990) are seen. In fact, such moments have also been noted in adolescents and adults (Hillburn-Cobb, 1998). More commonly, children who were disorganized as infants are described as adopting strategies in which they 'take charge' of the relationship and control the parent. These controlling strategies are either 'caregiving' or 'punitive.'

In the caregiving strategy, the child adopts a parental role towards his or her parent and focuses on entertaining, comforting or helping the parent. Such children may be inappropriately effusive and bright in their greetings, continue to exaggerate positive emotions throughout the episode, give advice, or 'teach' the parent. Despite the child's excessively cheery greetings or invitation, there may be little real mutual engagement. Conversation may be awkward and marked by *non sequiturs* from both parent and child. The parent's affect is usually subdued and markedly discrepant from the child's brightness.

Children whose attachment pattern is 'controlling-punitive' are overtly hostile towards the parent. They may violate the social rules by flagrantly ignoring the parent when they are well aware of a request or communication. In contrast to the dependent child, who makes outrageous requests in a whiny voice that indicates the expectation of being thwarted, the punitive-controlling child makes the same requests with an imperious air, fully expecting parental compliance. Indeed, the parent usually does comply, often with affectively flat resignation.

There is yet another attachment pattern described for preschoolers and 5 to 7-year-olds, namely 'insecure-other.' This category is reserved for children whose behaviour is indicative of insecurity but does not fit the other categories. The most common reason for assignment to this category is a mixture of the avoidant and dependent strategies. As in the infant system, the controlling and insecure-other categories are also assigned one of the remaining three patterns as an alternative 'best guess' at the primary attachment strategy.

The concept of 'disorganization' has also been criticized as inappropriate at any age (Crittenden, 1992, 1995). According to Crittenden, the behaviours considered to be disorganized are better interpreted as attempts to 'reorganize', or as a combination of two or more organized strategies. Thus the patterns described above as controlling-caregiving, punitive-caregiving, and the mixture of avoidant (defended) and dependent (coercive) termed 'insecure-other' above, are treated as atypical variants of the three main patterns, rather than as distinct classifications. Caregiving is considered to be a defended pattern, as the child ignores or fails to express his or her own attachment needs. The punitive pattern is considered to be an extreme form of coercion. The defended and coercive patterns can also appear in combined form.

In this classification system, described by Crittenden (1992, 1995), attachment patterns are considered in terms of two dimensions: (1) relative reliance on affective and cognitive information and (2) accuracy of information (see Figure 3.1). Thus the secure pattern represents a balanced reliance on objectively correct (true) information in both affective and cognitive domains, whereas defended patterns give more emphasis to cognition and coercive patterns rely more heavily on affect. The analogues of caregiving, punitive control and a mixed (coercive plus dependent) analogue of insecure-other fall within the range of patterns which rely on false or distorted information and are considered to be atypical.

Validation of observational measures for children

It is customary to validate such measures against a 'gold standard.' The strange situation was accepted as an important marker of the quality of parent–infant relationships because Ainsworth's early study, as well as later studies (see Chapter 4), showed that it was related to sampling of daily interactions in the home. In the case of behavioural observations for older children, there has not been clear agreement as to what the 'gold standard' may be. If we assume that patterns of attachment established in infancy should remain fairly stable, then the extent to which measures for older children match their infant attachment classifications can provide some validity. Two studies have reported high stability from infancy to early school age. Main and Cassidy (1988) reported that of 40 child–mother

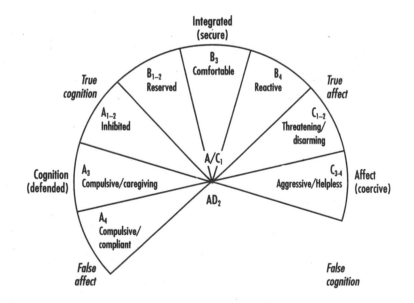

Figure 3.1 Representation of preschool attachment on the basis of reliance on cognition and affect. Adapted from Crittenden (1995) with permission.

pairs, 84 per cent were judged to use the same attachment strategy (avoidant, secure or disorganized) at both assessments, whereas in father-child pairs, the corresponding figure was 61 per cent. In the second study (Wartner *et al.*, 1994) 82 per cent of mother–child pairs showed the same patterns (avoidant, secure, dependent/resistant or disorganized) at 1 and 6 years. One published study (Howes and Hamilton, 1992b) used the scheme of Cassidy, Marvin and the MacArthur Working Group (1987, 1992) scheme and found 72 per cent of dyads to show the same pattern at 1 and 4 years, but several unpublished studies reported an absence of stability from infancy to the preschool years (Beckwith and Rodning, 1991; Goldberg *et al.*, 1998; Greenberg, 1997, personal communication; Sutton, 1994). Thus the evidence for agreement with infant classifications is inconsistent.

We can also ask whether this is, in fact, a good validity criterion. Many of these procedures were developed by identifying children who showed particular attachment patterns during infancy. Reliance on such procedures precludes the study of continuity of attachment – if we assume continuity, we cannot test for it (Crittenden, 1992). So while such agreements can show us that the methods for older children do what they were designed to do (that is, identify children who were secure, avoidant, resistant or disorganized as infants), we may not want this to be the primary basis for designing or validating attachment assessments at later ages. A more convincing demonstration of validity would be based on articulating how the attachment system functions outside the laboratory in these age periods, and comparison of home observations with the laboratory assessments.

Another approach is to show convergent validity – that these assessment schemes are linked to other measures in ways that attachment theory predicts. Thus securely attached children are expected to have higher self-esteem and better peer relationships than their insecurely attached peers, and demonstrations that an assessment of attachment is linked to such outcomes enhances the validity of the assessment. Each of the behavioural schemes for children has been shown to have reasonable relations with other developmental or family measures. For example, Hillburn-Cobb (1996) has shown relationships between her measures of adolescent attachment to each parent and family problem-solving style, and Greenberg and his colleagues (1991) have shown relationships between preschool attachment and clinic status. The shortcoming of this approach as the sole evidence of validity is that similar relationships may be predicted for aspects of parent–child relationships other than attachment (e.g. maternal warmth or teaching style). In the absence of validation against an agreed 'gold standard,' documentation of these relationships is supportive but inconclusive.

The Adult Attachment Interview

Origins, methods and classifications

Apart from the strange situation, the Adult Attachment Interview (AAI) is probably the most widely used and best-developed attachment measure. Like the strange situation, it has served as a touchstone for developing other measures for adults. It entails a very labour-intensive procedure. The adult participates in a semi-structured interview focused on childhood experiences (as early as can be remembered) with attachment figures. The participant is asked to provide general descriptions of relationships with their parents, give examples that support those descriptions, describe their parents' reactions to illness, hurt and emotional upset, explain why they think their parents behaved in the way that they did and, if appropriate, to discuss salient losses (e.g. deaths) and traumas (e.g. abuse). The interview is transcribed verbatim. A series of specific ratings are made and used to arrive at a classification that is based not on the content of the transcript, but on narrative coherence.

The concept of coherence is based on the notions of a linguistic philosopher (Grice, 1975) who identified coherent discourse as being co-operative and adhering to four maxims: (1) quality (be truthful and have evidence for what you say); (2) quantity (be complete but succinct); (3) relationship (be relevant); and (4) manner (be clear and orderly). Thus it is not what happened to an individual that is important for adult attachment, but how he or she thinks and feels about it as revealed in the coherence of the story that is told. The AAI is considered to assess what is described as the adult's 'state of mind' with respect to attachment.

Secure adults (termed 'autonomous' or 'free to evaluate', and hence indicated by 'F') value intimate relationships and acknowledge the effects of those relationships. Whether the specific experiences that they report are happy or troubled, they not only provide confirming detailed memories, but demonstrate an ability to reflect on those experiences with an understanding of both their own behaviour and that of their parents. Thus the secure adult might say that he or she felt rejected because 'my mother was always too busy for me,' but will also say 'I don't think my mother realized how much I missed her when she was at work. Now I realize how hard she had to work just to keep food on the table.' There is an ability to recognize the limitations of supportive figures as well as the positive aspects of inadequate attachment figures. Responses to the interview questions are clear, relevant and to the point.

Dismissing adults (termed 'Ds,' analogous to avoidant infants) usually have little to say about the attachment experiences of their childhood, and they provide relatively short transcripts. Their ability to recount specific incidents is limited, and they often assert that they cannot remember relevant information. They minimize the effects of important relationships in their lives ('I had a miserable childhood but it really hasn't affected me'). They also often idealize their relationships with their parents by using glowingly positive descriptions coupled with an inability to provide concrete supportive details. Thus a dismissing adult may describe his or her relationship with a parent as 'loving', but be unable to remember specific events to illustrate this and/or later describe distinctly unloving behaviour (e.g. being afraid to tell the parent about an injury for fear that the parent would be angry). Just as the avoidant infant or child makes the parent carry the responsibility for initiating contact, the dismissing adult forces the interviewer to bear the responsibility of the interview by giving short, minimally informative answers.

Preoccupied (or enmeshed, 'E') adults become so entangled in the details of early experiences that they are unable to provide an overview. They are still engaged in angry struggles with their parents over old issues. As a result, they provide extremely long, vivid but wandering narratives, and they often fail to answer the question they were asked. For example, when asked for 'five words to describe your relationship with your mother' the preoccupied adult may launch into a detailed description of an event but be unable to give a word or short phrase to convey the sense of what they have just described. Just as the resistant infant or the dependent older child struggles with the parent over control, the preoccupied adult forces the interviewer to struggle to maintain the interview on topic.

These three main patterns, each with several subgroups, were developed from interviews with parents of infants whose attachment patterns had been assessed in the strange situation. The autonomous pattern was most common among parents of secure infants, the dismissing pattern was most common among parents of avoidant infants, and the preoccupied pattern was commonest among parents of resistant infants. What characteristics identified the parents of infants with disorganized attachment? The parents of these infants were most often described as being 'unresolved' with regard to attachment losses or trauma.

Loss and trauma are inherently disorganizing events Normally, as people slowly recover, they develop new organizations of both behaviour and internal working models that reflect the painful experiences but allow them to move on with other aspects of their lives. Adults are considered to be 'unresolved' with respect to loss and/or trauma if, during the relevant parts of the interview, they give evidence that they have not succeeded in this reorganization. Thus they become briefly disorganized/disoriented when discussing these topics. For example, they may speak as if they are re-experiencing the loss or trauma, talk of a dead person as if they were still alive, describe the events of many years ago in great detail, or show dramatic changes in discourse style. Because these phenomena are limited intrusions, the unresolved classification is always coupled with an alternative classification that reflects predominant discourse characteristics in the remainder of the interview (autonomous, dismissing or preoccupied).

Validation, strengths, and limitations of the Adult Attachment Interview (AAI)

The narrative method used in the AAI is based on the assumption that, while some aspects of working models of attachment are available to consciousness and can be directly reported, some important features are not and must therefore be studied indirectly. The interview technique, in which the interviewer probes only minimally in order to elicit a coherent story, appears to succeed in Main's goal of 'surprising the unconscious' and allowing the individual's manner of thinking about attachment to emerge. However, the AAI is a very labour-intensive assessment. The interview takes one and a half hours to conduct, 7 to 10 hours to transcribe properly, and several more hours at least to code. Furthermore, while the administration of the interview can be learned in a few practice sessions with a trainer, skill in coding the transcripts requires prolonged and intensive training. Kobak (1989) has developed and used a Q-sort technique for coding which may offer some advantages in efficiency, but it has not yet been widely adopted by others.

Like the strange situation, the AAI yields classifications and it therefore has the same limitations for data analysis as any classificatory system. Nevertheless, it provides a rich and detailed picture of the 'state of mind' of the individual being interviewed, and despite its labour-intensive demands has immense appeal to clinicians because of the 'face validity' of its content.

Since AAI classifications are based on analysis of language, it is important to know whether the characteristics of language used during the interview are specific to the topic of attachment or simply reflect general cognitive and linguistic abilities or style. The three main patterns (autonomous, dismissing and preoccupied) are not generally related to measures of intelligence or memory (Bakermans-Kranenburg and van IJzendoorn, 1993; Sagi et al., 1994b). Furthermore, the discourse style used in the AAI does not necessarily correspond to that used for other topics (e.g. job history) (Crowell et al., 1996).

The AAI was originally developed by using the strange situation as a stepping-stone. As a result, there is an extensive literature examining the agreement between AAI classifications and those from the strange situation in parent–child pairs, as well as evidence that attachment patterns are maintained across three generations (Benoit and Parker, 1994). A statistical review of 18 studies which provided data on this type of predictive validity was conducted by van IJzendoorn (1995). When all four classifications for both infants and parents were considered, 63 per cent of dyads were matched as expected (autonomous-secure, dismissing-avoidant, preoccupied-resistant and unresolved-disorganized). When only the three main classifications were considered, 69 per cent of dyads were matched, and when only security/insecurity was considered, the rate of matches rose to 75 per cent. Thus if less stringent criteria are used for a match, the proportion of matches increases. A high proportion of the matches represent autonomous adults with secure infants. Each of these is the most common attachment pattern for the relevant age group. Thus spurious secure-autonomous matches may occur. Concordance for the other classifications is lower, with the preoccupied-resistant link being the weakest and showing little predictability. Nevertheless, these data demonstrate that for the most part, the AAI does what it was designed to do.

There are limited but mixed data on convergent validity showing links between attachment and some personality characteristics (Benoit et al., 1989; Zeanah et al., 1993), peer relationships (Kobak and Sceery, 1988) and marital conflict (Cohn et al., 1992). Similarly, there is some evidence that insecurity and unresolved attachment are associated with clinical status, but otherwise limited evidence that either dismissing or preoccupied attachment is associated with specific disorders (Stein et al., 1998).

Thus the validity of the AAI rests primarily on a substantial body of evidence that it predicts something about caregiving capacity, but is this the appropriate 'gold standard' for an assessment of adult attachment? Although the caregiving and attachment systems are related, they are not identical. Most definitions of adult attachment assume fulfilment of the same functions as attachment in childhood, namely protection and security when stressed (e.g. Crowell and Treboux, 1995; Stein et al., 1998; West and Sheldon-Keller, 1994). If so, a measure of adult attachment should reflect the manner in which adults use a small number of individuals as attachment figures – that is, sources of security in times of stress. Such data are lacking. However, despite this shortcoming, the AAI itself is often considered to be the 'gold standard' against which other measures of adult attachment are evaluated.

Other narrative measures

Several other interviews tapping attachment constructs are available for adults that focus on caregivers in childhood (Bartholomew and Horowitz, 1991), close friendships (Bartholomew and Horowitz, 1991) and romantic relationships (Bartholomew and Horowitz, 1991; Owens and Crowell, 1992). The Current Relationship Interview (Owens and Crowell, 1992) parallels the methods of the AAI in both structure and scoring. The Family Attachment Interview and the Peer Attachment Interview developed by Bartholomew and Horowitz (1991) focus on conscious aspects of experience with caregivers in the first case and friendships and romantic relationships in the second.

Both are scored directly from audiotape (rather than transcripts) and rely more heavily on content analysis than the previous measures. They are scored for four 'prototypes' that overlap to a great extent with AAI classifications, but are derived from a different interpretation of attachment constructs. Secure individuals exhibit positive evaluations of both self and other, preoccupied individuals evaluate the self negatively but the other positively, dismissing individuals evaluate the self positively but the other negatively, and fearful individuals evaluate both the self and the other negatively. All of these interviews show stability and some convergent validity with other personality and/or relationship-based measures. Because they are less cumbersome and labour-intensive than the AAI, the measures of Bartholomew and Horowitz (1991) are gaining currency for research with adult couples, while the AAI continues to be used for studies of adults as parents.

In contrast to the previous interviews, which ask about real experiences, there are assessments for both adults and children which use projective techniques, asking the individual to invent a story. The narratives produced by these methods are scored primarily for content. In such situations, it is assumed that the individual's personal interests and concerns provide the template for interpreting the stimulus materials used to elicit the story. Two such measures have been used with children. The first of these (Bretherton *et al.*, 1990) is appropriate for preschoolers and consists of four story items introduced in doll play. The items describe incidents where a child accidentally spills something, is hurt, frightened and separated from their parents. In each case the child is asked to complete the story. Although secure-insecure differences are identified, this method does not yield a full classification system. However, the types of stories that children tell are related to attachment classifications or attachment-relevant information based on concurrent or prior observational assessments.

The second measure, namely the Separation Anxiety Test (Klagsbrun and Bowlby, 1976), was originally designed as a clinical tool (Hansburg, 1972), but has been adapted and used in some research endeavours with children up to 12 years of age (e.g. Main *et al.*, 1985; Resnick, 1997). It consists of a series of family pictures involving separations (e.g. parents going away for the weekend, a child going to school for the first time), and in each case the child is asked about the feelings of the child in question and what he or she will do. Different sets of pictures have been developed for use with younger children (e.g. Shouldice and Stevenson-Hinde, 1992) and older children (Wright *et al.*, 1995). Scoring is based on the nature and focus of emotional expression as well as on elements of coping style (Slough *et al.*, 1988). As with the doll-play stories, there is evidence of a relationship between behavioural attachment classifications and attachment stories

(Shouldice and Stevenson-Hinde, 1992). There is also evidence that this method differentiates between clinical and non-clinical populations (Wright *et al.*, 1995).

A similar technique has been developed for adults (George *et al.*, 1999). It consists of seven line drawings depicting both children and adults experiencing potential attachment situations (e.g. illness, separation). In this case, the scoring is based on both content and coherency, and a classification scheme paralleling that of the AAI has been developed. All of these tools are still being developed and, although promising, none of them has yet emerged as a commonly used standard procedure for assessing attachment. Because other methods for older children (8 to 12-year-olds) are notably lacking, and because attachment representations are thought to become increasingly important during development, it is likely that narrative methods will contribute to filling this obvious gap. Narrative methods have been most often used in conjunction with other classification methods, and the findings of these studies will be discussed in Chapter 10.

Other measures of adult attachment

Although there have been efforts to develop questionnaires directly based on the AAI, the vast majority of adult attachment questionnaires were developed without reference to the AAI and from a different research tradition – that of studying relationships within mated couples. Two excellent reviews of these numerous measures and their relationships to the interviews discussed above are available (Crowell and Treboux, 1995; Stein *et al.*, 1998). These instruments vary in their psychometric development, assumptions and focus. For example, while all of them assume that attachment is a quality of particular relationships, some instruments assess a composite attachment style over different relationships (e.g. Sperling and Berman, 1991), others use separate interviews for different relationships (e.g. Bartholomew and Horowitz, 1991), and still others assume a generalized style (e.g. Feeney and Noller, 1990). Overall, in the studies which have compared one or more of these adult attachment measures, the correlations are not strong. It is clear that several different constructs are being assessed. In general, measures which are conceptually and methodologically similar and probe the same areas of functioning are correlated with each other and yield similar results (Stein *et al.*, 1998).

Stability and change in attachment patterns

Methods for assessing attachment beyond infancy have developed with the assumption that patterns analogous to those discovered in infancy will be detectable at later ages. Thus far, this assumption has been largely correct, although it is also evident that there are often more variants of the primary patterns at older ages. Given the emphasis of attachment theory on the propensity for early experiences to be carried forward, there is also the notion that the adoption of a particular attachment strategy in infancy marks the beginning of a specific developmental trajectory defined by continued use of that strategy.

The columns in Table 3.1 can be considered to outline these trajectories. Thus securely attached infants become secure preschoolers and, barring major changes in circumstances, they continue to be secure (or balanced) through childhood and adolescence, eventually becoming autonomous adults. Similarly, avoidant infants become avoidant (or defended) preschoolers and, unless provoked to shift by contradictory experiences, they remain avoidant (or limited, or defended) through childhood and adolescence and become dismissing adults. Resistant infants become dependent (or coercive) preschoolers and have a propensity to maintain this pattern through childhood and adolescence to become preoccupied adults.

The significance of the disorganized classification in infancy is less clear. First, as we have already noted, disorganization and its adult analogue, namely lack of resolution of trauma and loss, are not strategies, but rather the absence or failure of strategies. None the less, the controlling patterns described for 2 to 7-year-olds can be viewed as very specific strategies. The notion that, with maturing skills, disorganization eventually gives way to an organized pattern is easily understandable. While disorganized and controlling patterns may be the outcome of traumatic early caregiving experiences such as maltreatment, it is also clear that they occur in the absence of such obvious trauma. In the former case, the conditions for unresolved attachment status in adulthood exist. In the latter case they do not, and it is only in the context of subsequent trauma that individuals could become unresolved. Thus the very nature of the patterns described in this column seems to argue against a consistent developmental trajectory from infant disorganization to adult failure to resolve loss or trauma.

Nevertheless, continuity could occur if early disorganized or controlling attachment imposes limits on one's ability to recover from loss or trauma. Such a condition appears to be a plausible one and, coupled with the fact that significant losses inevitably occur in every life, may constitute the basis for linking these patterns across the lifespan. The notion that some attachment patterns are protective against inability to resolve loss or trauma is illustrated in a study by Ainsworth and Eichberg (1991). In a sample of 45 women, they found that unresolved status was more often associated with the preoccupied classification than any other alternative, and they speculated on the reasons why preoccupied attachment might limit ability to cope with loss.

Against this background, we can examine data on stability and change in attachment. Attachment theory emphasizes the proclivity for attachment strategies to persist. Initially, this view was supported by studies showing high stability (> 80 per cent) within infancy under stable life conditions (e.g. Waters, 1978) and predictable change under changing life conditions (Egeland and Farber, 1984). However, there is great variability in reported stability coefficients (Thompson, 1997), and some more recent data (Belsky et al., 1996a) showed very low stability (46 to 55 per cent) in infancy. Studying the maintenance of infant attachment patterns into the preschool years or beyond is dependent on the methods described above for assessing and classifying attachment in older children. These reflect a range of constructs, assumptions regarding continuity, and assessment techniques. Many of them still require further psychometric evaluation, and there is little clear consensus on the best instrument for any one age period.

We noted above that two studies which used the 5 to 7-year-old procedures and classifications reported high stability from infancy to early school age (Main and Cassidy, 1988; Wartner et al., 1994), and one published study (Howes and Hamilton, 1992b) showed high stability between 1 and 4 years when the Cassidy/Marvin preschool scheme was used. Several unpublished studies have reported an absence of stability (Beckwith and Rodning, 1991; Goldberg et al., 1998; Greenberg, 1997, personal communication; Sutton, 1994). Thus the evidence for stable attachment through early childhood is mixed.

There are an increasing number of studies in which children originally observed in the strange situation as infants have reached their late teens or early adulthood and participated in the AAI. In all of these studies it is evident that salient life changes contributed to changes in attachment patterns. One of these was a stable middle-class sample for which Waters (1978) reported high attachment stability in infancy. These highly stable families tended to remain stable. For example, for those who participated 20 years later (50 of 60 original families), 78 per cent of the original marriages were intact. In the entire group, 64 per cent of the subjects maintained the same secure, avoidant/dismissing or resistant/preoccupied attachment pattern over the 20-year interval. For the subgroups which had not experienced any major negative life events, this figure rose to 78 per cent (Waters et al., 1995). This is similar to the figure of 77 per cent stability reported by Hamilton (1994) over a 17-year period. In three other studies (Beckwith et al., 1995; Lewis, 1997; Zimmerman, 1994) the stability was lower, even minimal, and events such as parental divorce, illness, death or psychiatric disorder predicted adolescent attachment patterns.

In most of these cases, negative events contributed to changes to less secure patterns of attachment. Less attention has been given to ways in which those who were insecurely attached as infants or during a significant part of childhood might become secure/autonomous adults. Clearly this does occur. The scoring of the AAI assigns an individual with a chaotic or clearly traumatic early childhood to the secure/autonomous category if he or she is able to describe events and feelings from such a childhood in a coherent way and values intimate relationships. These adults are categorized as 'earned secure' to indicate that they are secure despite experiencing childhood events that should have engendered insecure attachments. In two studies that made this distinction within the secure group, 66 per cent (Pearson *et al.*, 1994) and 43 per cent (Phelps *et al.*, 1998) of the autonomous group were in the earned-secure category. These figures suggest that a considerable number of autonomous adults were most probably insecurely attached as youngsters. The factors that contribute to these shifts towards security have not yet been investigated.

Overview

The development of attachment beyond infancy has not been studied as intensively as infant attachment and its sequelae. In part, this has reflected a delay in developing appropriate assessment instruments. These in turn depend on careful elaboration of the functioning of the attachment system at later ages. Despite these limitations, some instruments have been developed, and evidence on attachment at later stages of the life cycle is beginning to accumulate. The extent to which attachment patterns are maintained over prolonged periods is controversial because the evidence is mixed. The examination of factors associated with stability and change in attachment patterns is likely to be a continuing area of research.

Suggested reading

Main, M., Kaplan, N. and Cassidy, J. (1985) Security in infancy, childhood and adulthood: a move to the level of representation. In Bretherton, I. and Waters, E. (Eds) Growing points of attachment theory and research. *Monographs of the Society for Research in Child Development*, 50, 66–104.
The first presentation of both the 5 to 7-year attachment procedures and the AAI with a rationale for studying attachment representations.

Kobak, R. and Sceery, A. (1988) Attachment in late adolescence: working models, affect regulation and representations of self and others. *Child Development*, 59, 135–46.
An elegant study of attachment and some of its concomitants in adolescents.

Marvin, R.S. and Britner, P.A. (1999) Normative development: the ontogeny of attachment. In Cassidy, J. and Shaver, P.R. (Eds), *Handbook of attachment theory and research*. New York: Guilford, 44–67.
A detailed account of the development of attachment set in the context of Bowlby's ideas concerning attachment and general systems theory.

Waters, E., Kondo-Ikemura, K., Posada, G. and Richters, J.E. (1991) Learning to love: mechanisms and milestones. In Gunnar, M. and Sroufe, L.A. (Eds), *Minnesota Symposium on Child Psychology. Vol. 23*. Hillsdale, NJ: Erlbaum, 217–55.
A critical developmental account of attachment which incorporates constructs from contemporary learning research and theory.

Part II

Antecedents of attachment

4 Caregiver influences on developing attachments

In this chapter we shall begin to examine factors that influence the development of early attachments. Since the emphasis of attachment theory has been on the role that caregivers play in the formation of attachments, we start with this perspective. In this chapter we shall review the theoretical origins of such a perspective and then consider the extent to which the available data confirm the influence of caregivers on early attachments.

Theoretical considerations

Since attachment is an aspect of relationships, both partners contribute to the nature of a shared relationship, but early work emphasized the role of the caregiver in shaping attachments. The view that parents play a formative role in their children's development has a long history and has been widely accepted. In 1969, Ainsworth published a theoretical review comparing and contrasting three then current approaches to the origin and development of the mother–infant relationship, namely psychodynamic theories of object relations, learning theories of dependency, and attachment theory. Each of the three approaches emphasized the role of the mother acting on the infant, albeit in a different way. The psychodynamic approach conceptualized the young infant as being at the mercy of basic physiological drives. According to this view, the infant forms an emotional bond with the mother based on the way in which she acts to reduce these drives, particularly through feeding activities.

Learning theorists of the time endorsed the notion that the infant–mother relationship is a pattern of learned dependency that can be accounted for by the same 'laws of learning' that account for all other behaviour. Whether emphasizing primary physiological drives (e.g. Dollard and Miller, 1950; Sears, 1963) or a broad range of reinforcers (e.g. Bijou and Baer, 1965; Gewirtz, 1969), learning theories focused on the infant as the learner and the mother as the provider of learning experiences.

In contrast to the psychoanalytical and learning approaches, which considered the infant to play a rather passive role in shaping the relationship, Ainsworth (1969) heralded attachment theory as an approach which credited the infant with active participation in the development of the first relationship. Rather than being an undifferentiated bundle of primary drives awaiting organization, or a blank slate on which experience is recorded, the infant of attachment theory is genetically biased towards the social interactions that lead to emotional ties with a caregiver. Even though the infant's behavioural repertoire is quite limited, it includes behaviours that are highly effective in drawing attention and eliciting caregiving behaviours from adults.

Despite this emphasis on infant contributions to the infant–mother relationship, Bowlby, Ainsworth and most other attachment theorists identify early experiences provided by the caregiver as the primary determinant of infant attachment patterns. This apparent contradiction may be understood in several ways. First, as noted in Chapter 1, Bowlby (1969) articulated a theory about the evolution and function of species-specific attachment behaviours, rather than a theory of individual differences. Thus there was more emphasis on why and how infants generally form attachments, rather than on how and why individual differences in attachment behaviours emerge.

However, as Ainsworth initiated the study of individual differences, she believed that maternal behaviour, particularly sensitivity to infant signals, would be the main influence determining the nature of attachment patterns. It is evident, even to the novice baby-watcher, that no matter how competent and sophisticated an infant may be, the adult caregiver is infinitely more so. The adult possesses cognitively complex abilities, including concepts of relationships, and has goals for the infant, whereas the infant does not have comparable cognitions with regard to the adult. It is natural to assume that infant cognitions regarding the primary caregiver, or caregivers in general, develop in the context of the first relationship. Thus when we examine maternal behaviour, we are in fact seeing something that reflects a dyadic relationship. It will change as the relationship evolves, but it is grounded in the notion of a relationship from the start. In contrast, when we examine the behaviour of young infants, it is simply infant behaviour. It will come to reflect dyadic experiences, but it begins as uncomplicated individual behaviour. Ainsworth emphasized that her definition of maternal sensitivity focused not on maternal behaviour in the abstract, but on a dyadic concept of maternal behaviour–sensitivity to infant initiatives.

With the emergence of the strange situation as a viable assessment tool, many individuals attempted to replicate Ainsworth's initial findings or to use her methodology for other purposes. Often this occurred within the framework of theories other than attachment and the general thinking of the day that mothers would be more influential than infants in shaping patterns of attachment. Thus the initial thrust of attachment theory and research highlighted the importance of maternal behaviour as a determinant of the quality of attachment. Research that reflects this approach will be reviewed in this chapter. The later consideration of the infant's contribution to individual differences in the first relationship is discussed in Chapter 5.

Early data: the Ainsworth studies

In both Uganda and Baltimore, Ainsworth carried out intensive home observations. In the Ganda sample she visited in the afternoon once every 2 weeks, and in the Baltimore study, 4–hour visits were made once every 3 weeks (Ainsworth, 1977). The Baltimore study built on the earlier Uganda study and involved more elaborate scoring schemes and statistical analysis, but many of the concepts and general findings were similar. Among the Ganda babies, Ainsworth described three attachment patterns, namely securely attached, insecurely attached and not-yet-attached. These descriptions paralleled the three groups later identified in the Baltimore study as secure, resistant and avoidant, respectively. In both studies, mothers were rated on scales that reflected availability, amount of physical contact, and sensitivity to infant signals. In the Ganda study, the measure which best discriminated between the three infant groups was the excellence of the mother as an informant. Mothers who were rated high volunteered a great deal of information with spontaneous details about the baby, and were most likely to have securely attached babies. The not-yet-attached group was characterized by low ratings of maternal availability and minimal physical contact.

In line with the initial theoretical emphasis on distress as an important attachment signal, Bell and Ainsworth (1972) undertook a detailed analysis of infant crying and maternal response to this in the Baltimore sample. They found no stability in the amount of infant crying until the second half of the first year, whereas maternal propensity to be unresponsive to cries was stable over the same period. In addition, maternal unresponsiveness in one quarter was correlated with infant crying in the subsequent quarters. Mothers who were more responsive early on had babies who cried less and had more varied communications (e.g. vocalizations and gestures) at later observations. They concluded that (1) the effect of maternal behaviour on infant crying is greater than the effect of infant crying on maternal behaviour, (2) early maternal responsiveness reduces the infant's tendency to cry in later months, and (3) babies who cry a great deal in the second half of the first year have a history of low maternal response in the early months.[*]

These conclusions led Bell and Ainsworth to suggest that by the fourth quarter of the first year infant crying is no longer a purely expressive signal, but is sometimes a substitute for other forms of communication. Because

---

[*] This report provoked a critical commentary from Gewirtz and Boyd (1977a), followed by a rejoinder from Ainsworth and Bell (1977) and a 'rejoinder to the rejoinder' (Gewirtz and Boyd, 1977b).

mothers who were responsive to cries were generally responsive to other infant signals, they considered how to code this more general sensitivity. A set of global rating scales was developed to reflect this aspect of maternal behaviour, namely sensitivity/insensitivity, acceptance/rejection, co-operation/interference and accessibility/ignoring. Ratings on these scales were strong predictors of infant attachment classifications in the strange situation (Ainsworth et al., 1978, chapter 8). It was these data which provided the validating groundwork for the broader use of the strange situation as an attachment assessment procedure.

The ideas that arose from this initial work went beyond the immediate data and included notions about patterns of maternal behaviour that would lead to each of the three main attachment patterns. Secure attachment was thought to arise from consistent and appropriate responsiveness to infant signals, particularly those relevant to attachment. Avoidant attachment was linked with consistent unresponsiveness to these same signals, and resistant attachment was considered to emerge when the maternal responsiveness to infant attachment signals was inconsistent. Thus secure infants learn that their signals of distress elicit a maternal response that is likely to reduce distress, avoidant infants learn that their distress signals will not enlist maternal assistance, and they develop strategies to comfort or distract themselves, and resistant infants learn that the mother is unpredictable, and they become preoccupied with maintaining her attention.

Replication and expansion

It was not long before numerous studies appeared in the literature examining links between maternal behaviour in the home and infant behaviour in the strange situation. Few of them explicitly sought to test theoretical ideas about the specific patterns of maternal behaviour associated with different forms of infant attachment. Because the usual distribution of infant attachment patterns yields relatively few cases of avoidant and resistant infant attachment, these two groups were often combined in order to test differences between secure and insecure groups.

Most of these studies did document links between maternal behaviour and infant attachment, but the effects were rarely as strong as those in the original study. Ainsworth's global ratings scales were extensively used, but other observation schemes were used as well. No one else could invest the large number of home observation hours that characterized Ainsworth's work. More characteristically, one to four visits of 1–4 hours in duration each were used to assess home behaviour. In some studies, observations of mother-infant interaction were concurrent with administration of the strange situation. In addition, whereas Ainsworth's original work was concerned with maternal response to infant initiatives and signals, some of the subsequent studies looked at broader aspects of maternal behaviour.

Because these studies are so numerous, the best way to review them is to turn to systematic statistical reviews of these findings. There have been two published meta-analyses of this body of work. In each case, reviewers searched out studies which used the strange situation and had one or more measures of maternal sensitivity as predictors. These measures vary widely in terms of the situations in which dyads were observed, the method of coding, and the actual definition of sensitivity. However, the art of meta-analysis is to develop a common metric that allows these diverse data to be aggregated in order to estimate the average effect size of a predictor variable (in this case, maternal sensitivity or responsiveness) on a dependent variable (in this case, subsequent attachment assessed in the strange situation). Effect sizes below 0.20 are considered to be small, those between 0.20 and 0.50 are regarded as moderate and those above 0.50 are considered to be large (Cohen, 1992).

In 1987, Goldsmith and Alanksy conducted such a review of 13 existing studies on maternal sensitivity and infant behaviour in the strange situation. The average effect size for maternal measures was estimated to be 0.30. Studies in which maternal measures were taken closer in time to the strange situation procedure were likely to have larger effect sizes. Ainsworth's Baltimore study was not included in this calculation, partly because it was exploratory and involved a small sample, and partly because it yielded large effect sizes well outside the range of all other studies. The most recent meta-analysis included 66 studies (De Wolff and van IJzendoorn, 1997) and yielded comparable effect sizes for maternal measures (ranging from 0.24 to 0.32 for different measures). Again, Ainsworth's original study was excluded as an outlier. Contrary to prediction, studies with methodologies closer to that of Ainsworth did not yield the highest effect sizes. However, even the studies that De Wolff and van IJzendoorn (1997) considered to be 'closer' to Ainsworth's methodology were significantly discrepant in terms of the features discussed above. The authors concluded 'that although our results appear to support the "orthodox" position that maternal sensitivity is an important condition of attachment security, the outcome of the Baltimore study itself cannot be considered to be replicated.'

Why has a clear replication of the Baltimore study proved so elusive? De Wolff and van IJzendoorn (1997) note that 'in the current set of attachment studies the concept of parenting is virtually limited to the parental domain of warmth and acceptance.' In a significant earlier paper, MacDonald (1992) spoke of the need to distinguish between warmth and attachment and Ainsworth herself (Ainsworth and Marvin, 1995) highlighted this distinction. In commenting on the findings of De Wolff and van IJzendoorn Thompson (1997) remarked, 'If attachment is only one aspect of the parent-child relationship . . . parental sensitivity may be most influential in situations directly related to the development of security in offspring.

Sensitivity when the child is fearful, anxious, or distressed might be more prognostic.' Since few of the studies included in these meta-analyses focused on such situations, a low to moderate effect may be exactly what is expected. The broadening of the concept of maternal sensitivity to include multiple aspects of parenting may obscure the originally postulated relationship between an infant's early experiences of being protected and secure base behaviour as observed in the strange situation.

A few studies explicitly focused on protective situations, namely infant distress. Crockenberg (1981) defined responsiveness as the 'average number of seconds before a mother responded to her infant's distress signals' during a 4-hour home visit at 3 months of age. She found that the effect of high vs. low maternal responsiveness was negligible. However, maternal responsiveness did interact with social support such that maternal responsiveness had a significant effect on attachment only when social support was low.

Belsky, Rovine and Taylor (1984) found significant differences between mothers of secure and resistant babies in maternal physical or verbal soothing of infant fussing and crying at 3 and 9 months of age, but no difference between the mothers of secure and avoidant babies. In a third study, Del Carmen, Pederson, Huffman, and Bryan (1993) focused on the frequency of interactions involving fussing and crying on the part of the infant, and calming and soothing on the part of the mother. Of three dyadic variables considered to be possible predictors of attachment (social/affective, object-related and distress-management interactions), only distress management differentiated between secure and insecure infants. When entered as the primary dyadic variable in a discriminant function with the best infant (negativity) and maternal (prenatal anxiety) predictors, distress management was the most powerful predictor of attachment security, with prenatal anxiety coming a close second.

These few studies give, at best, a mixed picture. In Bowlby's early discussion of the development of infant attachment (Bowlby, 1969), he lamented the fact that the two human studies available to him (Ainsworth's 1967 Uganda study, and that of Schaffer and Emerson, 1964) did not distinguish betweeen different aspects of the infant–caregiver relationship, particularly attachment and play. By and large, this distinction has not been made in subsequent studies. As a result, the focused concept of attachment as a protective phenomenon has implicitly been broadened to include other aspects of parent–child relationships.

Given this broader definition of attachment, the meta-analytical data show a reliable small to moderate effect of maternal sensitivity (variously defined) on infant behaviour in the strange situation, and indicate that maternal sensitivity plays 'an important but not exclusive causal role' (De Wolff and van IJzendoorn, 1997) in the development of infant attachment as assessed in the strange situation. However, for the most part these data are less clear in identifying patterns of caregiver behaviour that distinguish different types of insecurity.

Two studies approached the issue not by attempting to replicate Ainsworth's findings, but by conducting experiments in manipulating maternal behaviour. Like the studies described above, they focus on comparisons between security/insecurity and contribute little to distinguishing the antecedents of different types of insecurity. In the first study, low-income inner-city mothers of newborns were given either an infant seat or a cloth carrier for their babies (Anisfeld et al., 1990). The assumption was that the cloth carrier would increase physical contact between the mother and baby and result in greater maternal awareness and response to infant signals. Observations when the infants were 3½ months old indicated that there were indeed differences in maternal behaviour in the two groups, with the mothers who had the cloth carriers showing more contingent responding to infant behaviour. When attachment was assessed in the strange situation at 13 months, more babies who had experienced cloth carriers (83 per cent) were securely attached by comparison with those in the infant seat group (39 per cent).

A second experimental study was conducted in The Netherlands, where van den Boom (1990) initially selected 100 newborns who were rated as highly irritable on the Brazelton Neonatal Scales (Brazelton, 1973). On the assumption that these infants would be especially difficult to care for, the mothers of half of them received a brief intervention when the infants were 6–9 months old. The intervention consisted of three home visits that involved videotaping mother–infant interactions and viewing the tapes in order to help each mother to read her infant's cues and respond appropriately. Observations indicated that the mothers in the intervention group were indeed more consistently responsive to their infants, and when attachment was assessed at 1 year, 68 per cent of the intervention infants were secure, compared to 28 per cent of the control group.

Caregiver contributions to disorganized attachment

Interestingly, the type of insecurity for which specific links have been studied is disorganization. Since the discovery of the disorganized pattern took place over 20 years after Ainsworth's formative research, the roots of ideas about caregiver influences on disorganized attachment are much more recent. They lie, first of all, in work with maltreated infants where some of the disorganized behaviours were first noted (e.g. Crittenden, 1985; Radke-Yarrow et al., 1985) and secondly in the development of AAI classifications, where parents of disorganized infants often reported unresolved experiences of loss and trauma. This work gave rise to the idea that disorganized attachment develops when the caregiver cannot alleviate fear because he or she has become a source of fear (Main and Hesse, 1990). This places the infant in an insoluble dilemma when anxiety or fear is experienced, as he or she can neither approach nor move away. If such experiences are repeated with sufficient frequency, the infant either does not learn an organized strategy for managing this distress, or cannot successfully implement a previously learned strategy. It is under such conditions that the unusual behaviours which characterize disorganized attachment are thought to emerge.

What is the evidence to support this notion? First, rates of disorganization are disporprotionately high in maltreatment samples (48 per cent vs. 15 per cent in community samples), (van IJzendoorn, et al., 1997). Frank maltreatment, whether it involves abuse, neglect, or both, repeatedly exposes the child to uncontrollably frightening experiences. There may also be other clinical samples in which unpredictably frightening parental behaviour occurs, but this evidence is less clear. For example, some studies indicated high rates of disorganization among the children of depressed mothers (DeMulder & Radke Yarrow, 1991; Solomon and George, 1994). However, this effect is not a consistent one, and when the data from 16 such studies were aggregated, the combined effect size was quite small (0.06) (van IJzendoorn et al., 1997b). A single study of mothers with anxiety disorders (Manassis et al., 1994) also found a very high proportion of disorganized infants, but the sample was small and this study has not been replicated.

Three studies directly tested Main and Hesse's (1990) suggestion by observing parent behaviour in the home with disorganized and non-disorganized infants. All of these studies found elevated rates of behaviours that could be characterized as frightening, frightened or atypical (Jacobvitz, et al., 1997; Lyons-Ruth, et al., 1999; Schuengel in press). For the most part, these behaviours were subtle rather than obvious. They included behaviours such as sudden looming over the infant, failure to respond to clear infant signals, brief fear grimaces, or handling the infant in a timid manner (Lyons-Ruth, et al., 1999).

Two studies also examined parental reports of dissociative behaviour. Such behaviours are included in the scoring schemes for the above observational studies, and it is easy to imagine that a caregiver's sudden and unexplained unavailability when dazed, for example, would be frightening to an infant. One of these studies reported a large effect (0.31) (Lyons-Ruth and Block, 1996), but the second and larger study reported a smaller effect (0.17) (Schuengel et al., 1999).

Thus there is a rationale and preliminary evidence to support the notion that disorganized attachment is linked to caregiver behaviour that is frightened or frightening. Full confirmation of these ideas requires a larger body of consistent data.

Other caregiver characteristics

Researchers have also considered the possibility that the development of attachment is influenced by maternal personality characteristics. In Ainsworth's original studies, although maternal behaviour was the primary focus, Ainsworth also noted some personality characteristics that seemed to be related to infant attachment patterns. In the Ganda study, for example, the best predictor of attachment was the mother's 'excellence as an informant.' In addition, her descriptions of mothers in the Baltimore studies suggested, for example, that mothers of future secure infants were relatively flexible and emotionally expressive, while mothers of future avoidant infants were more rigid and less expressive. These were not systematic assessments of maternal personality, but rather clinical impressions summarized in the context of the original exploratory studies. Some subsequent studies used specific questionnaire assessments in an attempt to identify links between personality characteristics and attachment patterns. Most of the links uncovered in these studies were those related to maternal psychiatric disorders such as depression, drug dependence and anxiety. These studies will be reviewed in Chapter 8 as examples of extremely adverse conditions for development of attachment. Within the range of normal functioning, although there is consistently the suggestion that better maternal psychological health is likely to be associated with raising securely attached offspring (e.g. Belsky and Isabella, 1988), there has been little consistent evidence produced to indicate that specific personality traits are associated with either security of attachment or particular patterns of insecurity.

Transmission of attachment: predicting infant attachment from the AAI

There is a growing body of studies showing relatively strong links between parent classifications on the AAI (interpreted to mean attachment representations) and infant attachment to that parent. The original development of the AAI used a 'guess and uncover' methodology to develop descriptions of the narrative style of parents known to have secure, avoidant and resistant babies, referring to them as autonomous, dismissing and preoccupied, respectively. Disorganized attachment behaviour in infants was associated with unresolved responses to attachment loss or trauma in the parent's history (Main and Hesse, 1990). In this initial work, based on Main's longitudinal study in Berkeley, the parental AAIs were administered when the children were 6 years old, 5 years after the infants had participated in the strange situation. Subsequently, a considerable number of studies went on to show similar matches. Most of these studies were conducted with mothers; a smaller number also had infant–father data. Several of these were prospective studies in which maternal attachment during pregnancy predicted infant attachment more than 1 year later (Benoit and Parker, 1994; Fonagy *et al.*, 1991; Lyons-Ruth *et al.*, 1999; Ward and Carlson, 1995).

The data considered in Chapter 3, in discussing validity of the AAI, indicate that knowledge of parental AAI classification does predict infant attachment. Recall that van IJzendoorn's meta-analysis of 14 studies (18 samples) with both infant and parent attachment measures found relatively high levels of agreement between these two measures. In fact, the average effect size was large (> 1 for most comparisons) and was not affected by whether or not parental data had been collected before, concurrent with or after the strange situation assessment. This effect size is considerably larger than those discussed above. Thus, parental attachment status or attachment representations are considered to 'predict' infant attachment, even though the majority of studies were not prospective. The underlying assumption is that parental attachment status remains relatively stable over long periods of time and, as indicated in Chapter 3, there is evidence to support this notion. Recall also that a significant number of infant–parent matches are secure-autonomous pairs. In the cross–tabulation of nine studies using all four classifications, 77 per cent of autonomous adults had secure infants, 57 per cent of dismissing adults had avoidant infants, 21 per cent of pre-occupied adults had resistant infants and 52 per cent of unresolved adults had disorganized infants.

Since the AAI classifications were expressly designed to mirror infant behavioural attachment patterns, it is not surprising that there is a high level of agreement between infant and parent attachment classifications. The initial studies in which parent attachment was assessed 5 years after infant attachment allowed for the possibility that experience with a particular child influenced parent attachment representations. The demonstration that prenatal interviews predict subsequent infant attachment leaves no question about the direction of effects. How are caregiver attachment representations transmitted to infants so as to shape individual differences in attachment behaviour?

The transmission gap

Since it is difficult to imagine that infants have direct access to parental representations of attachment, these representations must be transmitted through some aspect of parent behaviour towards the infant. If this is the case, caregivers in each of the four attachment groups should be distinguished by their responses to infant behaviour. There were 8 studies (10 samples) in van IJzendoorn's meta-analysis which provided relevant data and showed effects of parental attachment on parental behaviour (van IJzendoorn, 1995). The average effect size was large (0.72), but not as large as that for the AAI–infant attachment link. Given the small to modest effect size linking caregiver behaviour and infant attachment, we find that the link between parental attachment and infant attachment is stronger than the links for the postulated processes that connect them. In van IJzendoorn's analyses, maternal sensitivity accounted for 23 per cent of the association between parent and infant attachment. This phenomenon has been described as a 'transmission gap' (Figure 4.1, from van IJzendoorn, 1995). Since it was first described, attachment researchers have naturally been concerned with 'closing the gap.'

What could account for this gap? One possibility already discussed concerns the nature of the parent–infant interactions that have been studied. To the extent that these observations reflect a relatively diffuse idea of 'good parenting' or something other than protection *per se*, they may yield smaller effect sizes than observations focused explicitly on attachment-relevant contexts (Goldberg *et al.*, 1999; Thompson, 1997).

Another methodological issue arises, in that only three of the studies in the van IJzendoorn meta-analyses actually included measures of all three components (adult attachment, parent–infant interaction and infant attachment). Thus the effect sizes shown in Figure 4.1 for different components of the model reflect different samples of individuals. However, the three studies that did include all possible measures yielded mixed results. Pederson and his colleagues (1998) set out to conduct a clear test of the relationships between these three key variables using well-validated observational measures of maternal sensitivity in the home.

A key feature of these measures was the use of a 'divided-attention task' in the laboratory. Unlike most parent–infant observations in which parents do something with their babies, the idea of the divided-attention task is to

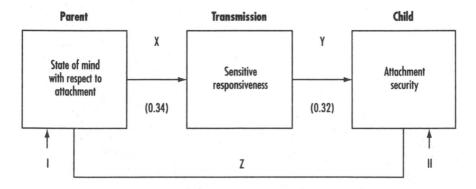

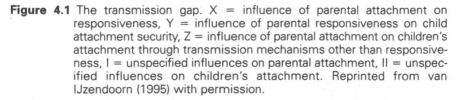

Figure 4.1 The transmission gap. X = influence of parental attachment on responsiveness, Y = influence of parental responsiveness on child attachment security, Z = influence of parental attachment on children's attachment through transmission mechanisms other than responsiveness, I = unspecified influences on parental attachment, II = unspecified influences on children's attachment. Reprinted from van IJzendoorn (1995) with permission.

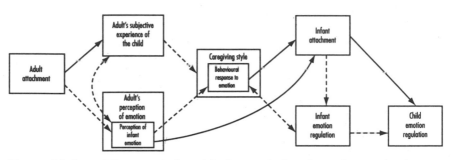

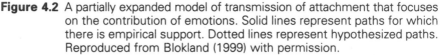

Figure 4.2 A partially expanded model of transmission of attachment that focuses on the contribution of emotions. Solid lines represent paths for which there is empirical support. Dotted lines represent hypothesized paths. Reproduced from Blokland (1999) with permission.

simulate a busy household in which the mother's attention must be divided between household tasks and infant behaviour. Thus the mother is involved in completing questionnaires or interviews with the infant in the room. In addition, the actual measure of sensitivity was based on a Q-sort that ranks maternal behaviour according to relevance for attachment (Pederson and Moran, 1995). Although Pederson and Moran found stronger links between maternal sensitivity and attachment than the average in the meta-analyses, maternal sensitivity again accounted for less than 25 per cent of the relationship between maternal attachment representations and infant attachment. Both maternal autonomy and sensitivity were strong predictors of infant security, but they were only modestly related to each other.

One useful approach to closing the 'transmission gap' is to recognize that Figure 4.1 is a very crude approximation of the transmission process. There are most probably intervening steps on both sides. For example, rather than influencing parental behaviour directly, adult attachment representations are probably related to representations of the infant. Such representations may then influence the way in which parents perceive, interpret and ultimately respond to different kinds of infant signals (see Figure 4.2). Infants may also differ in the signals that they present to caregivers and in their perception, interpretation and ability to react to caregiver behaviour. We began with the notion of attachment as an aspect of dyadic relationships, and the recognition that both partners contribute to the process of developing attachment. Thus far, the analysis of the transmission gap has been concerned only with the caregiver's role. We shall now consider the infant's contribution.

Suggested reading

De Wolff, M.S. and van IJzendoorn, M.H. (1997) Sensitivity and attachment: a meta-analysis on parental antecedents of infant attachment. *Child Development* **68**, 571–91.

A comprehensive meta-analysis of data on maternal sensitivity and infant attachment. See also the commentaries that follow.

Benoit, D. and Parker, K. (1994) Stability and transmission of attachment across three generations. *Child Development* **65**, 1444–56.
A unique study of mothers, infants and grandmothers.

MacDonald, K. (1992) Warmth as a developmental construct: an evolutionary analysis. *Child Development* **63**, 753–73.
An elegant discussion of the distinction between warmth and attachment.

5 Infant influences on the development of attachment

To the uninitiated observer, newborn infants may be indistinguishable from one another. Yet any parent who has raised more than one child will comment on how different they were 'right from the start.' Parents may even explain that they did their best to treat all of their children in the same manner, but found that their babies presented them with different demands, reacted differently to their interventions and developed differently. These early-appearing differences that persist and resist change are considered to be manifestations of infant temperament. Those who have studied temperament and emphasized its importance in development have been among the most vocal critics of attachment theory and research. This chapter focuses primarily on the controversy between temperament and attachment theorists, and reviews the relevant evidence and attempts at resolving the controversy. In addition, we shall briefly consider some other potential infant influences on early attachment.

Definitions of temperament

Thomas, Chess and Birch (1968) are generally credited with initiating interest in temperament in the modern research era. They were eager to counter the prevailing view that 'bad parenting' was the cause of most childhood behaviour disorders, and to make their colleagues aware that it is much more difficult to be a good parent to some children than to others. They defined temperament in terms of behavioural style, which included nine dimensions – such as activity level, predominant mood, readiness to approach new experiences, and so on. Their longitudinal study relied on parent interviews as the primary data. Later, Carey and his collaborators (e.g. Carey and McDevitt, 1978) developed parent questionnaires to provide a more systematic assessment of the temperamental dimensions described by Thomas, Chess and Birch (1968). As temperament gained credibility as a developmental factor, new questionnaires and then observational procedures were developed based on different models of temperament.

Temperament is often defined in terms of a biologically determined substrate of personality. This implies a predisposition to a behavioural style that is independent of experience. Thus Kagan (1994) defined temperament as 'any moderately stable, differentiating emotional or behavioral quality whose appearance in childhood is influenced by an inherited biology, including differences in brain chemistry.'

The predisposition itself does not change, but observable behavioural style is influenced by experience, including experience with caregivers. However, it is difficult to measure a 'predisposition' or to identify 'experience-free' components of behavioural style with simple observations or reports. Evidence that an aspect of behavioural style is persistent, resistant to change and linked with biological markers enhances the likelihood that we are truly assessing temperament. However, the most widely used temperament measures make inferences, either from observations of behaviour (e.g. Goldsmith and Rothbart, 1996) or from parent reports (e.g. Bates, 1980; Carey and McDevitt, 1978). In the first case, observed behaviour is not 'experience free,' and in the second, parent reports of behaviour or behavioural style have not only been shaped by experience but are also confounded by parent perceptions. However, the advantage of parent reports is that parents have access to more information about their infants' behaviour than any other observer. Studies relevant to the relationship between temperament and attachment use both types of measure.

Since temperament is traditionally defined in terms of direct physiological links, physiological measures such as heart rate (Kagan, 1994), salivary cortisol levels (Gunnar, 1990) or EEG patterns (Fox, 1994) are often studied as part of the temperamental complex. These measures are usually interpreted as markers of behavioural types rather than as measures of temperament *per se*. Behavioural, physiological and parent-report measures of the same temperamental trait are not necessarily highly correlated (Lamb and Fracasso, 1998), which raises further questions about potential 'gold standard' measures of temperament.

In summary, simple straightforward measures of temperament have proved to be somewhat elusive. For this reason, Bates (1987) suggested that temperament concepts should be considered as 'tools, not real entities' that enable us to 'see natural events in more productive ways.' For the purposes of this chapter, temperament refers to infant behavioural characteristics that are relatively consistent over time and resistant to change, even though the measures in specific studies may not be ideal indicators of these traits.

The controversy

Temperament and attachment theorists agree that relationships between parents and children are the outcome of child characteristics (such as temperament), parent characteristics, outside influences (e.g. family context, cultural expectations) and the synergistic effects of all of these factors. In focusing specifically on attachment, attachment theorists acknowledge a role for temperament (e.g. Sroufe, 1985) and temperament theorists acknowledge the contributions of caregiving experience (e.g. Calkins, 1994). However, these two groups disagree about the meaning of behaviour in the strange situation.

The intensity of the argument regarding interpretation of strange-situation classifications reflects the extent to which the assessment procedure has been reified. Observations in the strange situation are not 'attachment.' Rather, they are indicators of a relationship that is presumed to exist outside the laboratory. However, this assessment procedure dominates the literature, provides the foundation for central constructs and has been the 'gold standard' for other attachment measures. Thus, its interpretation is central to the field.

As discussed in Chapter 4, attachment theorists consider behaviour in the strange situation to reflect the outcome of an infant's repeated experiences of caregiver response to attachment needs. In contrast, temperament theorists (e.g. Chess and Thomas, 1982; Kagan, 1994) interpret behaviour in the strange situation as a reflection of infant characteristics. Infants differ in their vulnerability to distress, their style of expressing it, and their ability to modulate distress. Temperament theorists argue that it is these temperamental qualities which are being assessed in the strange situation.

Some infants – those who are termed 'avoidant' – simply do not become distressed in the strange situation and therefore do not need contact with their mothers during reunions. Others – those who are termed 'resistant' – readily become extremely distressed. It takes them a long time to settle once their mothers have returned. Hence they appear to resist comforting and do not easily return to exploring. It is not clear how temperament theorists explain attachment security because, as noted in Chapter 2, secure infants vary considerably in the amount of overt distress that they exhibit in the strange situation. Indeed, those who see the strange situation as an indicator of temperament often prefer to categorize behaviour in the strange situation primarily in terms of infant distress and contact-seeking, rather than the patterns relevant to security. The main point made by temperament theorists is that behaviour in the strange situation is determined less by caregiving history than by infant characteristics, particularly proneness to distress.

The evidence

For the most part, early studies did not find standard temperament measures to be systematically related to behaviour in the strange situation, although there were sometimes relationships between temperament measures and specific behaviours in the strange situation (see Bates, 1987, for a review of these early studies). Perhaps the clearest evidence that the strange situation is not a simple measure of proneness to distress comes from physiological assessments during and following the strange situation. Although avoidant infants are not overtly distressed, both heart rate and cortisol measures indicate that they are at least as physiologically aroused, if not more so, than other infants (Donovan and Leavitt, 1985; Hertsgaard et al., 1995; Spangler and Grossmann, 1993; Sroufe and Waters, 1977a). Thus, it is not distress per se that differentiates attachment patterns, but the infant's style of managing it. Attachment theorists would add that the strange situation assesses the way in which the infant uses the caregiver as part of this management strategy. Nevertheless, temperament theorists would not object to a description of the strange situation as a paradigm which assesses infants' style of managing distress. Ability to moderate distress is widely accepted as a temperamental trait.

Attachment theorists point to studies reviewed in the previous chapter in which maternal and infant behaviour were observed in the home and related to attachment classifications at the end of the first year. In most of these studies, maternal behaviours were better predictors of behaviour in the strange situation than were measures of infant behaviour. Temperament theorists point out that the effects of maternal behaviour are much weaker than attachment theory seems to require, and they note that infant characteristics and behaviours do afford predictive power in some studies.

It is worth noting that in Ainsworth's early work (Ainsworth et al., 1978, chapter 7), infant behaviour at home in the first and fourth quarter of the year was related to later attachment classifications. In the first quarter, infants who were later considered to be secure cried less and less often, and had more positive responses to being held as well as to being put down. In face-to-face interactions with their mothers, smiling and vocalizing did not distinguish attachment groups, but infants who were later secure were less likely to ignore their mothers and took more initiative in ending inter-actions than those who were later insecure.

In the fourth quarter, infants who were later secure cried less at home, took more initiative in making contact, were more compliant with maternal requests, and showed less anger than infants who were later judged to be avoidant or resistant. Ainsworth and her colleagues interpreted both sets of data as indicative of continuity of infant–mother relationships rather than as measures of infant effects on attachment. While the infant measures in both cases probably reflect experiences with caregiving, temperament theorists interpret these data as evidence of infant contributions to attachment.

The studies that are particularly interesting are those in which infant measures were recorded in the neonatal period and thus reflect minimal social experience. Several such studies found newborn behavioural measures related to later strange-situation classifications. Waters, Vaughn and Egeland (1980) reported that neonates later judged to be resistant were more motorically immature, less capable of orienting, and less capable of regulating arousal on day 7 than their counterparts who were eventually secure. Miyake, Chen and Campos (1985), and later Calkins and Fox (1992), found that neonates later judged to be insecure reacted to interruption of sucking with more intense and prolonged distress than those who were later secure. Finally, two studies indicated that newborns who were later insecure cried more in their first 48 hours (Holmes *et al.*, 1984) and were rated by nurses as more difficult to care for (Egeland and Farber, 1984) than those who later became secure. The data from these early behavioural observations support the position of temperament theorists.

One home-observation study in which infant measures predicted attachment classifications more strongly than maternal behaviours was conducted by Lewis and Feiring (1989). Mothers of infants in the three attachment groups differed significantly in both initiation and responsiveness to their infants in the home at 3 months, while infants differed in the amount of object- and person-oriented play in which they engaged. However, in an analysis designed to test methods of predicting infant attachment, only a composite measure of infant sociability was a significant predictor. Neither maternal initiation nor responsiveness discriminated between the groups. Although both infant and maternal measures were related to attachment classification, what is surprising about this study is that the data reverse the more typical pattern – infant effects were stronger than maternal effects. The authors are careful to point out that, although infant sociability can be considered to be an infant characteristic, it is impossible to rule out the effects of social experience with the caregiver. Indeed, since the observations were made in the context of the caregiver's presence, sociability may in fact be primarily a dyadic rather than an infant measure.

Some of the complexities in the controversy are indicated in the study by Crockenberg (1981) discussed in the previous chapter. Neonates recruited into Crockenberg's study were classified as either high or low in irritability based on their performance on the Brazelton Neonatal Scales. She defined maternal responsiveness as the 'average number of seconds before a mother responded to her infant's distress signals' during a 4-hour home visit at 3 months of age. Mothers were dichotomized into high- and low-responsive groups. In Crockenberg's study of infant temperament, social support and maternal responsiveness as predictors of attachment classification, the main effects of both temperament and maternal responsiveness were negligible. Instead, maternal responsiveness interacted with social support such that maternal responsiveness had a significant effect on measured attachment security only when levels of social support were low. Furthermore, low levels of social support were associated with insecure attachment classification only in the 'high-irritable' group. These data support neither the 'pure attachment' nor the 'pure temperament' story, but a more complex perspective on the determinants of attachment security. Two subsequent studies support this complex approach in finding both direct and indirect effects of temperament and maternal behaviour on behaviour in the strange situation (Seifer *et al.*, 1996; Susman-Stillman *et al.*, 1996).

In their 1987 meta-analysis, Goldsmith and Alansky reviewed the literature with a focus on measures of infant proneness to distress as well as maternal responsiveness. The average effect size for maternal influences was estimated to be 0.30. You will recall that the data from Ainsworth's original Baltimore study were excluded not only because they were of a different order of magnitude (4–13 times larger than that of other studies), but also because they were derived from a small hypothesis-generating study. The effect size for infant measures was 0.19. The latter, although small, was significantly different from zero. Indeed, these two effect sizes were not significantly different according to statistical criteria. Goldsmith and Alansky (1987) commented that 'An effect that many attachment researchers believe to be non-existent actually does seem to exist' and 'an effect that has enjoyed the confidence of most attachment researchers is not as strong as was once believed.' Unfortunately, the most recent meta-analysis examining the relationship between aspects of maternal care and behaviour in the strange situation (De Wolff and van IJzendoorn, 1997) did not explore infant measures as predictors. Thus we lack a recent and comprehensive view of the existing studies.

Rapprochement

An appealing 'empirical *rapprochement*' in this dispute was suggested by Belsky and Rovine (1987). They noted that the attachment classification system itself incorporates a temperament dimension – one which is evident when we examine the full range of classifications. Attachment patterns characterized by low distress and low contact-seeking (A1–B2 in Figure 5.1) form one temperament group and those characterized by high distress and high contact-seeking (B3–C2) form another. Each group includes both secure and insecurely attached infants. Thus, Belsky and Rovine suggested, caregiver behaviour determines whether infants are secure or insecure, while temperament (i.e. proneness to distress) determines the type of security or insecurity (i.e. high vs. low distress, biased towards limiting vs. exaggerating expression of attachment needs).

This argument was buttressed with data from three studies showing that some standard temperament questionnaires differentiated infants in these temperament-related groupings. Attachment classifications in the 'low-distress' grouping were associated with easy temperament and those in the 'high-distress' grouping with difficult temperament. Attempts to replicate these findings (e.g. Kochanska, 1998; Mangelsdorf *et al.*, 1990; Neuman and Goldberg, 1990; Susman-Stillman *et al.*, 1996; Vaughn *et al.*, 1989, 1992) were mixed. These mixed findings may reflect the 'rough approximation' of the continuum along which the attachment groups are shown to

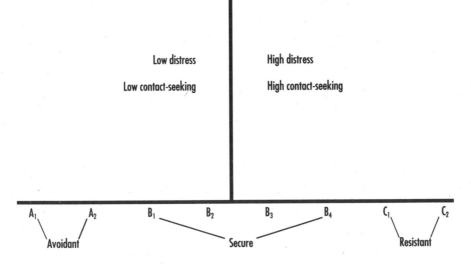

Figure 5.1 Attachment classifications and temperamental characteristics.

lie. For example, C_2 infants are not more obviously distressed than C_1 infants. Furthermore, it is unlikely that the B_3 pattern (supposedly optimal and most common) would be associated with difficult temperament (the least optimal and least common temperament type). Thus a simple match between attachment subgroups and temperament may not be as plausible as it first appeared to be.

In fact, Belsky and his colleagues (1995) later became convinced that this approach was incorrect. An important factor in changing their opinion was the previously discussed study by van den Boom (1995), in which 100 infants selected for high irritability as newborns were randomly assigned to intervention or a control group. The intervention was designed to enhance maternal sensitivity and responsiveness. In the intervention group, observations of mother–infant interaction showed that maternal responsiveness did increase over time. In addition, in the strange situation this group had a high majority of securely attached 1-year-olds. However, in the non-intervention group the predominant form of attachment was not resistance but avoidance. These data demonstrate that responsive maternal care can 'overcome' difficult temperament in determining behaviour in the strange situation. However, while the original suggestion was that difficult temperament should bias infants toward exhibiting resistant attachment behaviour, this study indicates that if such a bias exists, it is towards avoidance.

A trait or a dyadic characteristic?

Attachment theorists posit that attachment is both a trait and a dyadic characteristic. On the one hand, the strange situation provides us with a way of characterizing the infant–caregiver relationship (a dyadic character-istic) as inferred from the infant's behaviour. However, in order to do this, we assume that the infant has formed an internal representation of the relationship that filters and focuses perceptions and regulates behaviour (a trait). Yet in the argument between attachment and temperament theorists, attachment theorists emphasize the dyadic view, while temperament theorists focus on a trait view.

If attachment is a trait, then infants should show the same pattern of behaviour with a variety of caregivers. If attachment is a dyadic construct, then infants can show different patterns of attachment behaviour with different caregivers. It is clear that infants can and do exhibit different patterns of attachment with mothers and fathers (Fox et al., 1991a) or parents and professional caregivers (e.g. Goossens and van IJzendoorn, 1990). However, if there was to be a high degree of concordance between infant patterns of attachment to different caregivers, this would provide support for the temperament position.

Studies which included measures of attachment to both mother and father or parent and professional caregiver generally did not find significant concordance between them. However, Fox and his colleagues (1991a) pointed out that this could reflect lack of statistical power in single studies. As noted in an earlier chapter, the uneven distribution of attachment patterns requires large samples in order to obtain sufficient numbers of cases of the low-frequency patterns for analysis. Although parent/profes-sional caregiver data have not been subjected to meta-analysis, two meta-analyses of attachment to mothers and fathers have been performed. The first (Fox et al., 1991a, 1991b) found significant concordance for security/insecurity, whereas the second (van IJzendoorn and De Wolff, 1997), using a somewhat larger sample, did not. When data were analysed according to the high-distress/low-distress dichotomy, concordance was greater than would be expected by chance in the first analysis (Fox et al., 1991a, 1991b). That is, if an infant was on the 'limited-expression,' 'low-distress,' 'low-contact-seeking' side of the continuum with one parent, he or she was most likely to be on the same side of the continuum with the other parent. How-ever, security/insecurity within the split was not concordant – within the group of 'high-distress' infants, security with one parent did not predict security or insecurity with the other. The same was true within the 'low-distress' group. The second meta-analysis did not examine this type of concordance.

These observed concordances could reflect assortive mating patterns or similarity of parent behavioural styles that are either learned or reflect a shared context. However, they could also reflect a small but significant effect of temperament on behaviour in the strange situation. One study of infants on Israeli kibbutzim (Sagi et al., 1995) also showed significant concordance in attachment patterns with two different but co-operating caregivers.

Another study (Rosen and Burke, 1999) showed concordance in attachment to the mother and father for each of two siblings in the same family, often in the absence of concordance between attachments of the two children to the mother and to the father. Both of these recent studies provide evidence for child influences on attachment.

Genetic influences?

A limited number of studies explored another type of attachment concordance, namely that between twins. While twins share a highly similar caregiving environment, twins originating from two simultaneously fertilized eggs (dizygotic or fraternal twins) share no more genetic material than ordinary siblings. Twins originating from the same fertilized egg (monozygotic or identical twins) are genetically identical. If identical twins are more concordant in attachment patterns than fraternal twins, this would be indicative of a genetic contribution to attachment. Such evidence would support the notion that biologically determined infant characteristics influence attachment. It also provides one mechanism for the transmission of attachment patterns from one generation to the next.

Thus far, three studies with potential information on twin concordance of attachment have been conducted. The first involved a relatively small sample in which 3 of 4 pairs of identical twins and 2 of 4 sets of fraternal twins were concordant (Szajnberg et al., 1989). A second study (Ricciuti, 1992) combined data from three existing samples (two samples of 12-month-olds and one sample of 22-month-olds) in order to obtain 29 pairs of identical twins and 27 same-sex fraternal twin pairs. By using only same-sex fraternal twins, Riccinti controlled for potential within-pair variation attributable to gender among mixed-gender fraternal twins. Because there were age differences in some of the attachment measures, all of the analyses made statistical corrections for this effect. Ricciuti (1992) tested the fit of four different models to the data – one which included primarily non-shared environmental effects, a second with primarily genetic effects, a third based on shared environmental influences, and a fourth (full model) which included both genetic and environmental parameters. Secure/insecure concordance was low and non-significant for both groups of twins, and none of the models including a genetic factor fitted the data better than the pure environmental model. The findings for the high-distress/low-distress split were quite different. Here the intraclass correlation for identical twins was 0.58 and that for fraternal twins was 0.33. Although the difference between these correlations was not significant, adding the genetic parameter to the model significantly improved the fit. The best-fit model estimated 57 per cent of the variation to be attributable to genetic variation and 43 per cent to non-shared environmental variation and error. These data are consistent with Belsky and Rovine's (1987) proposal that the genetic effect is evident for the hypothetical temperamental component (high distress/low distress) but not for the secure/insecure component of attachment classifications.

Early data from the Louisville Twin Study with 34 identical pairs and 26 fraternal pairs used a procedure other than the strange situation for assessing attachment at 18 or 24 months of age. This procedure showed somewhat better agreement with the strange situation for the younger group than for the older group, but the level of agreement was high for both groups, and the difference between them was not statistically significant (Finkel *et al.*, 1998). It entailed separations and reunions involving both twins and the parent. During the first separation the twins were together. It was only during the second separation that each twin was alone and then with a stranger. Consequently, classifications were based only on the second reunion. For avoidant/secure/resistant classifications, the concordance for identical twins was 67.6 per cent, while that for fraternal twins was only 38.5 per cent – a significant difference. Interestingly, when divided into high-distress vs. low-distress groups, while the monozygotic twins were still more concordant (73.5 per cent) than the dizygotic twins (53.9 per cent), this difference was not significant. Thus there was clearer evidence for a genetic contribution to security than for the component thought to be related to temperament.

Subsequent data from the Louisville Twin study (Finkel and Matheny, 1998, unpublished data) examined a considerably larger sample at the 24–month assessments (99 identical and 108 fraternal pairs). Concordance for the tripartite attachment classifications continued to be higher for identical than for fraternal twins (62.6 per cent vs. 44.4 per cent). Interestingly, male identical twins contributed most strongly to this significant difference in concordance. Although the next highest concordance was for female identical twins, in this group and all three types of fraternal twins (male, female and mixed gender) the level of concordance was no greater than would be expected by chance. Quantitative genetic analysis further indicated that 25 per cent of the variability in attachment classifications was attributable to genetic factors and 75 per cent to non-shared environment. A difference in parental treatment is only one of many possible components of non-shared environment. This term includes error variance (e.g. measurement errors), differences in prenatal environment, differential treatment by other family members and different medical histories. Separate analyses for secure/insecure and high-distress vs. low-distress components were not performed.

Thus accumulating evidence indicates a significant genetic contribution to attachment patterns. It is possible, but not certain, that the route for this influence is primarily via genetic contributions to the temperamental component of distress proneness. There may also be a genetic contribution to security/insecurity.

Theoretical integration

There is indeed some evidence that behavioural dispositions measured in the neonatal period, particularly those associated with irritability, contribute to the development of attachment patterns as revealed in the strange situation. Attachment is a construct in which distress and its expression play a key role. Hence it is not surprising that an infant's temperamental traits – such as threshold for expressing distress – influence attachment-related interactions with caregivers. The evidence suggests that both caregiving and temperamental traits have both direct and indirect effects on attachment. Rather than argue about how much influence each of them has, it may be more useful to consider the way in which these two predictors interact in the development of attachment.

In 1985, Sroufe undertook this task. He reviewed the available evidence and concluded that attachment and temperament constituted distinct domains, the former being a dyadic construct and the latter a trait construct. He considered the following ways in which these domains may be related.

1. Attachment and temperament are orthogonal. Attachment and temperament measures represent different levels of analysis. Within this alternative, maternal care determines major attachment classifications, but temperament may play a role in determining which subgroup within major categories characterizes a particular parent–child relationship.
2. Security of attachment is determined by maternal care, but temperament determines the particular form in which insecurity is expressed.
3. Temperament determines the behaviours with which the caregiver is confronted, but these initial behavioural predispositions can be transformed by the type of care that is provided.

A fourth possibility (Rothbart and Derryberry, 1981; Seifer et al., 1996) is that temperament may determine the nature of appropriate care. Usually 'appropriate' implies 'tailored to the needs of the child'. What would be 'responsive care' for one infant would not necessarily be 'responsive' for another.

A fifth possibility is that temperament influences the way in which different infants experience particular aspects of care (Thompson, 1998). Thus an infant who is difficult to soothe and one who is relatively placid may interpret the same ministrations differently – the former as ineffective and the latter as comforting. An infant who is easily upset may have many more opportunities to experience caregivers' soothing efforts than one who is imperturbable, and may therefore develop different expectations of the effects of expressing distress.

Yet another possibility is that temperament influences how much an infant can be affected by differences in parental care. If this is the case, some infants will be securely attached regardless of caregiving conditions (as long as caregiving is well within the normal range), while others will be avoidant no matter what their care experience, and so on. Others will be extremely malleable and develop attachment patterns primarily on the basis of the care that they receive. Most infants will be influenced by some combination of inborn bias plus the care that they receive. Investigative efforts directed at exploring these possibilities promise to be more fruitful than previous attempts to determine the relative strength of temperament and caregiving effects on attachment.

Other infant characteristics

The temperament concept does not exhaust the list of infant characteristics that may influence developing attachments. The recent history of infancy research is populated with a series of studies devoted to the ways in which different medical conditions that occur in infancy may affect parent–infant relationships. A substantial number of these studies examined infant attachment as an important developmental outcome. Conditions which have been studied include premature birth, developmental delays, chronic illnesses such as cystic fibrosis, and malformations such as cleft palate. The general approach underlying all of these studies is that an infant's medical condition affects both the parents and the infant in ways that alter the nature of the parent–child relationship. The appearance and behaviour of such infants often differs from that of normally developing infants. This may reflect physical limitations, residual effects of medical treatment, or a unique developmental course. Medically compromised infants may be less active in signalling distress, less alert, have difficulty in feeding or be slow to develop, depending on the particular condition.

Whether it involves vigilant monitoring, extra medication, hospitalization or invasive procedures such as physiotherapy, parents must also provide additional care and meet somewhat different needs. Much initial and on-going care may be provided by specialized professionals. Relationships with these professionals can provide needed support, but can also undermine parental confidence in the ability to provide full care for their baby. Thus it is not surprising that many studies show that unique patterns of mother–infant interaction characterize dyads with infants and preschoolers born prematurely (see Goldberg and DiVitto, 1995, for a review), with Down's syndrome (see Hodapp, 1995, for a review), cleft palate (e.g. Speltz *et al.*, 1997) or other compromising medical conditions (e.g. Kogan and Taylor, 1973; Wedell-Monnig and Lumley, 1980).

Thus the expectation has been that medically compromised infants will be more likely to develop insecure attachments than their healthy counterparts. There are individual studies that support this prediction (e.g. Plunkett *et al.*, 1986; Vaughn *et al.*, 1994). However, a meta-analysis (van

IJzendoorn, *et al.*, 1992) which included samples selected for both infant and maternal clinical problems showed that infants' medical problems had very limited effects on attachment. The majority of infants in all diagnostic groups were securely attached to their mothers. Thus despite the general belief that an infant's medical condition may have direct and/or indirect effects on attachment, the available evidence does not confirm this expectation.

Conclusions

In this chapter we have considered two types of infant influences on development of attachment, namely those related to temperament and those related to medical conditions. While there is little evidence that medical conditions increase vulnerability to insecure attachment, as was originally predicted, there is clear evidence that temperamental character-istics exert both direct and indirect influences on attachment. Proposals regarding the ways in which infant temperament and caregiving combine to influence attachment point the way to future research in this domain.

Suggested reading

Chess, S. and Thomas, A. (1982) Infant bonding: mystique and reality. *American Journal of Orthopsychiatry*, 52, 213–22.
One of the early critiques of attachment work from the classic temperament perspective.

Susman-Stillman, A., Kalkoske, M., Egeland, B. and Waldman, I. (1996) Infant temperament and maternal sensitivity as predictors of attachment security. *Infant Behavior and Development*, **19**, 33–47.
An examination of the interplay between maternal sensitivity and infant temperament.

van IJzendoorn, M. H. (1995) Adult attachment representations, parental respon-siveness and infant attachment: a meta-analysis of the predictive validity of the Adult Attachment Interview. *Psychological Bulletin*, **117**, 343–87. Also the follow-ing critique by Nathan Fox, and van IJzendoorn's reply (*Psychological Bulletin*, **117**, 404–15).
A classical argument about the contributions of parental responsiveness and infant characteristics to the development of attachment.

6 Attachment in the family system

Thus far, we have focused on the development of a relationship between an infant and a primary caregiver, usually the mother. However, such dyads do not exist in a vacuum, but are nested within a family environment that influences the development and functioning of infants and their primary caregivers. Family members other than parents also serve as attachment figures, and each specific attachment is influenced by a network of surrounding relationships. As the size of the family increases, the complexity of this network escalates. In Figure 6.1 the top row of numbers indicates the number of pairwise (or dyadic) relationships (from 3 to 28) that exist in families of 3–8

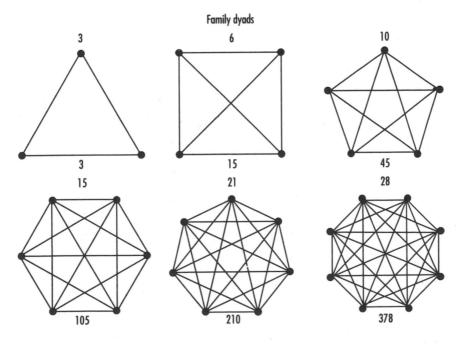

Figure 6.1 Family dyads and relationships between dyads. The number above each figure indicates how many dyads can be formed in a family of a given size. The number below indicates how many pairs of dyads influencing dyads can occur in the same context. Adapted from Emde (1991) with permission.

members. The second row of numbers shows the number of pathways by which dyads influence other dyads (from 3 to 378) in the same-sized families. Complex as it appears, this is an overly simplified representation of family networks because it only deals with dyads. Depending on the size of the family, there are multiple groupings larger than dyads, and each relationship (whether dyadic, triadic or larger) influences other relationships.

Attachment theorizing and research has been concerned primarily with dyadic relationships, which represent a very small part of this network. There has been some exploration of attachments other than the primary one, as well as study of the influence of sibling and marital relationships on primary attachments. However, in comparison to the plethora of studies on primary relationships, these are extremely limited. Nevertheless, there have been attemps to link attachment with theory and research on family systems. In the first part of this chapter we shall focus on family members other than the mother, the attachments that may be formed with them, and the way in which other family members or relationships influence infant–mother and/or infant–father attachments. The participants in these studies were most often traditionally organized families consisting of mother, father and one or more children. In the second part of the chapter we shall consider newly developing ideas concerning potential connections between attachment and family systems.

Other family members

Fathers

In their early interview study, Schaffer and Emerson (1964) discovered that for some infants the first attachment was to someone other than the mother. Most often, but not always, that person was the father. By 18 months, 80 per cent of the infants in their study were considered to be attached to their fathers. Not surprisingly, after mothers, fathers are the most frequently studied family members, both as influences on mother–child relationships and as attachment figures in their own right. Many of the early observational studies of infants and fathers were reactions to the predominant emphasis on mother–infant relationships, not only in attachment theory but also in other developmental theories. These investigators were eager to dispel the notion that the mother–infant relationship is the most important one in the infant's life and is the prototype for all subsequent relationships.

The first attempt to study fathers that incorporated Ainsworth's ideas regarding separations and reunions was conducted by Milton Kotelchuck (1976), but instead of using the strange situation, Kotelchuck constructed a more elaborate procedure which incorporated episodes with both parents (see Table 6.1). The design exposed the infant to all possible combinations

Table 6.1 Order of episodes for study of mother–father–stranger behaviour[a]

	Figures present	
Episode	Order 1	Order 2
1	Mother and father	Mother and father
2	Mother	Father
3	Mother and stranger	Father and stranger
4	Stranger	Stranger
5	Stranger and father	Stranger and mother
6	Father	Mother
7	Father and mother	Mother and father
8	Father	Mother
9	Father and stranger	Mother and stranger
10	Stranger	Stranger
11	Stranger and mother	Stranger and father
12	Mother	Father
13	Mother and father	Father and mother

and permutations of mother, father and stranger arriving and departing in the presence of each of the other participants. In total, 12 male and 12 female infants at each of five ages (6, 9, 12, 18 and 21 months) were observed during this procedure. Kotelchuck made no attempt to classify attachment patterns, but rather he tallied discrete infant behaviours in response to the arrivals and departures of the mother, father and stranger. Thus he examined change in play and crying and time at the door following the departure of each figure, as well as the mean duration of touching each adult on their return. In all cases, the largest differences were between responses to the mother and the stranger, with responses to the father falling in between these values. For the most part, responses to the father and mother were similar to each other, and both differed from responses to the stranger. These observations were used to argue that 'a monotrophic matricentric model of early infant interpersonal preference' (which Kotelchuck attributed to Bowlby and Ainsworth) 'is simplistic.'

Kotelchuck found little relationship between home caretaking and infant behaviour in his procedure on the basis of an interview about child-care activities with both parents. In fact, although behaviour towards mothers and fathers was quite similar, only 25 per cent of the fathers in this study had regular caretaking responsibilities, and fathers spent a greater percentage of their time with the infant in play than did mothers. Kotelchuck had only a very crude estimate of home behaviour in comparison to Ainsworth's extensive observations in Baltimore. Yet the data were similar to Ainsworth's finding that discrete behaviours in the laboratory could not be predicted from home observations (see Chapter 2).

The underlying assumption of classification in the strange situation is that the infant is being observed with a significant attachment figure. The low level of father involvement in this sample and the prominence of play as the primary activity provokes the question of how many of these fathers were actually significant attachment figures for their infants at the time of the assessment. Kotelchuck's findings with regard to father involvement are not unique in the literature. Although there are numerous studies documenting the ability of fathers to carry out the activities and responsibilities traditionally performed by mothers (e.g. Parke and Sawin, 1975), few fathers are primary caregivers of infants (Lamb et al., 1982), fathers are less available than mothers during infants' waking hours (Pederson and Robson, 1969; Richards et al., 1977; Russell. 1982), and fathers are more likely than mothers to read and to watch television (Belsky et al., 1984; Belsky and Volling, 1986) and to play (Lamb, 1977; Richards et al., 1977) than to engage in caregiving activities when they are with their infants.

In a relatively large study of the first 160 families from one city's birth registry that agreed to participate, the average father was found to be available to his 9-month-old for 2.75 hours daily, spent 45–50 minutes in direct interaction with the infant, and engaged in one caretaking activity per day (Ninio and Rinott, 1988). Of these fathers, 53 per cent engaged in no caretaking at all, and 46 per cent never took sole responsibility for the infant for as long as 1 hour during waking time. The average father was alone with his infant for an average of 8.8 minutes per day. In a sample selected for high levels of father involvement (Lamb et al., 1982), only 17 of 51 Swedish fathers had used their available parental leave to be primary caretakers for their infants for more than 1 month, few of the others used their parental leave, and all of the fathers reported themselves to be less involved than they had anticipated they would be when they were recruited for the study.

When engaged in similar activities, father–infant and mother–infant interactions are often qualitatively different. Videotaped interactions of mothers and fathers in face-to-face play with young infants suggest that fathers choose to engage in arousing playful interactions, while the activities of mothers are more likely to be directed towards reducing arousal and soothing the infant (Power and Parke, 1983; Yogman, 1983). To some extent, this difference is maintained even when the fathers are primary caretakers. In one study of face-to-face play, Field (1978) found that although fathers who were primary caretakers behaved more like mothers in some ways, several qualitative differences in interactive styles remained. Mother–father differences in interactive style were also observed in Israeli families where neither parent was the primary caregiver (Sagi et al., 1985). Thus responsibility for care does not appear to be the sole determinant of mother and father behaviour with infants.

In summary, although they are capable of serving as attachment figures, most fathers have limited opportunities to respond to attachment-relevant situations, and may be more oriented to the role of 'playmate' than that of 'protector.' Older infants and toddlers have been observed to direct more affiliative behaviour towards fathers and more attachment behaviour towards mothers (Clarke-Stewart, 1978; Cohen and Campos, 1974; Lamb, 1977), an observation which gave rise to the suggestion that fathers and mothers adopt different roles and influence different aspects of their children's development (Bridges et al., 1988).

If attachment is defined as a specific protective aspect of parent–child relationships, some fathers may not be attachment figures for infants. Although it seems likely that most fathers do become attachment figures for their children, these attachments may develop more slowly, if only because of the limitations on the amount of time that infants and fathers share together. I put forward such a suggestion on the assumption that attachment forms as the outcome of a series of repeated experiences that the infant and a caregiver share. On the other hand, if infant–father attachments develop concurrent with or very soon after attachments to mothers in traditionally organized families, we may need to revise our thinking about the basis of early attachments. One possible prediction is that infant–father attachment will develop more rapidly when the father is the primary caregiver.

Most of these speculations have not been explicitly tested. Among studies which used the strange situation to classify infant–father attachment, it has been surprisingly difficult to establish links to home behaviour. The first investigators to successfully do this (Cox et al., 1992) interviewed mothers and fathers individually about activities and responsibilities with their 3–month-old first-borns, and observed each parent with the infant for 15 minutes in a free-play situation. When the infants reached 12–13 months of age, each parent participated with the infant in the strange situation. These sessions were conducted 7–10 weeks apart (in order to reduce carryover effects) and counterbalanced – half of the infants were seen first with their mothers and half were seen first with their fathers.

In order to use correlational analyses, attachment classifications were assigned to a security scale developed by Main, Kaplan and Cassidy (1985). This scale ranges from a rating of 4 for most secure (B_3) to 1 for least secure (clearly avoidant, resistant or disorganized). The B_1, B_2 and B_4 classifications are given a rating of 3, and a rating of 2 is reserved for cases on the secure/avoidant and secure/resistant borders. This led to the interesting observation that, although the distribution of secure/insecure classifications was similar for the mother and the father (62 per cent secure in each case), more of the father–infant (32 per cent) than mother–infant (14 per cent) dyads were on the secure/insecure borders and were given a rating of 2. Most important, the infant's security of attachment to the father was predicted by the quality of interaction with the infant at 3 months, the time spent with the infant, and the father's attitudes to and reports about the infant.

For mothers in this same study, the quality of interaction and time spent with the infant predicted security of attachment, while attitudes to the infant and infant care did not do so. The authors suggest that, because fathers have a wider range of caretaking options than mothers, with infants in particular, the father's expectations and attitudes play a larger role (relative to those of the mother) in determining the nature of his relationship with the infant.

In a second study that established correlates of father–infant attachment, no home observations were made, but previously identified determinants of parenting (e.g. parent personality, marital quality, infant temperament) predicted attachment of 126 first-born infant sons to their fathers (Belsky, 1996). The more assets that the father, infant and family had, the greater was the likelihood that the infant would be securely attached. These two studies showing links between father–infant attachment and home conditions or interactions are balanced by attempts which either failed to link measures of father behaviour to later attachment (e.g. Volling and Belsky, 1992) or had mixed findings (e.g. Caldera et al., 1995).

In a meta-analysis of sensitive responsiveness as a predictor of attachment, van IJzendoorn and De Wolff (1997) included 8 studies with data for fathers and found that, in contrast to the reliable effect for maternal sensitivity, the effect for father sensitivity was not significant. Whereas there are multiple confirmations of links between home behaviour and infant–mother attachment, the validity of the strange situation for assessing father–infant relationships is not well established. The above reasoning suggests that one explanation for the mixed data on infant–father attachment is that the existing studies vary in the proportion of sample fathers who were attachment figures at the time of the assessment.

Thus those who observe fathers and infants in the strange situation make two assumptions that are not well supported empirically – first, that each father who participates is a significant attachment figure for the infant in question, and secondly, that infant behaviour towards the father in the strange situation reflects the quality of the infant–father relationship outside the laboratory in the same way it does for mother–infant relationships. Although these assumptions are logical, the failure of the limited data to support them indicates that caution is needed when interpreting the information we have about attachments to fathers. The same point can be made with regard to assessment of infant attachment to other family or extrafamilial caregivers who have been studied even less frequently than fathers. There are probably families in which the mother is not a significant attachment figure although, given the predominance of mother care, the number of such families is likely to be quite small.

The majority of studies which assessed father–infant attachment asked whether infant–mother and infant–father patterns of attachment are likely to be classified in the same way. In general, the distribution of attachment patterns with the mother and the father is similar, named about ⅔ secure, ⅕ avoidant and ⅙ resistant (few studies of infants with fathers included the disorganized classification). From Chapter 5 you will remember that infants can show different patterns of attachment with different caregivers, but attachment patterns with the father match those with the mother more often than would be expected by chance. Part of this concordance could be attributed to an infant temperament component that biased attachment patterns towards high or low expression of distress. What other factors might affect the configuration of attachment patterns to the mother and the father?

Marital relationships and child attachment

One possibility is that adult attachment patterns play a role in the choice of marital partner. Selection may be biased towards matches or towards specific types of mismatches. In one study of high-risk families (Crittenden *et al.*, 1991), although secure individuals had most often chosen secure partners, all but three of the remaining couples were described as 'meshed', such that one partner was dismissing and the other was preoccupied. A meta-analysis of five studies with both mother and father classifications on the AAI showed that matches in attachment pattern do occur more often than would be expected by chance (van IJzendoorn and Bakermans-Kranenburg, 1996). However, in a relatively homogeneous middle-class sample, such AAI matches did not account for concordance between infant–mother and infant–father attachment (Steele *et al.*, 1996). Instead, the model that provided the best fit with the data was one which included parents' influences on each other. In this case, the mother's attachment status was more influential than that of the father.

Thus parents may develop similar styles of response to their infants by influencing each other's pattern of child-care. Certainly there are many opportunities for this to occur as couples discuss child care, share the experience of rearing children, and learn through observation of each other. Because mothers generally spend more time with their infants and are assumed to be child-care experts (regardless of their training and experience!), fathers may take their cues from mothers more often than mothers look to fathers. Parents may also develop behaviour patterns that are complementary rather than similar. For example, one parent may relieve the other from infant care when exhaustion or preoccupation might lead to episodes of insensitive care. Similarly, one parent may take over non-parental tasks in order to free the other from distractions or stresses that interfere with sensitive care.

The birth of a couple's first child has been recognized as a major transition in adult life and in the development of the marital relationship. Living arrangements and daily activities are dramatically altered in order to accommodate infant care. A relationship that has previously been dyadic expands to include a dependent third individual. Couples have less time to spend with each other, and some of that time is devoted to infant-related topics (e.g. sharing information about the infant, negotiating arrangements for child care). In adapting to these changes, even when partners intend to share equally in child-rearing, it is common for couples to adopt relatively stereotyped sex roles, with the mother assuming primary responsibility for child care and the father adopting the 'breadwinner and protector' role (Cowan *et al.*, 1978; Entwhistle and Doering, 1981; Osofsky and Osofsky, 1984). This pattern emerges even when paternal leave is readily available (Lamb *et al.*, 1982). Typically, marital satisfaction is reported to decline following the birth of the first child.

The ability of the couple to adapt to these changes is the backdrop against which each engages with the infant, and this context most probably plays a role in the nature of the resulting attachments. Presumably marriages that are functioning well have a greater potential for supporting secure attachments with both parents. Although no study has generated data to the contrary, the data do not clearly support this prediction. Only a few studies have investigated the relationships between measures of marital quality and infant attachments, and the resulting data are inconsistent. For example, in one study, Lewis, Owen and Cox (1988) found that at 12 months, as expected, girls whose parents were in well-functioning marriages were more likely to have secure attachments to their mothers than those from poorly functioning marriages. However, this was not the case for boys. Furthermore, although the pattern for infant–father attachment was in the predicted direction for both girls and boys (secure attachment being associated with well-functioning marriages), the association was not statistically significant.

With older children, when marital adjustment was poor, toddlers were more likely to be insecure with one or both parents in the strange situation (Goldberg and Easterbrooks, 1984), and 3 to 5-year-olds were scored as less secure and/or more dependent on the Attachment Q-sort (Howes and Markman, 1989). However, at least two studies (Belsky and Isabella, 1988; Levitt *et al.*, 1986) failed to find these predicted relationships. Thus the evidence for the expected influence of marital relationships on attachment is equivocal.

Siblings

The birth of a second child heralds another transition in family development and associated changes in family relationships. The child-rearing resources that were once focused on a single child are now divided between two children characterized by different stages of development. Consequently, the parents once again revise their daily activities both to encompass the needs of the new baby and to reallocate their resources. Most commonly, fathers increase their responsibility and involvement with the older child while the mother devotes her attention to the baby.

Much has been written in the clinical literature about the first-born's experience of being 'dethroned,' and its possible implications for psychological development (e.g. Winnicott, 1964). Several studies which have assessed the amount of behavioural disturbance evident in the first-born following the birth of the second-born indicate that these reactions are related to the age and gender of the first-born, the quality of mother-first-born interactions, and the manner in which the mother prepared the first-born for the birth (e.g. Dunn and Kendrick, 1982; Gottlieb and Mendelson, 1990). Although multiple factors are implicated, at the very least this is a time when the first child's attachment to each parent is vulnerable to change.

Accordingly, Teti and his colleagues (1996) visited 194 two–parent families expecting a second child when their first child was 1 to 5 years old. A second visit was made 4–8 months after the new baby had arrived. On both occasions, the first child's attachment to their mother was assessed on the Attachment Q-sort completed by trained home visitors. Although security scores from time 1 to time 2 were correlated, average security scores declined following the birth of the baby, and this decrease was larger if the first-born was more than 2 years old. Attachment security at both time periods was related to the mother's affective involvement with the first-born (as assessed during a puzzle task) and a questionnaire measure of marital harmony. Increased affective involvement and greater marital harmony were related to higher security scores. Although maternal psychiatric symptoms were not related to initial security scores, they became more important in predicting security at the second assessment, as well as the decrease in security. First-borns whose mothers reported more psychiatric symptoms showed larger decreases in security.

These data provide a first look at family determinants of attachment during the changes marked by the birth of a second child. The fact that maternal psychiatric symptoms are more influential after the second birth is consistent with the common notion that vulnerabilities become more evident as conditions become more demanding or stressful. It also seems possible that, depending on the older child's preparation for the new family organization, confusion regarding changed parental responsiveness might be accompanied by transient disorganization in attachment. This might be even more likely if other changes (e.g. a move to a new bed or bedroom or to totally new living quarters, introduction of an alternative caregiver) accompany the birth. This is purely speculative, as there are as yet no empirical data to consult on this point.

In an earlier chapter we noted that a parent's state of mind with respect to attachment, as assessed by the AAI, consistently predicts the quality of infant attachment to that parent. If adult attachment status is a powerful predictor of infant/child–parent attachment, we should find that siblings in the same family exhibit similar attachment patterns to each parent. Although this has not yet been studied with respect to child–father attachments, in Chapter 5 we considered child–mother attachment in the special case of twins. There we considered concordance of attachment patterns in twins from the point of view of what they might tell us about genetic contributions to attachment. Identical twins were more likely to have similar attachment patterns than fraternal twins, particularly if they were boys. In these studies it was estimated that 25 to 57 per cent of variation in attachment patterns may reflect a genetic contribution.

Twins, of course, also experience a unique caregiving arrangement in that they share the attention of their parents from the very beginning of life. Whereas most children grow up in families with older and/or younger siblings, only twins have a ready-made, same-aged peer. Thus the case of twins may not provide a good basis for estimating general similarity in attachments between different-aged siblings.

One study examined two successive siblings in 65 families at 12 months in the strange situation with their mothers, and also observed the mother in a series of problem-solving tasks with each child at 24 months (Ward *et al.*, 1988). In this study of low-income, high-risk families, concordance of sibling attachment was 57 per cent (similar to that noted earlier for fraternal twins). Measures of maternal and child behaviour in the puzzle tasks were related to attachment concordance. When mother and sibling behaviours were similar, attachments were also likely to be similar. A second study (Rosen and Burke, 1999) assessed concurrent attachment to both mother and father in a 4 to 5–year-old (using the Attachment Q-sort) and a toddler (in the strange situation), as well as concurrent parent–child interaction in each of the dyads. In each family, with both mother and father, attachment of the younger and older children was independent. While mothers' caregiving behaviour was related to attachment of the younger child, neither mother behaviour with the older child nor father behaviour towards either child was linked to child attachment. Thus, while there might be a slight bias toward siblings forming the same kind of attachment to the mother, the addition of siblings can also alter family circumstances sufficiently to result in different maternal caregiving patterns and different attachment patterns with different children. The limited data on fathers are consistent with the previous discussion concerning the difficulty in linking paternal caregiving behaviour with child attachment to the father.

Parents' time and energy are increasingly divided as subsequent births add to the family. Depending on the age of the older children when these additions occur, some caregiving responsibilities are carried out by siblings. Attachment theorists have suggested a number of ways in which the older child's attachment experiences influence their ability to care for a younger sibling. For example, internal working models of attachment are thought to include representations of relationships with caregivers, as well as the role played by each participant (child and caregiver). Thus, as children mature, they are predisposed to re-enact elements of the kind of care that they themselves experienced (Bretherton, 1985; Sroufe and Fleeson, 1986). A simple modelling explanation makes a similar prediction. Children learn how to behave towards others, including younger family members, by following the behavioural models that their caregivers provide. Those who experience care that generated a secure attachment should thus be more capable of providing similar care for siblings. In addition, the confidence that a child has developed regarding parental availability in times of distress may affect the extent to which a new sibling is viewed as a threat to their own well-being. Children who are unsure of the parent's availability and have developed insecure attachment strategies may be more likely to react negatively to a new sibling.

Information on how a first-born's attachment influences caregiving behaviour with younger siblings is quite limited. The first such study examined the behaviour of 18 to 32–month-old first-borns when alone with an infant sibling as a function of attachment as measured with both the strange situation and the Attachment Q-sort. Securely attached older siblings directed more positive behaviour and less negative behaviour towards the infant sibling both at home and in the laboratory (Bosso, 1985).

A second study observed the behaviour of first- or second-born 2 to 7-year-olds in two–parent families with a 1 to 2–year-old sibling (Teti and Ablard, 1989). In this case, the attachment of each of the children was assessed, as well as the attachment behaviours of the infant towards the older sibling. Prior to the first of two laboratory visits, the mother received a copy of the Attachment Q-sort for the older child, and was asked to think about how each item was or was not characteristic of that child. On the first visit to the laboratory, only the mother and the younger child came and participated in the strange situation. Then the mother completed the Q-sort for the older child with the help of a research assistant. On the second visit, the mother and both children participated in a session designed to assess the interaction between the siblings as well as the behaviour of each of them towards the mother. This session consisted of a series of episodes during which the mother first attended to both children, then attended selectively first to one child followed by the other (instructing the other to play alone), and then left the room. During her absence, the two children were first alone, then with a female stranger, and finally the stranger left the room with the older child. Before the mother's return, the older child rejoined the infant to provide an opportunity to observe the infant's potential attachment behaviours toward the older sibling (see Table 6.2).

Table 6.2 Sequence of episodes for sibling study[a]

Episode	Participants	Description
1	Mother, infant and 2 to 7-year-old	Warm-up
2	Mother and both siblings	Mother attends to one child, and instructs the other to play alone (counterbalanced)
3	Mother and both siblings	Mother switches attention to the other child
4	Both siblings	Mother departs
5	Stranger and both siblings	Stranger enters, responds but does not initiate contact with children
6	Infant	Stranger leaves with older child
7	Infant and 2 to 7-year-old	Older child returns
8	Mother and both siblings	Mother returns

[a] Based on Teti and Ablard (1989).

Older siblings with higher security scores were more likely to attempt to soothe and comfort distressed infants. Older siblings who were insecure were sometimes nurturing towards their infant siblings, but only under extreme circumstances – that is, when the latter were very distressed. These relationships were not moderated by the age or gender of the older child. Furthermore, infants whose older siblings had higher security scores were less likely to be distressed when alone with the sibling. Although infants generally did not direct attachment behaviours towards the older sibling, they were more likely to do so when the older sibling was more secure. Furthermore, infants who were secure with their mothers were less likely to protest when the mother directed attention towards the older sibling, but a similar pattern was not found for the older children. Thus there is some evidence to support the notion that children's care of younger siblings is influenced by their existing attachments to the mother, and that infant attachments to older children may reflect the older child's attachment status. However, it is less clear whether an older child's attachment status predicts reactions to loss of maternal attention.

Family systems and attachment

Theories

The phenomena discussed above illustrate the functioning of attachment within family systems. Attachment theory is relatively unique among developmental theories in being a theory about systems. This is not surprising, as Bowlby deliberately incorporated biological thinking concerning living organisms as systems and reflected themes from what is called 'general systems theory' in his work. The basic notion of systems theory is that phenomena cannot be fully explained by analysing their component elements – rather, the whole can only be understood when the relationships between the elements are taken into account.

Thus attachment itself cannot be fully understood by looking only at the individual. Any attachment relationship is a 'goal-corrected' biobehavioural system featuring mutual regulation of two partners in order to fulfil a specific function (protection of one member by another). Furthermore, attachment in such a dyad operates concurrently with other systems (e.g. for the infant, the exploratory system, the affiliative (or sociable) system, the fear-wariness system). In fact, we characterize attachment patterns in terms of relationships among systems. We say, for example, that secure infants exhibit a balance between exploration and attachment behaviour that is flexibly moderated by environmental circumstances. Each of the other patterns is considered to be less flexible and characterized by a bias towards relying more heavily on a particular system. Avoidant infants are biased towards activating exploratory activities under conditions that are expected to activate attachment behaviour, whereas resistant infants are disposed to engage in attachment behaviours under conditions that are expected to activate exploration.

A number of thinkers have pointed out that, among the array of psychological theories, attachment theory is uniquely suited to be integrated with family systems theories precisely because it is a theory about systems to begin with (e.g. Byng-Hall, 1990; Byng-Hall and Stevenson-Hinde, 1991; Marvin and Stewart, 1990; Stevenson-Hinde, 1990). These developments reflect Bowlby's early interests in the role of the family in the aetiology and treatment of childhood behaviour problems (see Chapter 1). Theories about family systems have been developed primarily by sociologists and by clinicians engaged in therapeutic work with families. The family is characterized as consisting of many subsystems, with each family member participating in different subsystems both sequentially and simultaneously. Thus families include a spouse subsystem, a parenting subsystem, multiple parent–child subsystems, sibling subsystems and, depending on the family situation, subsystems, that include varying numbers and kinship statuses of other relatives. Each subsystem has its own implicit rules to govern interactions and relationships between members as well as relationships with other subsystems.

The transitions described above as adaptations that families make as new members are added can be described as additions of subsystems, changes in subsystem membership, and realignments in the boundaries of subsystems. We have discussed the beginnings of attachment research on these phenomena. Changes also occur in response to other significant internal or external events, such as loss of family members, family moves, and change in employment conditions of one or more members. Well-functioning families are able to make these changes readily, whereas others are either hampered in their efforts or unable to implement change. It is in these latter cases that families develop 'symptoms' that may require therapeutic intervention. John Byng-Hall (1990) articulated the notion of family therapy as a process in which the family therapist serves as a transitional attachment figure who is able to 'open' the family system for development of adaptive realignments.

Several family systems theories identify different types of family systems in terms that strongly resemble patterns of attachment. We shall consider two of these. Marvin and Stewart (1990) outline Minuchin's (1974) descriptions of three types of family systems or subsystems thus:

1. adaptive: 'mutually sensitive, openly communicative and supportive, while respectful of developmental and situationally appropriate autonomy;'
2. disengaged: 'avoidant, or under-involved, angry and insensitive;'
3. enmeshed: 'over-involved, intrusive, ambivalent, and disrespectful of appropriate autonomy and boundaries.'

From the above descriptions it is easy to see the similarities between adaptive family systems and secure attachments, disengaged family patterns and avoidant/dismissing attachments, and family enmeshment and resistant/preoccupied attachment patterns. These apparent analogies lead to the conjecture that there is a propensity for secure attachments to occur in adaptive families, for avoidant/dismissing attachments to occur in disengaged families and for resistant/preoccupied attachments to characterize enmeshed families. Thus far, there are no empirical data available to test this hypothesis.

However, there is at least one example of an attempt to test similar predictions arising from another family systems theory, namely David Reiss's (1981) theory of family paradigms. Reiss characterized family problem-solving styles as organized by shared group constructions of reality which he called 'paradigms.' These paradigms have many features in common with Bowlby's notion of working models. In fact, Reiss's paradigms might be considered to be family 'working models' with family rules and rituals as the content (Hillburn-Cobb, 1993).

Reiss described three types of family paradigms:

1. environmentally sensitive: there is a shared perception of the environment as masterable and reliable. Family members openly exchange information and do not feel pressured to arrive at solutions until all of the evidence has been logically examined. Hillburn-Cobb (1996) consid-

ered this paradigm to be analogous to secure (or in her adolescent system, balanced) attachment, and expected that families with secure or balanced attachments would share this family paradigm;

2. distancing: the environment is viewed as complex yet masterable, but affects each individual in a unique way. Collaboration is viewed as introducing more problems than advantages, and individual initiatives are preferred. There may be a strong emphasis in the family on achievement and autonomy. Such families settle quickly for less complex problem solutions. Families with distancing paradigms were expected to have dismissing (or limiting) attachments (Hillburn-Cobb, 1996);

3. consensus-sensitive: family members view the environment as chaotic and unknowable, and prefer their own shared view of events. These families focus on solidarity among themselves, and give minimal attention to environmental cues. They often reach a quick consensus without thoroughly evaluating the information. This paradigm was predicted to characterize families with preoccupied (or involving) attachments (Hillburn-Cobb, 1996).

An empirical test

Hillburn-Cobb (1996) tested these predictions by studying 62 family triads (mother–father–adolescent) in order to obtain multiple measures of attachment of the adolescent to each parent as well as a measure of family problem-solving. The latter was based on a task developed by Reiss and his colleagues to assess family paradigms. Family members sort two sets of cards containing alphabet letters arranged so as to allow many different ways of grouping the cards. These groupings can be objectively ranked in terms of complexity. While engaged in the sorting task, individual family members are situated in separate booths and must communicate via microphones and signal lights. For the first card sort, each member works alone, and for the second, participants are encouraged to confer with each other, although they are told that they are not required to do so. On the basis of scores for the actual sorts and behaviour during the sorting process, families can be identified as using one of the three paradigms described above.

Configurations of adolescent–parent attachment in the triad were compared with family scores on the Reiss Card Sorting Procedure. The majority of adolescent attachments to the mother and the father were congruent – that is, the adolescent showed the same attachment pattern with both parents. These congruent configurations were related to the family paradigms inferred from the card sorting task in much the same way that Hillburn-Cobb (1996) predicted. This study stands as one of the few investigations that empirically support the notion that specific types of family systems will be linked with particular attachment patterns. Do family paradigms emerge as a result of the configuration of existing attachment patterns? Or are attachment patterns shaped by pre-existing family paradigms? Probably the influence is bidirectional, but these are questions that require further empirical research.

Overview

In this chapter we have taken a 'first look' at some of the family figures other than the primary caregiver to whom an infant or child might be attached, and we have considered both the ways in which attachment relationships can influence one another and ways in which attachments may be influenced by the more complex family environment. Because fathers and siblings have been the primary subjects of study, these were the figures we have considered. This does not mean that grandparents, aunts, uncles and cousins are not attachment figures or cannot influence primary attachment relationships – only that we lack the relevant information to discuss them in detail.

Just as attachments are developed and maintained within the family system, the family exists within a broader context. Young children may be cared for by adults outside their household and develop attachments to these individuals. Furthermore, the cultural context in which the family is embedded affects significant aspects of the family system, including the extent to which extra familial adults serve as caregivers. In the next chapter we shall consider these influences on attachment.

Suggested reading

Marvin, R.S. and Stewart, R.B. (1990) A family systems framework for the study of attachment. In Greenberg, M.T. Cicchetti, D. and Cummings, E.M. (Eds), *Attachment in the preschool years*. Chicago: University of Chicago Press, 51–86.
An excellent discussion of the relationship between attachment theory and family systems theories.

Teti, D. M. and Ablard, K.E. (1989) Security of attachment and infant–sibling relationships: a laboratory study. *Child Development* 60, 1519–28.
A solid study and one of the few to examine infant–sibling relationships.

Crittenden, P.M., Partridge, M.F. and Clausen, A. H. (1991) Family patterns of relationship in normative and dysfunctional families. *Development and Psychopathology* 3, 491–512.
Some provocative analyses of attachment in couples and families, with data comparing well and poorly functioning families.

7 Beyond the family

In the previous chapter we assumed that children live in households consisting of a mother, father and their children, and that these were therefore the available attachment figures. In fact, if we did a world survey, this household arrangement would not be the most common. Even in the industrialized Western world where this is considered to be the norm, there are numerous variations in household composition. An increasing number of children are reared in households with one parent, two partners of the same gender, multi-generational families, or households that include a non-familial resident.

In addition, many children, even during infancy, regularly spend time in the care of someone other than a household member, either in their own homes or in a centre organized for that purpose. Although arrangements with professional live-in caregivers are routine in wealthy families in many cultures, the use of extrafamilial caregivers so that mothers can engage in paid work outside the home has been highly controversial. The first part of this chapter will examine some of the issues in and data on that controversy.

The second part will focus on the cultural context of child-rearing and its implications for family organization and child-rearing goals. Bowlby's vision of attachment theory was concerned with features that are universal for our species. However, most of the development and exploration of his ideas is the work of predominantly middle-class academics in highly industrialized countries. The underlying assumptions regarding child-rearing goals and children's needs may not be equally applicable to all of the varied conditions in which child-rearing occurs on our planet. For example, in some cultures (e.g. the Efe foragers in Zaire; see Tronick *et al.*, 1992), in contrast to emphasis on a single unique caregiver for young children, multiple simultaneous caregivers are the norm. Infants may sleep in the same bed with their mothers (e.g. Japanese and Mayan infants), in a separate bed but in the same room, in a room of their own, or in a special children's house away from their parents (as on some Israeli kibbutzim). These variations in caregiving practice and child-rearing expectations may have implications for attachment. Although the secure pattern is considered to be optimal, there may be cultures in which another pattern is more advantageous. For example, Belsky, Steinberg and Draper (1991) argued that under relatively benificent conditions, where it can be taken for granted that offspring will survive to reproduce, it is adaptive to delay childbearing, limit the number of offspring and invest heavily in individual offspring. These are conditions under which secure attachment is both likely to occur and desirable. Under adverse conditions, where the survival of offspring is less certain, it is more adaptive to produce many offspring in order to increase the likelihood that at least some will reach adulthood. Thus it is desirable to begin reproduction early, produce many offspring, and invest minimally in each of them. In these circumstances, avoidant attachments are more adaptive. Do cultural variations influence the distribution of attachment patterns and, if so, how? These issues will be discussed in the second part of the chapter.

Maternal employment and alternative care

Bowlby and those who followed him emphasized the importance of a prolonged period of consistent care by a primary caregiver for optimal early development. Although Bowlby noted that this figure did not have to be the biological mother, the majority of infants world-wide are cared for by their biological mothers. Thus both research and theorizing assume biological motherhood, and the term 'mother' is used generically to mean 'primary caregiver.' In industrialized nations, an increasing number of families rely on two incomes for economic survival or comfort, and limited (or no) maternity leave means that many mothers return to work while their infants are still young. There is evidence to suggest that, for preschoolers and older children, maternal employment has some benefits (see Hoffman, 1979, 1989), but there is less confidence about alternative care for infants. None the less, in the 1990s well over 50 per cent of 1 to 3-year-olds in Canada, for example, were living in families with mothers working outside the home (Statistics Canada, 1996).

What does this mean for developing attachment relationships? One set of implications is related to the impact of maternal employment on family life and infant attachment to each parent. A second set focuses on the relationships that infants form with professional caregivers.

Attachment to the mother: hypotheses

The negative consequences of maternal employment have received considerable attention. Both popular and professional thought is marked by the implicit belief that mothers should be solely responsible for infant care. At the same time, there are cultures where this is not the norm. Furthermore, most professionals are themselves working mothers or fathers, eager to reassure both themselves and other families. The literature in the field is marked by tensions between these conflicting personal concerns.

The more time a mother spends outside the home, the less available she is to the infant. Fewer attachment-relevant situations occur while the infant is in her care, and more of these situations occur in the care of someone else. This is just as true for stay-at-home mothers (who employ occasional or regular babysitters) as for those who regularly work away from home. In the latter case, separations are frequent, regular, and follow a predictable pattern. Thus the infant of a mother working outside the home experiences departures and returns more often, more regularly and more predictably than one whose mother is usually at home. It is also likely that for a mother with a major commitment outside the home, work and child care compete for her available energy and enthusiasm.

How do these different experiences of maternal availability affect the infant? One suggestion is that low availability and repeated separations lead the infant to view the mother as unavailable and unresponsive, and will be associated with an increase in insecure attachments. In the light of the issues raised in the previous chapter, we must also consider the possibility that repeated and prolonged separations are linked with slower development of attachment and/or choice of someone else as the primary attachment figure.

An alternative prediction is that repeated separations and reunions, particularly those that are regular, help the infant to learn that separations are temporary and that the mother always returns. These conditions should increase confidence in the mother's return in comparison to peers with a stay-at-home mother. If this is the case, the brief separations of the strange situation may not activate attachment behaviour reliably. If the substitute caregiver's style of infant care echoes that of the mother, this could support more rapid generalization of the infant's representational models of adult behaviour. It seems likely that parents choose other caregivers whose attitudes and styles of infant care are similar to their own. If so, we would expect to find similar patterns of attachment to parents and professional caregivers.

Yet a third possibility is that the use of substitute care on a regular basis has no effect at all on attachment to the mother. Mothers who routinely work during an infant's waking hours are usually available full-time at weekends and in the evenings. This may provide ample opportunity to support formation of the first attachment. For example, there is some evidence that responses to night waking are especially salient in the formation of attachments. On Israeli kibbutzim where infants slept at home, the rate of secure attachment to the mother was higher than it was in kibbutzim where infants slept in the children's house (Sagi *et al.*, 1994a). We shall review this particular study in more detail when we compare cultural differences in caregiving.

Even the best of other caregivers, including relatives, differ from parents in the level of emotional investment that they make in any particular infant. In some child-care arrangements, caregivers have several or many infants to care for simultaneously. In others, although there is only one infant to be looked after at any given time, the caregiver knows that eventually this child will be replaced by another. In fact, in many day-care settings, high turnover of staff is common. This differential involvement and possible lack of consistency is likely to be detected by the infant. Thus the first attachments may be biased towards the parents even when they are not available full-time. The age of the infant when alternative care begins, the quality and consistency of that alternative care, and the relationship between the parents and other caregivers probably moderates any of these predictions.

Of course, identical issues can be raised with regard to infant attachments to fathers, the majority of whom regularly leave home for paid employment. Yet it has rarely been suggested that low availability of the father and repeated infant–father separations will have a detrimental effect on infant development. The effects of other caregivers on attachment to the father have not been widely studied, although such effects would be predicted.

For example, when a mother works regularly outside the home, the balance between care by the mother and the father may alter. In some cases, the father is the main caregiver during the mother's time away from home. Mothers who are at home full-time with their infants often consider evenings to be father–infant time. When both parents are away in the daytime, parents may be more likely to spend the evenings together with the infant, or agree that it is more important for the mother and baby to be together. In fact, some studies that examined the effect of maternal employment found that attachments to the father were affected more than those to the mother (e.g. Belsky and Rovine, 1988; Chase-Lansdale and Owen, 1987).

The controversy and the evidence

In the 1970s when out-of-home care was on the increase but was still considered unusual, there was a wave of studies examining the effects of centre-based care on infants. These studies were conducted in centres that provided exceptionally good-quality care. Most of them were attached to academic institutions, had carefully selected staff, low infant–caregiver ratios, and carefully designed developmental programmes. Investigators were eager to demonstrate the worth of these centres and their programmes. For example, a large study comparing Anglo- and Chinese-American infants at home or in day care provided exemplary centre-based care and a stimulating developmental programme, and ensured that each infant had both a consistent primary caregiver and a regular alternative of matching ethnicity (Kagan et al., 1978). In this study, there were no significant developmental differences between infants in day care and those at home. Reviews of these early studies (e.g. Belsky and Steinberg, 1978;

Clarke-Stewart and Fein, 1983) indicated few negative effects of centre-based day care. In fact, in some cases the centres serving disadvantaged infants were found to confer certain advantages (e.g. Ramey and Mills, 1977).

These studies provided some data on infant–mother interactions, but did not assess attachment *per se*. Even more important, the centres in these studies were a far cry from those available to most parents seeking facilities for their infants. Thus, while they demonstrated that high-quality care is benign if not beneficial, these studies revealed nothing about the typical experiences of infants in non-parental care. The wide variety of social experiences that infants and toddlers encounter in non-parental care is illustrated by a UK study comparing care by relatives, family day-care and day care centres (Melhuish *et al.*, 1990). These varied in the number of children in the setting, the ratio of adults to children and the age and experience of the caregiver, as well as in the amount of physical contact, attention, affection, joint activity and communication that the child experienced.

In the 1980s, as out-of-home infant care became more common, an increasing number of studies used the strange situation or the Attachment Q-sort to assess the effects of 'maternal employment' on attachment. In these studies, the independent variable was usually the amount of time that the mother spent working away from home, or the age at which care began. A wide variety of care arrangements were aggregated in these categories. For example, one study of 97 infants in two-parent middle-class US families described the circumstances of those infants whose mothers began work outside the home before they were 6 months old as follows: 44 per cent in family day care, 16 per cent cared for by a non-relative in their home; 9 per cent cared for by their fathers; 9 per cent cared for by another relative; and 21 per cent experiencing a combination of care arrangements (Chase-Lansdale and Owen, 1987). In a second study of 136 infants of working and middle-class families with mothers in outside employment before the infant reached 9 months of age, their care arrangements were as follows: 36 per cent were in family day care; 17 per cent were cared for by a non-relative in their homes; 9 per cent were cared for by fathers; 11 per cent were cared for by other relatives; and 9 per cent were in day-care centres (Belsky and Rovine, 1988). Thus, whereas early studies focused on centre-based care, later studies with representation of actual child-care conditions found only a small minority of families using this type of care.

Among these 'second-generation' studies, conducted primarily in the USA, several which directly assessed attachment suggested that although the majority of infants whose mothers had paid employment away from home were securely attached to their mothers, there was a noticeable decrease in the percentage of secure attachment and a corresponding increase in avoidant behaviour in the strange situation (Clarke-Stewart, 1989; Lamb and Sternberg, 1990).

Although he had co-authored an earlier review that adopted a positive attitude towards day care (Belsky and Steinberg, 1978), Jay Belsky was concerned about these shifts in infant–mother attachment associated with maternal employment. In part, this concern was based on research (which we shall examine in Chapters 11 and 13) that linked avoidant attachment with later difficulties, such as aggressive behaviour in school settings. Belsky was outspoken about these concerns, arguing that using some forms of non-maternal care for more than 20 hours per week in the infant's first year was detrimental both to early attachments and to development (Belsky, 1986). He was roundly criticized by some of his colleagues (Phillips et al., 1987). Further elaborations by Belsky (1988) and replies by colleagues followed as the 1980s drew to a close (see Fox and Fein, 1990).

Although the data pertained to maternal employment (rather than a specific type of alternative care), the term 'day care' figured prominently in the debate in both professional and popular publications. Many feared (with reason) that this attention to negative effects would allow policy-makers to ignore the earlier studies with good outcomes in high-quality care, and to recommend cuts to child-care programmes. Since an increasing number of families in the USA were finding paid work to be an economic necessity and good-quality child care facilities were already limited, any deterioration in the amount and/or quality of care facilities was an ominous prospect.

Given that researchers generally agreed on the evidence, what were the disagreements with Belsky's interpretation? First, critics pointed out that the strange situation was not standardized for infants experiencing daily separations from their parents. Familiarity with separations might make the strange situation inherently less stressful, engender less distress and therefore not activate attachment behaviour. In support of this position, one follow-up study noted that strange-situation classifications did not predict later socio-emotional outcomes for children whose mothers had outside employment during their infancy, but did predict such outcomes for children who had been in full-time maternal care (Vaughn et al., 1985). However, other data showed that infants in alternative care (including those judged to be avoidant) were just as distressed by separation, if not more so, than their counterparts in full-time maternal care (Belsky and Braungart, 1991; McCartney and Phillips, 1988; Thompson, 1988).

Secondly, critics suggested that differences in attachment associated with non-maternal care could reflect pre-existing differences in families. Mothers who chose to work might already be different kinds of mothers to those who chose to stay at home. Moreover, among those who did work away from home, pre-existing maternal or family differences could influence the type and amount of alternative care chosen. Thus the data might not reflect the effects of maternal employment at all. The available studies provided only minimal information for addressing this possibility.

Thirdly, although the differences between full-time mother care and other care were statistically significant in aggregated large samples, they were actually very small in magnitude – possibly not small enough to engender differences in developmental trajectories. For example, in one meta-analysis the average ratings for avoidance differed by only half a point, with both groups scoring between 2 (very slight) and 3 (slight isolated avoidance) on the avoidance scale (Lamb *et al.*, 1992). Finally, precisely because these differences were so small, concern was expressed about the number of studies that remained unpublished because of failure to find differences (Roggmann *et al.*, 1994).

A major response to this controversy was the formation of a consortium in the USA to study early child care and its effects in a broad fashion with a sample large enough to allow examination of interactions between child, family and alternative care variables. This group, the National Institute of Child Health and Development (NICHD) Early Child Care Research Network, comprised most of those who had previously conducted research on this question, including both Belsky and his antagonists. In 1997, this group published their findings on infant–mother attachment, based on a sample of 1153 infants drawn from 31 hospitals in nine of the United States, with each subsample representative of its area (NICHD Early Child Care Research Network, 1997).

This study had many strengths. It used a prospective longitudinal design in which families were recruited at the time of birth and followed for 3 years. They were visited at home when the infants were 1, 6 and 15 months old in order to collect information about the home environment and mother–infant interactions. The study took advantage of naturally occurring variations in maternal work plans and use of alternative care. Infants who were regularly cared for by others were visited for 2 half-days in their usual alternative-care setting at 6 and 15 months in order to assess the characteristics of care. Additional information on caregiving conditions, such as the number of changes in arrangements, was also noted. Infant–mother attachment was assessed in the strange situation at 15 months.

First, the data showed no differences in the amount of distress in the strange situation between infants in alternative care and those at home full-time with their mothers. In addition, there were no differences in rater estimates of confidence in the classifications for these two groups of infants. Thus there was evidence to support the validity of the strange situation for infants in alternative care. There were no significant effects of any of the alternative child-care variables on attachment to the mother. As expected, maternal sensitivity/responsiveness was related to attachment security. Infants were more likely to be secure when their mothers were rated higher in sensitivity/responsiveness. However, child-care experience and maternal behaviour did combine to affect attachment. Poor-quality alternative care, increased hours of care, and changes in care arrangements were associated with insecure attachment when combined with low ratings of maternal sensitivity/responsiveness.

This large-scale study appears to be the last word on the US controversy in the 1990s. A subsequent smaller but parallel study in Canada substantially replicated many of these findings (McKim et al., 1999). Nevertheless, we should not lose sight of the fact that attitudes toward maternal employment, social policy and availability and quality of care facilities change with time and place. The prominent public debates and the data from the studies of the 1970s and 1980s may well have influenced changes in patterns of infant care in the 1990s that are reflected in the NICHD and Canadian studies. Later decades may bring their own changes which are not well represented in the literature at this time.

Attachment to professional caregivers

When infants are regularly cared for by hired caregivers, whether in the home or in centre-based care, we can also ask questions about the relationships they form with such caregivers. Are these attachment relationships? If so, are they influenced by the same factors that affect their relationships with parents? Do infants form attachments of similar quality to parents and professional caregivers?

Studies conducted before the development of the strange situation generally relied on separation protest to indicate the existence of an attachment relationship. Such studies provide ample evidence that attachments can be formed to non-familial caregivers in both infants (e.g. Schaffer and Emerson, 1964) and older children (e.g. Maccoby and Feldman, 1972). Fox (1977) adapted the method that Kotelchuck (1976) used with fathers to study the behaviour of 122 infants between 8 and 24 months of age towards their mother and their regular primary caretaker (metapelet) on 7 Israeli kibbutzim. Like Kotelchuck, he made no attempt to classify attachment, but focused instead on infant behaviours at departures and reunions with three figures – mother, metapelet and stranger. All of these infants routinely spent more time with the metapelet than with the mother. Although they protested at departure of both familiar figures when left in the presence of the stranger, on reunions infants were more positive and, if distressed, more likely to settle with their mothers. Factors related to individual differences such as birth order and gender influenced reunion behaviours but not separation behaviours. These observations are consistent with the principles underlying classification in the strange situation, namely that reunion behaviours capture individual differences more readily than do separations.

Several studies used the strange situation to evaluate attachment to one or both parents together with attachment to a regular alternative caregiver. In The Netherlands, Goossens and van IJzendoorn (1990) conducted strange-situation observations in counterbalanced order for mother, father and professional caregivers from day-care centres for 75 infants in families where both parents worked for more than 15 hours per week. Observation sessions were spread over a 6 to 7-month period starting when the infants were 1 year old. Before implementing the strange-situation procedures, separate observations were made in order to obtain data on the sensitivity of each potential attachment figure to infant behaviour, and professional caregivers also completed a questionnaire in order to provide information on the characteristics of each infant's day-care experience.

The overall distribution of attachment patterns was similar with each of the three caregivers. The majority of attachments were secure, the next largest group was avoidant, and there was a small number of resistant attachments. In addition, when individual infants were considered, 28 per cent had three secure attachments, 43 per cent had two secure attachments, 20 per cent had only one secure attachment and 9 per cent were insecure with all three caregivers. Although there was a significant correspondence between attachment patterns with the mother and father, attachment to the professional caregiver was independent of both. Infants were more likely to be securely attached to their professional caregiver if they spent more time in her care and had a younger and more sensitive caregiver.

A second study followed infants through toddlerhood and preschool age using the Attachment Q-sort to assess attachment to day-care teachers, and both the Q-sort and the strange-situation coding scheme to evaluate attachment to the mother based on reactions to her arrival and departures from day care. In infancy, 85 per cent of this sample were in centre-based care, while the rest were in family day-care homes. By preschool age, all of them were in centre-based care. Instead of using only traditional continuous Q-sort measures, Howes and Hamilton (1992a, 1992b) also used a scheme that they had developed for extracting standard classifications (secure, avoidant or resistant) from the Q-sort.

Security scores with the mother were significantly higher than security scores with the teacher, but the distribution of classifications was similar. Approximately 75 per cent of attachments were secure in each case. Compared to those that were insecure, children in the secure category with their teacher were the recipients of more intense and responsive involvement by their teachers (Howes and Hamilton, 1992a). Furthermore, classifications with teachers were more likely to be stable over time if the child remained with the same teacher. However, there was no concordance between mother and teacher attachments.

Two separate studies of infants reared on Israeli kibbutzim focused on slightly different information regarding infant attachments to the metapelet who was their primary caregiver (Sagi *et al.*, 1985, 1995). In part, because these studies were separated by an interval of 10 years, the differences reflect secular changes in the organization of child care on the kibbutz. The first study included only infants who slept in the children's house at night – the traditional kibbutz arrangement. Because of an increasing shift to family sleeping, the second study was able to compare those remaining in the children's house with those who slept with their families at night, reflecting different policies on different kibbutzim.

In the first study, although there was no similarity in security/insecurity between the mother and the metapelet, there was a significant relationship between attachment to the father and to the metapelet. Security with the metapelet was related to the age at which the infant moved into the children's house, the length of time for which the infant had been with this specific metapelet, and whether the metapelet had chosen or was assigned to her job. In addition, for metaplot observed with more than one child, there was evidence that children in the care of the same metapelet formed similar attachments to her.

The second study used both the strange situation and the Attachment Q-sort (completed by metaplot). The main questions were whether children with the same metapelet would form similar attachments to her, and whether the same child would form similar or dissimilar attachments to two different metaplot. Children with the same metapelet formed congruent relationships with her more often than incongruent ones on the kibbutzim with family sleeping arrangements. On kibbutzim where children slept in the children's house, only about half of the pairs formed congruent attachments. In two of three subsamples, there was a significant association between the pattern of attachment that a child formed with two different caregivers.

In general, these studies indicate that infants do form attachments to professional caregivers, and that these are influenced by factors similar to those thought to influence infant–parent attachments, namely the amount, quality and consistency of care. Although the majority of the studies suggest that attachment to professional caregivers is independent of attachment to parents, there is some evidence of an infant effect, with some studies showing concordance between infant attachments to different caregivers. Thus the general pattern of these findings is similar to those reviewed in Chapters 4 and 5 – there is evidence of both caregiver and infant effects.

Attachment hierarchies and the question of monotropy

Given that many infants have multiple figures to whom they can form attachments, is there any evidence to support the existence of a hierarchy of preferences as Bowlby postulated? Is there, in fact, evidence for the principle of monotropy – that is, a strong preference for one attachment figure over all others? Surprisingly, these questions have not generated many relevant studies.

Several sets of naturalistic observations in traditional societies are consistent with the concept of monotropy. For example, in her initial observations in Uganda, Ainsworth noted that babies did tend to focus most of their attachment behaviour on one particular person when they were tired, hungry or fearful. More recent observations of Efe infants (Morelli and Tronick, 1991) showed that, although multiple individuals provided sensitive care for each infant, primary attachments were usually formed with the mother. The main task that was exclusive to the mother was taking care of the infant during the night. The unique significance of night care was also discussed above with regard to studies of infants raised on Israeli kibbutzim. However, the preferred figure is not necessarily the mother. In a setting in Nigeria where two or more mothers live together and share child care, Hausa infants appeared to become attached to whichever caregiver held and interacted with the infant most. In 8 of 14 cases observed, that person was not the mother (Marvin *et al.*, 1977).

Experimental evidence is also relatively scarce. The studies by Kotelchuck (1976, see Chapter 6) and Fox (1977, discussed above) compared specific behaviours towards the mother, father, and stranger, and mother, metapelet and stranger, respectively. Kotelchuck emphasized the similarities rather than the differences between behaviour towards the mother and the father. However, Fox noted that, if distressed, infants were more likely to settle with their mothers than with the metapelet, although they spent more time with the latter. In an experimental paradigm designed to compare attachment preferences between the mother and the father, Colin (1987) reported that as stress increased, most infants were more likely to direct attachment behaviour towards their mothers, but 12 (of 50) babies showed a greater preference for their father and 6 babies showed no clear preference. Although the mother was almost always the primary caregiver, less preference for the mother was shown in families where fathers spent a substantial amount of time with their infants and engaged in regular caregiving (as opposed to only play).

These data are relatively consistent in suggesting that infants are likely to have a preferred caregiver, and that it is not always the mother or the person who spends most time with the infant. They are less clear in establishing necessary and sufficient conditions for the development of preferences, and are limited in investigating the full scope of possible attachment hierarchies.

Cultural context and attachment

The above discussion has already provided evidence that contemporary and historical differences in the organization of child care influence attachments. Parent–child relationships and child development have been studied in remarkably diverse cultural settings. We shall begin this section by considering three contrasting examples, namely the Israeli kibbutz and Japanese and German homes. These examples will be used to generate and test ideas about how different cultural attitudes and patterns of child care may influence attachment.

Kibbutz care in Israel

Kibbutzim are co-operative farms, mostly founded in the early days of Israel's nationhood. Because their arrangements for child care differ radically from those which most psychologists consider to be ideal (i.e. primary care by the mother), the development of kibbutz-reared children has been of great interest. Children are cared for communally in a children's house, usually with two caregivers (metaplot) for a group of 6–8 young children. Between 6 and 12 weeks after an infant is born, the mother returns to her regular job while continuing to feed the infant. Most mothers increase their work hours gradually, and infants spend increasing amounts of time in the children's house until, by the end of the first year, they are in full-time care. Regardless of age, all children routinely spend the hours between 4 and 7 p.m. with their families. However, parents may visit their children in the children's house at other times during the day.

When children return from family time to the children's house, they are put to bed by their parents, but during the night they are in the care of special night watchwomen who may or may not sleep close by. In some cases the night watchwoman is responsible for regularly checking several different locations. Many different women take turns at night duty, and an infant may or may not be familiar with the person providing care in response to night waking. More recently, because parents were increasingly dissatisfied with these arrangements, the majority of kibbutzim have shifted to family sleeping arrangements. Under these conditions children go to their homes at 4 p.m. for family time and do not return to the children's house until the following morning (Sagi et al., 1985, 1995).

Japan

Japan is an example of a highly industrialized, urbanized non-Western country that has retained methods of child care that share many features in common with rural non-industrial societies. The mother is the primary caregiver, but the expectations and goals of Japanese mothers differ considerably from those of their Western counterparts. The majority of Western mothers view young infants as highly dependent, and focus on promoting autonomy and independence. In contrast, Japanese mothers consider the young infant to be a relatively independent creature who must be socialized into interdependence with others. The first of these interdependent relationships is with the mother herself. Consequently, Japanese infants are carried on the mother's back for much of the time, sleep with her and bathe with her. Even older children continue to sleep in the same room as their parents, and are readily taken into the parents' bed for comforting. Thus the infant is rarely separated from his or her mother, and it is unusual for infants to be cared for by others, especially those outside the family (Miyake *et al.*, 1985).

Northern Germany

This provides a sharp contrast with the practices and expectations in Japan. Although the mother is the primary caregiver, there is a very high demand for early independence and the development of coping strategies that do not rely on assistance from others. As soon as infants are mobile, they are discouraged from staying too close to their mothers. To carry an infant who is capable of locomotion or to respond to cries by offering contact is considered to spoil the child. 'The ideal is an independent, nonclinging infant who does not make demands on the parents but rather unquestioningly obeys their commands.' (Grossmann *et al.*, 1985, p.253). In comparison, for example, to Ainsworth's Baltimore sample, infants in Bielefeld, Germany, were picked up twice as often but held on average for only half as long, and Bielefeld mothers were less tender, careful and affectionate while holding the infant. Although holding the infant was most effective in terminating distress, the majority of mothers were likely to try distracting techniques before resorting to picking up when their infants when they were crying (Grossmann *et al.*, 1985).

Some questions and answers

What kind of attachment relationships would we expect these infants to form with their mothers? We might predict that the highly available and relationship-focused Japanese mother would lead her infant to develop a secure attachment. We might expect that infants in Northern Germany would experience lack of attention to their signals and discouragement of contact as rejection, and be more likely to develop avoidant attachments. Finally, we might anticipate that kibbutz infants who experience regular prolonged periods of relatively undivided attention during family time coupled with unpredictable responses at night would be more likely to develop resistant attachments to their parents. The evidence shows that some but not all of these predictions are confirmed.

First, in each of these settings the distribution of attachment patterns differs from that found in low-risk samples in North America. In the first study in Northern Germany (Grossmann *et al.*, 1985) 49 per cent of 49 infants showed the avoidant pattern, compared to 26 per cent in the

Baltimore study and 21 per cent in a meta-analysis of cross-cultural samples (van IJzendoorn and Kroonenberg, 1988). Furthermore, among the secure infants the B_2 pattern (which includes some avoidance) was more common than the B_3 pattern. Nevertheless, the relationship between ratings of maternal behaviour and attachment classification was similar to that found in Ainsworth's sample. Mothers of infants classified as secure were rated as more sensitive, tender and responsive to their babies than were mothers of avoidant or resistant infants. Nevertheless, the investigators suggested that mothers who were rated low on sensitivity were not necessarily inherently 'insensitive' but rather they conformed to cultural expectations regarding infant care. When this sample was combined with two other German samples, one from Berlin and one from Regensburg, avoidant attachment was found to be over-represented in the German samples (van IJzendoorn and Kroonenberg, 1988).

In a study of 86 kibbutz-reared infants, insecure attachments to all figures (mother, father and metapelet) were also more common than they had been in the Baltimore sample, with the increase evident in the resistant category (22–33 per cent were resistant, compared to 12 per cent in Baltimore). Two other features were notable. First, there was an unusually large group of infants in the B_4 category. Secondly, a disproportionate number of assessments (35 per cent) were curtailed or modified (no second separation) because of extreme infant distress. Finally, attachment patterns in a comparison sample of 36 city-reared Israeli infants were significantly different to those of the kibbutz group, and were more like those of the Baltimore sample (Sagi et al., 1985).

One set of Japanese data came from Sapporo and did not conform to the above predictions. Although the majority of infants were secure, the expected increase in secure attachments did not occur. Furthermore, Miyake, Chen and Campos (1985) found no avoidant infants and an increase in the number of resistant attachments. In addition to infants who were considered to be unambiguously resistant, this team also identified a group of infants who were considered to be 'pseudo-resistant.' These were infants who behaved like secure infants in every way until the final episode of the strange situation, when they behaved like resistant infants, with much crying and inability to be soothed. Resistant and pseudo-resistant infants accounted for 38 per cent of this sample of 31 infants. In contrast to some of the previous studies, earlier maternal behaviour was not a good predictor of infant attachment classifications, but several aspects of infant temperament (such as neonatal crying and early irritability) discriminated future secure from future resistant infants. Although there were also data from Tokyo which had a more typical distribution (13 per cent avoidant, 61 per cent secure, 18 per cent resistant, 8 per cent unclassifiable) and showed some links between infant attachment and maternal reports of spousal support (Durrett et al., 1984), the Sapporo data were more provocative and received more attention.

These cultural differences, and in particular the Japanese data, which not only failed to confirm the predictions but also failed to detect relationships between maternal care and attachment, gave rise to prolonged discussion regarding the cross-cultural validity of the strange situation. Just as some proponents argued that experiences of regular alternative care may render separations in the strange situation insufficiently stressful to activate attachment behaviour, it was suggested that the absence of separations between Japanese mothers and infants renders the separations of the strange situation excessively stressful (i.e. well beyond the moderate stress assumed by the classification scheme).

One approach to interpreting the Japanese data is to place them in the context of a comprehensive meta-analysis of infant attachment studies from around the world (van IJzendoorn and Kroonenberg, 1988), which included nearly 2000 strange situations from eight different countries. At that time, 18 of 32 samples were from the USA, and all other countries were represented by 1–4 samples. The authors noted that where it was possible to estimate this, the 'within-country' variation was larger than the 'between-country' variation. This observation, coupled with the small number of studies from some countries, highlighted the importance of exercising caution in considering any one sample to be representative of its country or culture. Nevertheless, secure attachments were dominant in every country.

The Israeli and Japanese samples contributed heavily to the overall variation, but the US samples contributed minimally. In fact, it was noted that the global distribution would hardly change if the US samples were omitted. On this basis, it was suggested that there is no reason to doubt that the validity data collected for the strange situation in the USA could be generalized to cross-cultural use. However, the Sapporo data had already suggested a failure to generalize.

In a later Sapporo study, Takahashi (1990) confirmed the observation that many infants classified as resistant follow the pattern described by Miyake, Chen and Campos (1985). Until the very last episode, they appear like secure babies. If classified only on the basis of the first separation, the proportion of infants classified into the resistant group is comparable to that found in US samples. Furthermore, Takahashi (1990) suggested that at later ages, when separations become more common, Japanese infants should behave more like American 12-month-olds. Consistent with this expectation, at 12 months of age, 68 per cent of 60 Japanese babies were secure and 32 per cent were resistant, and at 23 months of age 81 per cent were secure and 19 per cent were resistant. The latter data are more consistent with our first predictions above. The absence of avoidant attachments is remarkable in the context of the global distribution of attachment categories, but perhaps not so remarkable when we consider the goals of Japanese socialization described above. Furthermore, given the Tokyo data, these findings are not necessarily typical of Japan.

The observed shifts and the discussions which they initiated suggest that, although one may use the strange situation in a variety of settings and learn something about the nature of infant attachments, it is wise to think carefully about how the data should be interpreted. Valid interpretations require intimate knowledge of child-rearing customs and goals.

Cultural concepts of early relationships

In one attempt to evaluate cultural consistencies in views of attachment behaviour, mothers in seven countries (China, Colombia, Germany, Israel, Japan, Norway and the USA) used the Attachment Q-sort to rate both their own children (infants through preschool age) and their 'ideal child' (Posada *et al.*, 1995). In addition, 104 professionals used the Q-sort to rate the 'optimally secure' child. Mothers' ratings for their ideal child and expert ratings were highly correlated across countries. Furthermore, although there were some cultural differences, both mother and expert ratings indicated that security, as defined by the US-based Q-sort, was considered desirable in all countries, suggesting that developmental researchers are not unrealistic in thinking that secure attachment is generally advantageous. Nevertheless, the issues discussed above suggest that the strange situation does not necessarily have the same meaning to infants reared in different cultural settings.

In order to investigate such a possibility, Harwood and her colleagues (Harwood, 1992; Harwood *et al.*, 1995) focused on ascertaining the meaning that mothers from different cultures attribute to the same patterns of behaviour. To do this, they examined the child-rearing values of Anglo and Puerto Rican middle-class and working-class mothers in the USA. In addition to answering questions about child-rearing goals and conceptions of desirable and undesirable child behaviour, mothers were presented with six vignettes chosen to illustrate specific patterns of behaviour in the strange situation.

Mothers in both groups preferred secure toddlers, but apparently for different reasons. Anglo mothers' attitudes generally endorsed the mainstream goals of individual development and achievement. Their ideal toddler was one who was competent and active but interested in social relationships. Thus they did in fact focus on the balance between relatedness and autonomy that the strange situation is thought to assess. Puerto Rican mothers adhered to goals that valued group coherence over individual achievement. They were concerned about 'proper demeanour,' the qualities necessary to being admired by others, namely *obediente* (obedience), *respeto* (respect), *tranquilo* (calm) and *amable* (politeness, goodness). Their ideal toddler was quiet and co-operative and obediently stayed close to his or her mother. Thus the Puerto Rican mothers focused on issues that are not particularly relevant to attachment theory.

Nevertheless, both groups of mothers preferred toddlers who fitted the description of the secure pattern to those who showed either of the other patterns. Anglo mothers' negative view of the resistant pattern was primarily attributable to their dislike of dependency. Puerto Rican mothers rated the same patterns negatively to reflect their dislike of such a child's inability to exercise the self-control required to restrain angry behaviour. Furthermore, within the secure group, Anglo mothers showed more preference for the B_1 and B_2 patterns, namely those reflecting more independence. In contrast, the Puerto Rican mothers preferred the B_4 pattern and its greater dependency. There were also social-class differences in both groups, with working-class Anglo mothers being more ambivalent than their middle-class peers about endorsing the US mainstream ideal of individual achievement. Among Puerto Rican mothers, the working-class women were more emphatic about the importance of proper demeanour than their middle-class counterparts. These data suggest that, while the securely attached child is valued in most cultures, the reasons for this may differ and may not be related to the constructs of attachment.

Overview

In this chapter we have considered factors outside the family that can influence the formation of attachments. Many such factors exist, but we have considered only two, namely the effects of maternal employment outside the home, and the broader cultural context in which families live. These two factors are not independent. In settings where maternal employment outside the family is highly valued, as in the kibbutz, the social structure is organized to provide other forms of care for children. Where exclusive maternal care is valued by the culture (e.g. in Japan and Germany), there are few alternatives to full-time mothering. However, there may be supports to ensure exclusive maternal care, such as paid maternity leave. In Germany, for example, government financial support is available for the first 2 years of the child's life (Spangler and Schieche, 1998). Although the pattern traditionally considered to indicate secure attachment appears to predominate in all of the cultures that have been studied, there are shifts in the type of security and insecurity that are related to cultural expectations and interpretations of desirable child care and behaviour. In addition, although most cultures appear to value secure attachment, different cultures may value it for different reasons.

Suggested reading

Fox, N.A. and Fein, G. (1990) *Infant day care: the current debate*. Norwood, NJ: Ablex.
A collection of articles about the day-care and attachment controversy, plus additional articles about the effects of day care.

Harwood, R.L., Miller, J.G. and Irizarry, N.L. (1995) *Culture and attachment*. New York, NY: Guilford.
A detailed account of a unique approach to the cross-cultural study of attachment which raises some thoughtful questions.

NICHD Early Child Care Research Network (1997) The effects of infant child care on infant–mother attachment security: results of the NICHD study of early child care. *Child Development*, **68**, 860–79.
The most comprehensive study of maternal employment, alternative care and infant attachment.

van IJzendoorn, M.H. and Sagi, A. (1999) Cross-cultural patterns of attachment: universal and contextual dimensions. In Cassidy, J. and Shaver, P.R. (Eds), *Handbook of attachment*. New York: Guildford Press.
A recent and comprehensive view of research on cultural differences in attachment.

8   Attachment under adversity

Bowlby argued that because attachment and the caregiving behaviours which support it are central to the survival and well-being of young infants, humans evolved in such a way as to ensure that infants will become attached to their caregivers. Infants are equipped with neural structures that predispose them to solicit protective care, and adults are likewise predisposed to provide such care. However, there are conditions under which these predispositions may be impaired, overridden or suppressed. These are conditions that would be extremely adverse for the development of attachment. This chapter will illustrate some of these situations and their effects on the formation of attachments – infant limitations or disabilities, social disadvantage, parental disorders, maltreatment and institutional care. In most of these cases, the available data raise both theoretical and empirical questions regarding attachment and its assessment.

The compromised infant

In Chapter 5 we referred to an extensive body of work on infants with medical or developmental problems. We shall reconsider some of these studies here as exemplars of situations in which infants are limited in their ability to solicit care. As specific examples, we shall consider infants born prematurely and those with Down's syndrome, these being the two groups for which we have the most extensive data on attachment. When interpreting the results of these studies, a caution is in order. Although the strange situation has now been widely used with children experiencing a variety of disabling conditions, there are few studies providing home-observation data to validate the strange situation as an attachment assessment in these groups. The focus on prematurity and Down's syndrome in part reflects the availability of potential validity data for these groups.

Prematurely born infants

When an infant is born prematurely, he or she is not well adapted to life outside the womb. Modern technology has succeeded in forcing back the age of viability so that many infants born at 25 or 26 weeks' gestation (compared to the normal 38–40 weeks) do survive. These are infants who would not have survived in our 'environment of evolutionary adaptedness.' Hence it is not surprising that their capacities for signalling differ from those of full-term infants. Preterm infants are less alert and less responsive, and their cries are initially weaker than those of full-term babies (Goldberg and DiVitto, 1995). Since many aspects of development proceed on a timetable that is based on time of conception and independent of the time of birth, the appearance of behaviours that the full-term infant uses to achieve and maintain contact with a caregiver, such as smiling, clinging, reaching and following, are slow to appear in prematurely born infants. For infants who are extremely small and vulnerable to the medical complications associated with premature birth, a prolonged period in hospital is routine. During this time, interactions with caregivers are limited, and are often restricted to medical procedures.

Many observations have documented subsequent alterations in home interactions in dyads with preterm infants. Specifically, infants are described as less alert, responsive and initiating, as well as more irritable, and their mothers are noted to be more active, more directive and less sensitive (Goldberg and DiVitto, 1995). Although some reports suggest that these differences diminish with age (e.g. Alfasi *et al.*, 1985; Brachfeld *et al.*, 1980; Crawford, 1982) others note differences as late as 2 years of age (Barnard *et al.*, 1984). Some observers (e.g. Field, 1977) suggest that these mothers are being inappropriately intrusive with their preterm infants, while others (e.g. Goldberg, 1982) suggest that these differences in maternal behaviour represent unique adaptations to the needs of preterm infants. To the extent that the evidence shows normal development of attachment in this group, we can argue that maternal behaviour is more likely to be appropriate rather than maladaptive.

At least one study (Goldberg *et al.*, 1986) has documented the expected links between home observations at four age points in the first year and assessments in the strange situation for preterm infants. Thus there is some limited evidence for the validity of the strange situation with this group. However, at least one adaptation needs to be made. Because the development of these infants is notably behind that of their chronological age-mates, assessments need to be delayed in order to allow the requisite skills (e.g. person permanence and locomotion) to emerge. Thus instead of assessing preterm infants at 12–18 months after birth, they are assessed at ages that represent 12–18 months plus the number of weeks it took them to reach term after their birth.

As we noted in Chapter 5, although a few studies suggest minor differences in the distribution of attachment patterns, the majority of preterm infants are securely attached to their mothers by 12–18 months corrected age (van IJzendoorn *et al.*, 1992). It is generally argued that unless other adverse conditions arise, the majority of parents are able to compensate for infant limitations imposed by premature birth (Goldberg and DiVitto, 1995).

Down's syndrome

Nowadays, Down's syndrome is generally identified early in the infant's life, often before initial discharge from the hospital. Whereas it was once recommended that such infants should be institutionalized, current practice is for the majority of children with Down's syndrome to be reared at home. As a result, there is a wide range of abilities and outcomes among these children. In addition to marked facial features, these infants are slower than normal to develop and, of particular significance for attachment, they are described as having muted emotional expressions (Emde et al., 1978). Because their musculature is not capable of the same level of tension as that of other infants and children (Cicchetti and Sroufe, 1978), their smiles are described as less bright, and their facial expressions and cries of distress as less intense. This suggests the possibility that caregivers miss some infant attachment signals or have difficulty in decoding them. In addition, it raises the possibility that observers may have difficulty in interpreting attachment behaviours (Vaughn et al., 1994).

Cicchetti and his colleagues conducted a series of developmental studies of infants and toddlers with Down's syndrome, including observations in the strange situation. In these studies the emphasis was on description of behaviour, and there was no attempt to make attachment classifications. Youngsters with Down's syndrome showed clear evidence of reactions to separation through change in the amount and quality of play as well as expressive behaviour, although they were less likely to become overtly upset than normally developing children (Cicchetti and Serafica, 1981; Serafica and Cicchetti, 1976; Thompson et al., 1985). In addition, they responded positively to the return of their mothers. This led Cicchetti and Beeghly (1990) to conclude that by the time children with Down's syndrome achieve the capacities of normal 12 to 24-month-olds they have also succeeded in constructing attachment relationships with caregivers that are normatively secure. That is to say, most children with Down's syndrome are using their primary caregivers as a secure base for exploration and as a haven of safety by the time they have reached the developmental age of 1–2 years.

Nevertheless, classification of children with Down's syndrome has proved to be somewhat difficult, particularly in younger samples. Vaughn and his associates (Vaughn et al., 1994) examined classifications for three different samples of children with Down's syndrome. They reported that, particularly for children who were younger (of mean chronological age approximately 2 years), a large proportion (in some samples close to 50 per cent) of children had to be considered 'unclassifiable.' Secondly, the reliability of classifications for the Down's syndrome samples was generally lower than that for a comparison normal sample, and this was attributable to the occurrence of many mixed behaviour patterns (i.e. the rater considered several alternative and often unrelated classifications as possible fits). If the 'unclassifiable' cases were considered to be insecure (as recommended by Main and Solomon, 1990), then the Down's syndrome groups were characterized by higher rates of insecurity than the normal comparison group. When the 'unclassifiable' cases were eliminated, these differences disappeared. However, Vaughn *et al.* (1994) suggest that it is unclear whether the strange situation can be interpreted for children with Down's syndrome in the same way that we routinely use it for normally developing children. In particular, the level of stress that the strange situation engenders in the Down's syndrome group may not be consistent with the assumptions underlying the classification scheme. Furthermore, the validating home data are equivocal.

Two studies provided data on links between home behaviour and attachment classifications in the strange situation for children with Down's syndrome. In the first (Vaughn and Seifer, 1989), the security index based on the Attachment Q-sort was not related to strange-situation classifications. However, the second study (Atkinson *et al.*, 1999a), which used a somewhat older group of children (developmental age approximately 2 years), did find a significant association.

What is the bottom line here? Can the strange situation be used reliably for children with Down's syndrome? And what can we say about the development of attachment in this group? What is consistent about the above findings is that there is evidence that attachment, like other developmental phenomena, is slower to emerge in children with Down's syndrome. The strange situation seems to be more useful and easier to code and the distribution of attachment more normative as children with Down's syndrome get older. The large number of 'unclassifiable' children may in fact be not yet attached. Alternatively, it may be useful to make a further study of such cases in order to see whether new attachment patterns can be discovered. Further conceptual and empirical work is required for a full understanding of the meaning of attachment behaviours not only in children with Down's syndrome, but also in other groups of children with disabling conditions.

Social disadvantage

Some of the basic early studies of attachment considered infants living under disadvantaged conditions, such as low-income, minority-status and single-parent households. Often (but not always) conditions of social disadvantage cluster together making it difficult to discern which one(s) might influence the formation of attachments. Some of these disadvantages have direct deleterious effects on infants. For example, extreme poverty is likely to be associated with poor nutrition, poor medical care and inadequate housing, and hence with poor health and developmental problems. A disproportionate number of premature infants are born into families that are already coping with these kinds of multiple disadvantages. In addition to direct effects on the infant, these disadvantages encumber the primary caregiver with problems that impinge on the time and energy required for normal care of the infant. In such situations, overburdened parents may be forced to compete with their children for scarce resources, and the stability of family life is threatened. Thus multiple social disadvantages create environments in which development is more likely to go awry than in more comfortable circumstances. For this reason, they are characterized as 'high-risk' environments. Nevertheless, a significant proportion of children who grow up in high-risk circumstances receive good care from their caregivers and have good developmental outcomes.

In general there is evidence that, under conditions of high social risk, attachment is less often secure and less likely to be stable than in low-risk conditions (Spieker and Booth, 1988). However, a review of four relatively large studies of high-risk samples (Spieker and Booth, 1988) led to a striking conclusion. When known cases of maltreatment and inadequate care were removed from these samples, secure attachment was just as frequent as in more advantaged samples. Furthermore, this was true even in the presence of risk factors such as poverty and single parenthood.

For example, Egeland and Sroufe (1981) divided their Minnesota sample of low-income mothers and infants into groups characterized by 'excellent care' ($n = 33$) and 'inadequate care' ($n = 31$). The excellent-care group included relatively high proportions of secure infants at both 12 (75 per cent) and 18 (76 per cent) months. In the group receiving inadequate care, 62 per cent were insecure at 12 months and 44 per cent at 18 months.

Data such as these suggest that social disadvantage does not inevitably compromise infant attachment. Rather, the extent to which multiple risks are present and the resources and supports that are available to meet such challenges determine whether the mother (or other attachment figure) is able to provide good care. When the available resources and support are insufficient to surmount multiple problems, inadequate care is the result.

Maltreatment

The term 'maltreatment' covers a variety of conditions under which children receive inadequate care. The most common way of characterizing maltreatment differentiates between abuse (in which needed care is generally provided, but is accompanied by excessive anger, harshness or hostility) and neglect (where normal and necessary care is lacking), although it is not unusual to find abuse and neglect coexisting. Crittenden (1988) also speaks of 'marginal maltreatment,' namely conditions in which lack of foresight and planning for the child's needs periodically provokes brief crises during which some abuse or neglect surfaces. The emotional dynamics of abusive and neglecting relationships are thought to differ in important ways. Abusive parents show strong emotional involvement with their children, while neglecting parents are more likely to be withdrawn and detached.

What types of relationships do children form when their primary caregivers are unable to provide adequate care? Every introductory psychology student probably has strong memories of Harlow's 'motherless monkeys' who were highly abusive to their first infants. Yet, remarkably, these infants continued to show strong contact-seeking towards their inadequate mothers. If child protection is the primary function of the attachment system, the caregiver's failure to perform this function, whether through abuse or neglect, should somehow be reflected in the child's attachment behaviour. However, some of the early work showed that, while the majority of maltreated children were insecurely attached, some did behave like securely attached children in the strange situation (Main and Solomon, 1990).

As discussed earlier (in Chapter 2), such puzzling findings contributed to the eventual development of the disorganized/disoriented classification. In fact, it is notable that many of the early studies of maltreated children found it necessary to invent new classifications to describe unusual attachment behaviours that were observed. In the earliest of these studies, Egeland and Sroufe (1981) used a 'D' category that included infants who were clearly anxiously attached but could not be considered either avoidant or resistant – for example, infants who were apathetic or disorganized.

Crittenden (1988) described combinations of avoidance and resistance (A/C) that appeared in children in the most problematic families in her samples. For example, such children might show strong avoidance by moving away from or ignoring the caregiver, but instead of showing the neutral affect that usually accompanies avoidance, they were extremely distressed and failed to settle. Thus they also had to be given high scores for resistance. Another version of this combination would be a child who showed strong avoidance during the first reunion, ignored the caregiver with little show of affect, but then broke down shrieking and wailing at the door when the caregiver departed. In Crittenden's groundbreaking work, 50 per cent of physically abused and 58 per cent of abused and neglected children fit into the A/C pattern (Crittenden, 1988).

Lyons-Ruth and her colleagues (Lyons-Ruth *et al.*, 1987) used the term 'unstable avoidance' to describe attachment patterns where extreme avoidance in the first reunion gave rise to behaviours that looked secure in the second reunion. According to the coding instructions, these children would normally be considered to be secure. However, 21 per cent of maltreated infants and only 2–4 per cent in the comparison groups showed this pattern.

In somewhat older children, Crittenden (1988) described 'compulsive compliance.' These were toddlers who were unusually accomodating and co-operative with their mothers, who showed extreme insensitivity and an absence of positive affect towards them. Their histories revealed severe or pervasive maltreatment. Crittenden (1988) suggested that these children had learned that vigilant compliance was safer than either avoidance or passivity.

In all of these studies, a substantial number of children in the maltreatment group could not be adequately classified in the existing schemes for classifying attachment. Thus, in addition to finding some children who would have been classified as secure in the standard classification scheme, all of the early studies of maltreated children noted unusual behaviours or patterns of behaviour that had not been described in previous community samples.

More recent studies have made use of classification schemes that included new categories designed to encompass the unusual observations made in the early maltreatment studies, most notably the disorganized disoriented classification of Main and Solomon (1990). In one study, for example, over 80 per cent of maltreated infants, compared to 20 per cent of the comparison group, could be placed in the disorganized/disoriented attachment classification (Carlson et al., 1989). A follow-up of this sample showed that 60 per cent of children with disorganized attachments at 12 months were also disorganized at 24 months of age (Barnett et al., 1992).

Cicchetti and Barnett (1991) used the Cassidy/Marvin (1987) scheme for coding preschool attachment to examine the stability of attachment from 30 to 48 months in a maltreatment sample. At all ages, maltreated children were more likely to be insecurely attached than were children in the comparison sample. Furthermore, while secure attachment was highly stable in the comparison group, it was not stable in the maltreated group. From 30 to 36 months, 80 per cent of securely attached children in the comparison group remained secure, compared to 22 per cent in the maltreatment group. The corresponding figures from 36 to 48 months of age were 93 per cent and 33 per cent for the comparison and maltreatment groups, respectively.

Although standardized attachment procedures are notably lacking for middle childhood, Lynch and Cicchetti (1991) reported that about 30 per cent of 6 to 12-year-olds in a maltreatment sample displayed 'confused' patterns of relatedness with their mothers. These children reported feeling emotionally positive and secure, but also felt that they needed more closeness than they received. In sixth grade, in response to a projective story-telling task, children with a history of maltreatment revealed more negative expectations for relationships than their non-maltreated peers (McCrone et al., 1994). These two studies of older maltreated children suggest that there are long-lasting effects of early maltreatment on internal working models of relationships.

In summary, studies of maltreated samples identified patterns of attachment that are not generally seen in low-risk samples, and when the disorganized classification was available, a substantial number of maltreated cases fell into this category and tended to remain disorganized on subsequent assessment. In contrast, those who appeared to be anomalously secure often did not maintain their secure status as they developed.

Maternal disorders (depression)

The presence of a psychiatric disorder is likely to interfere with normal caregiving and thus influence the development of attachment. Clinical depression is the most widely studied such disturbance, partly because it is relatively common among the mothers of infants and young children. Not surprisingly, mothers who are experiencing multiple disadvantages are particularly vulnerable to depression. Thus maternal depression frequently coexists with other risk factors such as marital discord, high stress and low social support (Cicchetti *et al.*, 1998), and indeed many parents in the maltreatment samples described above were probably also depressed.

Approximately 10–20 per cent of mothers experience significant symptoms of depression in the postpartum period. During depressive episodes, a parent's emotional availability is limited. Thus the child is likely to perceive the caregiver as being inaccessible and unresponsive (Cummings and Cicchetti, 1990; Cummings and Davies, 1994). Furthermore, affective disturbance in the parents exposes the developing infant to episodes of sadness, irritability, hopelessness, helplessness and confusion, and in bipolar depression these alternate unpredictably with periods of euphoria and grandiosity (Cummings and Cicchetti, 1990). As early as 3 months of age, the interactions of the infants of depressed mothers reflect a depressed mood style not only with their mothers but also with others, and this pattern persists if the mother's depression continues (Field, 1992).

When Radke-Yarrow and her colleagues (Radke-Yarrow *et al.*, 1985) first examined attachment in the toddlers of depressed parents, they found it necessary to add a new category to the coding system, namely a mixed avoidant/resistant category similar to that described by Crittenden (1988). Like Crittenden (1988), they also found that the A/C pattern was associated with the most extreme caregiving conditions. Their project assessed 99 toddlers and their mothers. In total, 14 mothers had been diagnosed with bipolar depression, 42 mothers with unipolar depression, 12 mothers with minor depression and 31 mothers with no depression. It was predominantly in the bipolar group that the occurrence of insecure attachment escalated dramatically, with 79 per cent of the toddlers being insecure. DeMulder and Radke-Yarrow (1991) later confirmed that the rates of insecure attachment in children of mothers with unipolar depression did not differ from those in a non-depressed sample.

In contrast, Cicchetti, Rogosch and Toth (1998) found that when attachment was assessed with the Q-sort, the toddlers of mothers with unipolar depression were significantly more likely to be insecure (43 per cent) than were those in the comparison group (18 per cent). The relationship between maternal depression and toddler insecure attachment could not be explained by the presence of other contextual risk factors such as marital discord, stress or lack of social support.

Some studies have suggested that the rate of disorganized attachment is especially high in samples with depressed mothers, but a recent meta-analysis found only a very small association (0.06) between maternal depression and disorganization (van IJzendoorn *et al.*, 1997) However, the association between depression and insecurity produced stronger effect sizes, with a mean of 0.27 (Atkinson *et al.*, 1999, unpublished data). Thus there is clear evidence that the presence of maternal depression increases the likelihood that an infant will develop insecure attachment, but the evidence for an increase in a particular type of insecurity is inconsistent. Questions regarding the effects of particular types of depression, severity, timing of its occurrence and the pattern of recurrence all merit more detailed examination.

Recovery from early deprivation/inadequate care

To what extent can some of the potentially negative effects of early adversity be overcome? In most cases, the experiments that would be needed to answer such questions cannot be conducted, as children cannot be randomly removed from conditions of adversity and placed in more advantaged environments. However, we do have some examples where such changes occur naturally. In the first case, involving children adopted after institutional care, early deprivation has usually been far more extreme than any of the examples discussed above. In the second case, namely placement into foster care, protective services have intervened to remove children from some of the most extreme conditions considered above.

Orphanage Care

We noted previously (in Chapter 1) that observations of the detrimental effects of institutional care on children's development figured heavily in early formulations regarding infant–mother relationships. These observations also contributed to the general demise of institutional care in much of the Western world, in favour of foster-care arrangements. The early studies (e.g. Bender and Yarnell, 1941; Goldfarb, 1943a, 1943b; Skodak and Skeels, 1949; Spitz, 1945, 1946) did not have the benefit of systematic methods for assessing attachment, but universally reported unusual social behaviours in institution-reared children. These children did not seem to form close relationships, and were often described as indiscriminately friendly.

Some years later, Tizard and her colleagues (Hodges and Tizard, 1989a, 1989b; Tizard and Rees, 1974; Tizard and Hodges, 1978) reported similar findings at 4, 8 and 16 years of age from a residential institution in London where children received excellent physical care and adequate cognitive stimulation. Many of these children were eventually adopted or restored to their natural parents. Although mothers sometimes reported that the children were indeed attached to them, teachers reported many social problems with peers. This was especially true for children who stayed in the institution for the first 4 years of their lives.

It was data such as these that suggested there might be a sensitive or critical period for the formation of attachments. The implication of a sensitive period is that, while conditions conducive to the formation of the first attachment exist primarily in the early years of life, the first attachment can develop at a later stage, albeit with some difficulty or a need for additional support. The notion of a critical period for the formation of attachment implies that failure to form the first attachment in the opening years of life cannot be remedied by later interventions.

Unfortunately, there have been opportunities to revisit questions concerning institutional care and attachment in the 1980s and 1990s using more recently developed assessment tools. Nations wracked with wars and political and economic struggles took abandoned and orphaned children into institutional care, and media attention to these conditions led to a run of international adoptions. The situation which received most publicity in both North America and Europe was that of children in Romanian orphanages. Several studies focused on the ability of these children to recover from their extremely depriving early experiences, after adoption into families outside Romania.

One of the largest of these studies was conducted in British Columbia, where Elinor Ames and her colleagues located 92 per cent of children adopted from Romania into families in British Columbia between 1990 and 1991. They were able to study three groups of children longitudinally: first, those who had spent at least 8 months in an orphanage in Romania ($n = 46$); secondly, Romanian children adopted before 4 months of age directly from families or hospital who would have gone to orphanages if they had not been adopted ($n = 29$); and thirdly 46 Canadian-born children matched to the orphanage group with regard to gender and age. The children were assessed after adoption at two different times, once when they had been in their homes for approximately 11 months and again when most of them were approximately 4½ years old.

When they were first adopted, 78 per cent of the orphanage group were developmentally delayed in all areas of development (fine motor, gross motor, personal-social and language areas). They were small and malnourished, and many of them had serious medical problems. In other words, they were children with special needs who were likely to be a challenge to their adopting parents (Chisholm *et al.*, 1995).

At both times, attachment was assessed with a questionnaire based on salient items from the Attachment Q-sort. On this measure, the orphanage children were rated as less secure than those in the other groups at the first assessment but not the second one. At the second assessment only, an adaptation of the strange situation was administered in the home and scored using Crittenden's (1992) classification scheme for preschoolers. Whereas 58 per cent of the Canadian-born and 67 per cent of the early-adopted children were judged to be securely attached, only 37 per cent of the orphanage group were considered to be secure. In addition, 33 per cent of the orphanage group, compared to 7 per cent and 4 per cent of the Canadian-born and early-adopted groups, respectively, showed atypical forms of insecure attachments. All of these were described as either defended-caregiving or mixed (defended/coercive) attachments. In addition, the children in the orphanage group engaged in more indiscriminately friendly behaviour than those in either of the other two groups (Chisholm, 1998). Interestingly, the attachment patterns of the orphanage group were not related to specific aspects of orphanage care (e.g. length of stay, size of group), but rather to child and adoptive family characteristics. The orphanage children who were insecurely attached had more behaviour problems and more developmental delays, and their parents reported more stress.

A second Canadian study of Romanian adoptees in Ontario used the Cassidy/Marvin (1987) preschool attachment scheme, and similarly found that 40 per cent of the adoptees showed atypical (disorganized) attachment patterns (Marcovitch *et al.*, 1997). Like the previous study, insecure attachments were associated with behaviour problems and developmental delays. A third study in the UK also found a decrease in security and an increase in atypical attachments among adoptees from orphanages, with longer periods of institutionalization exaggerating these trends (Marvin and O'Connor, 1999). Thus although a substantial minority of children with prolonged orphanage experience succeeded in forming secure attachments, the majority did not do so, and many of the insecure attachments took atypical forms that are not usually seen in low-risk samples. Associations between attachment and child and family problems may have reflected pre-existing conditions that interfered with the development of secure attachments. However, at present it is impossible to distinguish this possibility from the alternative, namely that insecure attachments contributed to developmental and behavioural problems as well as to family stress.

Thus with more sophisticated tools and larger, more systematic observational data, the findings of these recent studies echo those of the early research. All of the orphanage children formed attachments and made remarkable developmental and behavioural gains, and were able to have better lives than those they left behind in the orphanage. However, a substantial number of them developed problematic attachments.

Indiscriminately friendly behaviour and attachment

Both the early and more recent studies of children with early institutional experience noted the occurrence of indiscriminately friendly behaviour, and some researchers have speculated that such behaviour is evidence of failure to form attachments (Lieberman and Pawl, 1988; Provence and Lipton, 1962) or of an attachment disorder (Zeanah, 1996). Tizard (1977) defined indiscriminate friendliness as behaviour that was affectionate and friendly towards all adults (including strangers) without any evidence of the fear or caution that is seen in normal children. Furthermore, behaviour towards caregivers was not distinguished by any evidence of a special relationship. In Tizard's studies, such behaviour was reported by the adopting parents of institutionalized children at 2, 4½ and 8 years of age, although there was some decline by 8 years (Tizard and Hodges, 1978). Chisholm's (1998) study of Romanian orphans relied on parent responses to five questions: (1) whether the child wandered without distress; (2) whether they were willing to go home with a stranger; (3) whether they were friendly with new adults; (4) whether they were ever shy; and (5) how the child reacted to new adults. The first two items were considered to represent extreme forms of indiscriminate friendliness. When measured in this way, indiscriminate friendliness characterized the orphanage group (but not the comparison groups), and did not decline over the 4-year period during which the children were followed. Indiscriminately friendly behaviour was more characteristic of insecurely rather than securely attached children, and was significantly associated with behaviour problems, parental stress, and having been a favourite of orphanage staff. However, indiscriminately friendly behaviour (predominantly the less extreme forms) did occur among those orphanage children who were judged to be securely attached, and therefore Chisholm argued that it was unrelated to attachment.

A different view of attachment and indiscriminately friendly behaviour emerged from two other studies. Sabbagh (1995) assessed indiscriminate friendliness by examining behaviour towards the stranger in the salient episodes of the strange situation for a group of Romanian adoptees and controls living with their biological parents and matched for age, gender and attachment status. Again, indiscriminately friendly behaviour was more common in general among children who were insecurely attached, but adoptees who were considered to be securely attached were more likely to show indiscriminately friendly behaviour than their matched controls. These data are supported by those from the UK study showing that indiscriminately friendly behaviour was most common among children with atypical attachments, but there was also an unexpected increased frequency of such behaviour in the secure group (Marvin and O'Connor, 1999).

Sabbagh (1995) reasoned that truly indiscriminately friendly behaviour is dangerous for young children and is therefore an indication that the attachment behavioural system cannot be functioning properly. The observation of such behaviour in children who are otherwise considered secure suggested to her that attachment classification systems for older children, which typically ignore behaviour towards the stranger in the strange situation, should be revised to include such considerations. Clearly there is much further work to be done in order to understand indiscriminately friendly behaviour and its meaning for attachment. Indiscriminately friendly behaviour is also familiar to child-care workers who work in protective services and observe children experiencing repeated foster placements. Although this aspect of rearing in foster care has not been studied systematically, there have been recent attempts to study the way in which infants and toddlers adjust to foster care and form attachments with foster mothers (Stovall and Dozier, 1998).

Foster care

Children are removed from their parents only when to remain with them would threaten their well-being. Thus even very young infants taken into foster care have already experienced inappropriate care. Mary Dozier and her colleagues made regular home observations of infants placed in foster care to see how attachment behaviours towards the new caregiver begin to emerge. In addition, they considered the attachment status of the foster mother, predicting that – as for infants raised by their biological parents – the foster parent's state of mind with regard to attachment should predict the type of attachment the infant develops. For infants who were placed in care before 12 months of age, a stable pattern of attachment behaviours usually emerged within 2 weeks (Stovall and Dozier, in press), and in most cases (71 per cent), eventual attachment quality was concordant with the foster mother's attachment status (as measured with the AAI). This is quite similar to the levels of concordance reported for infants and their biological parents (see Chapters 3 and 4).

However, when infants were placed in foster care after 12 months of age, the length of time before stable attachment behaviour emerged extended up to 2 months. More importantly, those children who were placed in care later than 12 months of age were more likely than those placed earlier to develop insecure attachments to their new caregivers, even when the foster mother was secure/autonomous with regard to attachment. Thus, even when placed with a secure parent who would normally be expected to support the development of a secure attachment, the late-placed infant was more likely than the early-placed infant to develop an avoidant, resistant or disorganized attachment to the caregiver.

According to foster mothers' reports, infants in the early-placement group had significantly fewer attachment-related difficulties than those in the late-placement group. Babies placed before 12 months of age expressed needs in more direct ways than did those who were placed later. Later-placed babies were more likely to act as if they did not need or want care, or were unsoothable, and even autonomous foster mothers were likely to ignore or lose patience with them (Dozier and Stovall, 1999; Stovall and Dozier, in press; Tyrrell and Dozier, in press).

Dozier and her colleagues suggested that, by the end of the first year, infants who have received inappropriate care develop patterns of relating to caregivers that are designed to counteract and protect themselves against the insults they experienced and anticipate receiving again. These behaviour patterns interfere with the formation of a secure attachment, even if the infant is paired with a mother who is otherwise capable of providing responsive care. Thus these infants need more than good care in order to establish normal attachments. They require therapeutic care, and even autonomous foster parents require support and guidance in caring for these infants. Such interventions are currently being studied, but it is still too early to evaluate their impact.

Overview

In this chapter we considered a variety of conditions of extreme adversity for the formation of attachment. Several were notable for their lack of influence on attachment. Conditions affecting the infant (prematurity and Down's syndrome) were not marked by an increase in insecure attachment, although in the latter case there was evidence of difficulty in making classifications. Poverty on its own was also found to have little specific effect on attachment. In all of these cases, parents who are not encumbered by other disadvantages are usually able to meet the challenges of providing good care and supporting the development of secure attachments. However, multiple risks were noted to contribute to the likelihood of insecure attachment. Research in most of the areas surveyed led researchers either to question the validity of standard procedures or to elaborate classification schemes in order to capture the unusual attachment behaviour patterns shown by children whose first attachments developed under extremely adverse conditions.

What little data we have on possible recovery from early adversity suggests that some children do recover sufficiently to form attachments within the normative range. This evidence is consistent with a sensitive (rather than critical) period for formation of the first attachment. However, a significant minority of children who experience early deprivation fail to develop normal attachments, and show atypical attachment patterns. By the time they are placed in more optimal care conditions, many children who experienced severe early adversity have developed a protective repertoire of behaviours that interferes with the normal development of attachment. Thus they require more than good care – they need therapeutic intervention.

Suggested reading

Chisholm, K. (1999) A three-year follow-up of attachment and indiscriminate friendliness in children adopted from Romanian orphanages. *Child Development*, 69, 1092–106.
Data on recovery from early institutionalization from an intensive study in British Columbia.

Cicchetti, D., Rogosch, F.A. and Toth, S. (1998) Maternal depressive disorder and contextual risk: contributions to the development of attachment insecurity and behavior problems in toddlerhood. *Development and Psychopathology*, 10, 283–300.
A relatively sophisticated and complex examination of the effects of maternal depression on attachment.

Crittenden, P.M. (1988) Relationships at risk. In Belsky, J. and Nezworski, T. (Eds), *Clinical implications of attachment*. Hillsdale, NJ: Erlbaum, 136–74.
A summary of some of Crittenden's early work with maltreatment samples.

Goldberg, S. and DiVitto, B. (1995) Parenting children born preterm. In Bornstein, M.H. (Ed.), *Handbook of parenting. Vol. 1. Children and parenting*. Mahwah, NJ: Erlbaum, 209–32.
A review article on the challenges of caring for preterm infants and early attachment outcomes.

Tizard, B. and Hodges, J. (1978) The effect of early institutional rearing on the development of eight-year-old children. *Journal of Child Psychology and Psychiatry*, 19, 99–118.
One of the classic reports on early institutionalization.

Part III

Correlates and effects of attachment

9 Attachment and emotion regulation

In the previous section of the book (Chapters 4 to 8) we were concerned with factors that influence the development of attachment. This chapter is the first in a new section in which we shall consider how attachment influences other aspects of development. Bowlby's basic notion was that the early experiences which shape attachment behaviour are encoded in internal working models, and it is through these models that early experiences are carried forward to influence later personality and behaviour. These models include information that is both cognitive and affective, and both conscious and unconscious, and they become increasingly complex as new experiences contribute to both their content and their organization. In Chapters 9 and 10 we shall examine the processes of emotion regulation and information-processing that are fundamental to the operation of internal working models. Chapters 11 and 12 will examine the behavioural and physiological outcomes of attachment.

Emotion and emotion regulation

Virtually all theories of emotional development agree that emotional expressions undergo transformation in the course of development. Contemporary research documenting these changes shows that the expression of some emotions is evident in the newborn period, whereas others appear in the repertoire later in development (Izard and Malatesta, 1987). Emotional expressions become more differentiated, subtle and complex as children get older (Demos, 1986). At some time in the preschool years children begin to understand implicit rules about displaying emotions (Lewis and Michalson, 1983) and to exercise deliberate control of facial expressions (Cassidy and Kobak, 1988; Cole, 1985). One of the most difficult emotional feats is that of 'masking' emotions, particularly negative emotions – for example, to pretend pleasure by exhibiting a smile during a negative experience such as receiving an unattractive gift. While children as young as preschool age can enact happiness on request (Cole, 1985), even school-age children find it difficult to display pleasure during a negative experience (Saarni, 1979).

Historically, the management of negative emotions was a central issue in the study of emotional development, and discussions of emotion regulation focused on negative emotions and their control (e.g. Dodge, 1989). However, knowledge of when and how to express and inhibit positive emotion is also learned. Positive emotions play an important role in social interactions and are also subject to regulation. For example, one might inwardly experience satisfaction or glee when a rival experiences failure, but outwardly offer condolences. To incorporate this notion, Thompson (1994, p.27) suggested the following definition of emotion regulation: 'Emotion regulation consists of the extrinsic and intrinsic processes for monitoring, evaluating and modifying emotional reactions, especially their intensive and temporal features, to accomplish one's goals.'

Psychological views of emotions are changing. Where emotions were once viewed as 'noise in the system' that disrupts higher-order cognitive functions, the current view is that emotions are themselves organizers of behaviour and regulators of interactions with the environment (Thompson, 1994). In infancy, caregiver response to infant affect provides a template for the infant's acquisition of self-regulatory abilities (Feldman et al., 1999; Kopp, 1989). Central elements of this template are the adult's ability to read, interpret and respond to infant affect. Furthermore, through processes such as selective reinforcement, modelling and emotion-focused discourse, caregivers (and later peers) channel emotional expression into forms that are consistent with cultural expectations.

Attachment theory has been concerned with two aspects of emotional development. First, the manner in which attachment figures respond to affect is considered to be a focal aspect of the experiences that shape attachment patterns. Secondly, because attachment theory makes predictions about relationships between early experience and later features of personality, researchers have studied the way in which early or concurrent attachment is related to individual differences in emotional expression and regulation.

Attachment as a theory of emotion regulation

Historical perspective

Attachment is usually defined in terms of an emotional bond between two individuals based on the expectation of one (or both) members of the pair that the other will care for and provide protection in times of need. Bowlby's original exposition emphasized the evolutionary function of infant–caregiver attachments as that of enhancing the likelihood of survival. The infant's propensity to seek proximity to the caregiver in times of danger and the behaviour of seeking the caregiver when frightened were described as the quintessential features of attachment. In the opening chapters of *Patterns of Attachment*, Ainsworth and her colleagues (1978) described security of attachment thus: 'The opposite of feeling afraid (whether alarmed or anxious) is feeling secure or, according to the Oxford Dictionary, feeling "untroubled by fear or apprehension." ' Thus the idea of linking attachment and emotions is not new. From the outset, at least one emotion, namely fear, figured prominently in the development of the theory.

If we seriously consider the protective role of the caregiver, it can be parsed into a proactive and a reactive component. The proactive component encompasses removing hazards in the environment and removing the infant from hazards when necessary. These actions prevent the infant from experiencing distress. Hence, unless it is grossly deficient, the infant is unlikely to be unaware of this aspect of the caregiver's protective activity. The second component involves responding to the infant's perceptions of danger and the resulting emotions. Because infants may perceive danger in conditions that adults consider to be objectively safe (e.g. an unfamiliar friend of the parents wants to play with the infant), the success of the caregiver in this domain is related to their ability to see things from the infant's perspective and to read affective cues accurately. It is here that differences in caregiver behaviour are likely to arise and have implications for differences in the infant's emotional development. Thus Ainsworth emphasized caregiver response to infant signals as the primary determinant of early differences in attachment patterns.

In designing the strange situation, Ainsworth wanted to operationalize the construct of the attachment figure as a secure base for exploration. An underlying assumption of the procedure which she adopted was that being in a strange room with a strange person and experiencing separations from the attachment figure gives rise to fear or anxiety in 12- to 18-month-old infants. How the infant uses the caregiver as a resource for regulating the emotional discomfort that arises under these moderately stressful conditions is the key to identifying behavioural patterns of attachment.

In fact, each of Ainsworth's patterns can be conceived as a strategy for regulating and expressing emotions. Secure infants can be described as expressing their needs for protection and comfort freely and directly, avoidant infants as limiting their expression of attachment needs, and resistant infants as exaggerating their attachment needs. These descriptions diverge somewhat from the classic ones, but they serve to highlight the role that emotions play in basic attachment constructs. When classifying attachment patterns, the secure infant is identified by positive affective sharing with the caregiver before the separations, varying amounts of distress during the separations, and a rapid return to positive affect during reunions. The avoidant infant is identified by a distinct lack of affective expression (either positive or negative), and the resistant infant is distinguished by the predominance of negative affect before, during and after separations. Infant distress and parent response to it are considered to be key events that guide the development of these emerging differences.

Descriptions of attachment patterns in preschoolers and older children also include information about emotional expression. In mother–child dyads with secure children, the two partners show matching patterns of affect. Among dyads with avoidant or defended children, the child's affect is relatively flat while the caregiver is often described as 'overly bright.' One might draw the inference that the parent is working to 'brighten' the child's affective state. In dyads with a dependent or coercive child, both pair members express predominantly negative affects towards each other. While the punitively controlling child is repeatedly negative and hostile towards the caregiver, the caregiver's affect is flat. Finally, a child is most likely to be judged as controlling-caregiving when he or she is 'overly bright' and the caregiver is emotionally flat. In the latter case, it appears that the child is trying to 'brighten' the parent's mood.

When assessing adult attachment, the AAI can be interpreted as a procedure to reveal the way in which a person expresses and regulates emotions related to early childhood experiences. Remember that in this interview adults are asked to describe childhood experiences with important attachment figures, to tell how they think they have been affected by these experiences, and to explain why they think their parents behaved as they did. They are also asked to describe how each parent reacted to them when they were ill, physically hurt or emotionally upset.

Whether their childhoods were happy or not, adults classified as secure or autonomous tell a coherent story supported by detailed memories with appropriate affect. Dismissing adults idealize their childhoods, have few supporting memories, describe painful experiences without appropriate affect, and dismiss the emotional effects of these experiences. Finally, the narratives of preoccupied adults are suffused with such anger over old issues that they become mired in details and are unable to tell a coherent story. It is clear from these descriptions that emotion regulation during the course of the interview is a key feature of these patterns.

Thus even without an explicit focus on emotion development or emotion regulation in early theory, the expression and regulation of emotions played an important role in characterizing attachment patterns of infancy, childhood and adulthood.

Current theory

The germ of the idea that attachment theory is a theory of emotion regulation was introduced in a now classic paper by Sroufe and Waters (1977b), which described attachment as 'an organizational construct' and emphasized the regulation of 'felt security' as a central component of attachment. According to this view, the parental response to the child's affective signals provides the critical context within which the child organizes emotional experiences and regulates his or her felt security. Outside attachment theory other developmentalists focus on the adult–infant dyad as a system for mutual regulation of affect (e.g. Tronick, 1989), and this notion has been imported by some attachment theorists. For example, the origins of felt security and the expectation that a caregiver will be a secure base for exploration can be located in prior experience of the caregiver as consistently able to reduce infant arousal and minimize states of negative affect (Seifer and Schiller, 1995).

In his research with adolescents, Kobak (e.g. Cassidy and Kobak, 1988; Kobak et al., 1987, 1993; Kobak and Sceery, 1988) has amplified and pursued the idea that affect regulation is an important feature of the attachment system. He describes secure attachment as organized by rules that 'allow acknowledgement of distress and turning to others for support,' avoidant attachment as organized by rules that 'restrict acknowledgement of distress,' and ambivalent/resistant attachment as organized by rules that 'direct attention towards distress and attachment figures in a hypervigilant manner that inhibits development of autonomy and self-confidence.' Thus an individual's working models of attachment figures are linked to or include concurrent rules for regulating distress.

Furthermore, attachment strategies in childhood can be elaborated in the following manner. When a child's working model includes the expectation that the caregiver will respond effectively to signals of distress, the experience of distress leads to active attempts to contact the caregiver. Main (1990) called this strategy 'primary' because it is a direct and effective way to restore felt security and allows the child to return quickly to other activities. When the child's model includes the expectation that emotional signals will elicit only selective responses from the caregiver, he or she is forced to use secondary strategies. There are two such strategies, namely deactivation and hyperactivation (Kobak et al., 1993). Deactivation involves attempts to suppress information associated with attachment needs, including affect, and is characteristic of avoidant or dismissing attachment. Hyperactivation involves exaggeration of attachment behaviours and emotions, and is characteristic of resistant or preoccupied attachment (see Figure 9.1).

Cassidy (1994) propounds a similar view, that considers emotion regulation to be an aspect of attachment strategies. Security is associated with open and flexible emotional expression. With a parent who has been responsive to a wide range of emotions, the child learns that expression of emotion is useful in relationships and that negative affect alerts the caregiver in times of distress. Avoidance is associated with minimizing emotional expression. In this case, it is assumed that the caregiver has previously ignored or rebuffed expressions of negative affect, and the child has learned to restrain or falsify such expressions in order to prevent painful rejections. Positive emotions are also restrained because they signal readiness to interact, and enthusiasm for a relationship that has in fact been disappointing. Resistance is associated with heightened expression of emotions. This is

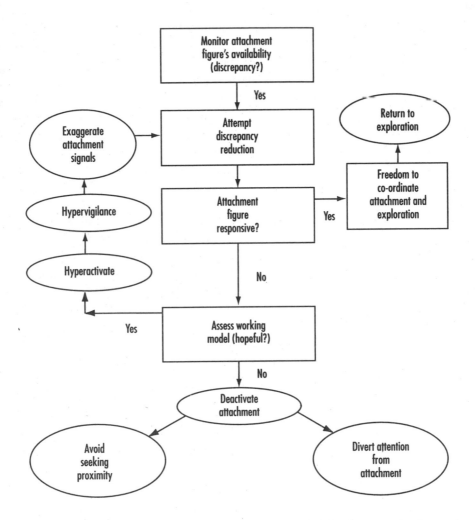

Figure 9.1 An analysis indicating the processes underlying hyper-activating and deactivating attachment strategies. The secure strategy is represented by an early return to exploration. Reproduced from Kobak *et al.* (1993) with permission.

thought to reflect the child's previous experience of a selective and inconsistent response to negative affect. Thus to relax involves the risk of losing the caregiver's attention.

A somewhat different approach to the role of emotions in attachment is described by Crittenden (1995). In her view, different attachment strategies are best described in terms of the extent to which they rely on affective and cognitive information. Avoidant, defended or dismissing attachment is characterized by reliance on cognitive information with the exclusion of a significant amount of affective information. Resistant, coercive or preoccupied attachment is characterized by reliance on affective information at the expense of excluding salient cognitive information. Security is marked by an appropriately balanced approach that integrates both affective and cognitive information.

Common to all of these views is the assertion that different attachment patterns are associated with experiences in which caregivers convey distinct messages about the rules for emotional expression and, as a result, correspondingly distinct styles of emotional expression and regulation develop. However, it is notable that little is said about a role for disorganization (or lack of resolution of loss and trauma) in the development of emotions or emotion regulation. This may partly reflect the relatively late arrival of these constructs on the attachment agenda. On the other hand, since these classifications are not strategies in and of themselves, and are always associated with another attachment strategy, it may be the case that they do not involve any particular pattern of emotional expression or regulation. What evidence is there of links between attachment patterns and either differential socialization experiences or patterns of emotional expression?

Socialization of emotion

Several studies have shown that attachment is linked with parental behaviour towards emotional expression by their offspring. First, Grossmann and Grossmann (1984) identified three conversational styles used by mothers in the home when infants were 2, 6 and 10 months old. The 'tender' style featured intermediate speech tempo, many quiet expressions of pleasure, few directives, prompt responses to infant vocalizations, prompt soothing in a calm tone of voice, and no impatience or tension. The 'lighthearted' style was characterized by fast tempo of speech, extremely exaggerated variation in loudness and pitch, much laughter and mock surprise, and intermittent – often delayed – responses to infant vocalizations. The 'sober' style was characterized by a slow speech tempo, few and short utterances, an uneven rate of response to the infant, a long reaction time, and delayed soothing with signs of resignation. While the sober style was common in all attachment groups, 50 per cent of mothers whose babies were later secure used the tender style, compared to 11 per cent and 10 per cent in the avoidant and resistant groups, respectively. The lighthearted style was used mainly by mothers of infants who were later judged to be insecurely attached.

Haft and Slade (1989) observed autonomous, dismissing and preoccupied mothers interacting with their infants, and recorded maternal 'attunements' to the infant. 'Attunement' is used to describe actions in which one person captures the emotional quality and form of another's behaviour without necessarily imitating or repeating it. Thus an infant may bang a toy in a particular rhythm and the mother may attune to this behaviour by saying 'Bang! Bang! Bang!' with matching intensity and rhythm. Haft and Slade (1989) found that autonomous mothers attuned to the full range of the infant's emotional expressions, mothers who were dismissing did not attune to negative emotions, and preoccupied mothers showed a random pattern of attunement.

Finally, Goldberg, McKay-Soroka and Rochester (1994) reviewed the strange-situation videotapes of 30 12-month-old infants selected to include 10 secure, 10 avoidant and 10 resistant infants. A coder who knew nothing about attachment identified salient emotional events from the episodes in which both mother and infant were present. These events were of three types: (1) affect that would be evident to the mother; (2) events that would be occasions for emotion (e.g. a fall is assumed to engender unpleasant feelings); and (3) occasions when the mother said or did something that indicated she had made an inference about emotion (e.g. she said, 'You're in a good mood today!'). These were classified according to the baby's behaviour as positive, negative or neutral events, and maternal responses were then coded.

Of course, if you consider the familiar descriptions of behaviour in the strange situation, you will know that this was not an equal-opportunity experiment for the mothers – avoidant babies showed little negative emotion and resistant babies showed a lot. Therefore the analyses considered the percentage of events to which mothers responded, and classified responses into categories (e.g. comfort, distract, encourage, imitate, verbal comment). Mothers of secure babies were observed to be most responsive, and were equally responsive to all three types of infant events. Mothers of avoidant babies were least responsive, and were particularly ignoring of the little negative emotion that their babies expressed. Mothers of resistant babies were moderately responsive, but particularly ignoring of positive emotions.

An unexpected finding was that mothers of avoidant infants were most likely to comfort and distract them when there was no objective evidence of emotional cues from their babies. In a similar observation from another study, mothers of avoidant infants joined them in play when the infants appeared to be content, but withdrew when the infants expressed negative affect. In contrast, mothers of secure infants were more likely to interact when the infant expressed distress and to leave the infant alone when he or she was content (Escher-Graeub and Grossmann, 1983).

When Goldberg, MacKay-Soroka and Rochester (1994) examined verbal comments, mothers of secure babies were most likely to make emotion-relevant comments (to 50 per cent of the events), and these comments frequently expanded beyond labelling the emotion, most often giving a reason for it (e.g. 'you really missed me'). In the other two groups, only 20 per cent of the emotional events elicited comments, and these were usually restricted to simple labels.

These few studies suggest that, even in infancy, attachment patterns are linked with distinctive messages from caregivers regarding the expression of emotions. Secure infants are told that all emotions are acceptable and that emotions are a topic for conversation. Avoidant infants receive the message that emotions, especially negative ones, are ineffective in recruiting help from the caregiver, and that emotions are not for discussion. Furthermore, when their mothers comfort and distract them in the absence of emotional cues, avoidant infants may also learn that 'it doesn't matter how I feel; someone else will tell me.' Resistant infants receive the message that the effects of expressing ·emotions are unpredictable, but intense negative emotions are most likely to provoke attention. Nevertheless, emotions are not a topic for discussion.

By the preschool years, caregivers are more likely to make conscious attempts to manage children's expressions of emotion. Among the mothers of preschool children, those whose children had been avoidant infants reported more attempts to subdue or control their child's negative expressions, whereas mothers of those who had been resistant infants reported few such attempts (Berlin and Cassidy, 1996). In general, the above studies are consistent in suggesting that there is pressure to mask or subdue negative emotional expressions in avoidant infants and young children. The evidence for pressures to heighten or exaggerate negative emotions in association with resistant attachment is less consistent.

Furthermore, mothers offer different attachment-related approaches to help their children to cope with emotionally arousing experiences. For example, Nachmias and her colleagues (Nachmias *et al.*, 1996) conducted a study in which toddlers and mothers participated in a 'coping session.' This included three novel experiences – a mechanical robot, a clown who tried to engage the child, and a puppet show. Mothers of secure children encouraged them to approach these novel stimuli, but also offered comfort, whereas mothers of insecure children more often demanded that the child should approach the stimuli and did not offer comfort.

Another route via which children learn the rules for affective discourse is by observation. Differences in the emotional expressions of mothers are observed to be associated with different infant attachment patterns. In Ainsworth's Baltimore study, mothers of secure infants were described as expressive and flexible, while mothers of avoidant infants were described as relatively unexpressive and rigid. Later studies supported these early observations with detailed assessments of mothers' emotional expressions. Unfortunately, most of these studies made comparisons only between secure and insecure children. The insecure children were predominantly avoidant, and although we learn something about the differences between security and avoidance, such studies provide no information about important theoretically predicted differences between the experiences of avoidant and resistant infants.

Nevertheless, the data are consistent in showing that the mothers of insecurely attached toddlers are less expressive not only with their own infant (Gaensbauer *et al.*, 1985: Main *et al.*, 1979; Malatesta *et al.*, 1989) but also with another adult (Main *et al.*, 1979). In addition, mothers of insecurely attached toddlers expressed more anger towards their children compared to mothers of securely attached toddlers (Gaensbauer *et al.*, 1985; Main *et al.*, 1979), and were rated as more fearful and less happy than the mothers of securely attached infants (Gaensbauer *et al.*, 1985).

In an attempt to remedy the general lack of information about resistant attachment, Cassidy and Berlin (1994) reviewed all of the available litera-ture to provide a summary of what is known about the origins and sequelae of the insecure-resistant attachment pattern. While this review showed that mothers of insecure-resistant infants were less available to their infants than mothers in other groups, there was no consistent information regarding either general emotional expressiveness or the expression of particular emotions.

In summary, the data provide most information on differences in early socialization experiences between children who develop secure and avoidant attachment patterns, with some limited information on those in the insecure-resistant group. If we can extrapolate from this information, we would predict that as children develop, those who are securely attached will express emotions of all kinds freely and openly, and those who are avoidantly attached will inhibit their emotional expression, particularly with regard to negative emotions. It is less clear whether those who are resistantly attached will exaggerate their emotional expressions, although this is what is predicted theoretically. In addition, securely attached children should develop and use a richer emotional vocabulary than those in the other two groups. Is there any evidence to confirm these predictions?

Attachment and emotional expression

We have already noted that the behavioural patterns from which attach-ment strategies are inferred are marked by distinct affective characteristics. However, in order to conclude that these unique styles of emotional expres-sion are persistent personality features, we need to know whether they are carried over to other situations and social interactions.

The most detailed study of the development of facial emotional expres-sion was conducted by Malatesta and her colleagues (1989), who followed 58 mother–infant pairs with assessments at 2½, 5, 7 and 22 months of age. The last observation included the strange-situation procedure. All of the sessions were videotaped, and facial expressions were coded from the tapes with a system that examined detailed changes in the activity of the facial musculature in order to identify particular emotions. In addition, several signs of emotional suppression (compressing the lips, lip-biting and knitted brow) were coded.

These procedures showed differences between securely and insecurely attached children. In general, insecurely attached children were emotionally more negative than their securely attached peers. However, during stressful situations, when it would be adaptive to communicate negative affect to an attachment figure, insecurely attached children displayed more positive emotion (primarily interest) together with the 'compressed lips' expression. This was interpreted as revealing 'a pattern of emotion suppression and vigilance' (Malatesta *et al.*, 1989, p.72).

Similar attempts to control emotion were observed among 3-year-olds (Berlin and Cassidy, 1996) in the presence of their mothers, and among 4-year-olds in response to mood-induction vignettes (Lay *et al.*, 1995). When the vignettes involved the mother and were intended to induce a negative mood, children with high security scores on the Attachment Q-sort were more likely to give negative responses, while insecure children were more likely to give positive responses. Attempts to minimize negative affect are also seen in 3-year-old children's responses to winning and losing in a game with an unfamiliar adult (Lutkenhaus *et al.*, 1985). Although avoidant children manifested sadness at losing during the game, they expressed positive affect towards the adult when the game was over and there was an opportunity to communicate more freely. Securely attached children were more likely to show their sadness at loss after the game.

One study which did distinguish between those who had been avoidant and resistant in infancy observed 45 3-year-olds (15 children who had been secure as infants, 15 who had been avoidant and 15 who had been resistant) in free play and in a clean-up session with their mothers. Those in the avoidant group spent more time expressing negative emotions than those in the other groups, but expressed these emotions with less intensity and were judged to be restraining these expressions, while children who had been secure or resistant infants were judged to be more spontaneous and displayed more intense negative expressions. As predicted, the resistant group were rated as exaggerating their negative emotions (Blokland, 1993). Surprisingly, children in the resistant group also spent more time expressing positive emotions than those in the other groups. Observations of 12 to 16-month-old infants also showed that resistant infants responded to both positive and negative maternal behaviour with positive affects (Tarabulsy *et al.*, 1996). As we shall see later, there are parallel data from adults to indicate that the propensity of children who had been resistant infants to express positive emotion inappropriately is unlikely to be a chance finding.

Kobak and his colleagues examined self and peer ratings of personality traits (Kobak and Sceery, 1988) and observed adolescents in a conflict resolution situation with their mothers (Kobak *et al.*, 1993). Peers rated secure adolescents as less anxious and less hostile than they rated those in other groups, and the adolescents themselves reported relatively little distress and high levels of social support. Adolescents whose attachment interviews identified them as dismissing received relatively high peer ratings for hostility, and reported more loneliness and less social support from their families than those in the other attachment groups. Finally, peers rated preoccupied adolescents as more anxious than those in the other groups, and the adolescents themselves reported high levels of personal distress, but viewed their families as more supportive than did adolescents in the dismissing group (Kobak and Sceery, 1988).

In problem-solving sessions with their mothers, secure adolescents expressed little dysfunctional anger and showed willingness to engage in discussing the problem. In contrast, problem-solving sessions with mothers and their adolescents who used deactivating (dismissing) attachment strategies were marked by the expression of dysfunctional anger by the adolescent (Kobak *et al.*, 1993).

In summary, although the evidence is not extensive, it is relatively consistent in showing differences between attachment groups at several different developmental stages. As expected, information about emotional expression in resistant/preoccupied attachment patterns is less plentiful than that about avoidant/dismissing attachment. The evidence indicates that the avoidant/dismissing group experiences more negative feelings than they express, and that these negative emotions are dampened or suppressed.

Attachment, emotional perception and emotional language

Another important domain of emotional development concerns acquisition of the ability to perceive, interpret and label accurately the expressed emotions of others. Although there is evidence that children begin to use labels for inner states almost as soon as they begin to talk (Bretherton *et al.*, 1986), there has been little study of children's use of emotional language within the framework of attachment. However, if the predominant experience associated with secure attachment is that emotions are openly expressed and discussed (Bretherton, 1990), we would expect secure attachment to be associated with more realistic perception and interpretation of the emotional experiences and expressions of others. If insecure attachment is associated with discrepancies between what is felt, expressed and discussed, we would predict that insecure attachment would be associated with more difficulty and confusion in interpreting and describing the emotional expressions of others. Indeed, there is evidence to suggest that this is the case.

Among 2½ to 6-year-olds responding to puppet-show vignettes, attachment security as assessed with the Attachment Q-sort was related to accuracy of inferences about the emotions of others (Laible and Thompson, 1998). These children viewed vignettes in which the key character expressed either 'stereotyped' or 'non-stereotyped' emotions. In the stereotyped situations, the key character showed the emotion that most people would experience under the circumstances. In the non-stereotyped vignettes, the emotion portrayed was consistent with each mother's prior prediction of how her own child would feel in that situation. At the end of each vignette, the child was asked to pick one of four faces, portraying happy, sad, angry and fearful expressions, to show how the key character felt. In addition, trained observers visited the children's preschool or day-care centres and interviewed the target children about discrete expressions of emotion among their classmates. Although older children generally showed a more accurate understanding of emotional expressions than did their younger counterparts, children with higher security scores obtained higher scores for emotional understanding than those with low security scores. Further analyses indicated that the contribution of attachment status was predominantly for negative emotions and emotions in the stereotyped stories.

Contrasting findings were obtained from a Finnish study (Silven and Laine, 1996) in which there was no evidence that attachment influenced 3 to 4-year-olds' ability to explain congruent or incongruent emotions in others. However, children categorized as defended by Crittenden's preschool scheme were more skilled than coercive children in explaining incongruent emotions.

Adult responses to infant emotions also reflect differences in attachment status. The IFEEL pictures (Emde et al., 1993) are close-cropped photographs of facial expressions of 1-year-olds with predominantly complex emotional expressions that are used to ascertain emotion perception biases. The viewer's task is to provide a brief label to describe the main emotion that the infant is feeling. Afterwards, a standard lexicon is used to categorize these labels. For example, happiness, glee and joy are all placed in the same category. When responses to a subset of clear positive, clear negative and mixed emotions were analysed, the mothers of secure, avoidant and resistant infants differed in their choice of labels. There were no differences in the responses to clear positive emotions, but mothers of avoidant infants consistently chose lower-intensity labels for negative emotions. For example, whereas the other two groups most often chose labels in the 'distress' or 'anger' categories, mothers in the avoidant group most often chose labels from the 'sad' category. In addition, in response to mixed emotions, the mothers of secure and resistant infants were equally likely to choose labels from all of the possible categories, while the mothers of avoidant infants limited their choices to the category of 'interest,' a low-intensity positive emotion (Goldberg et al., in press). Thus, the mothers of avoidant infants reported seeing less intense infant emotions than did the mothers in the other groups.

To follow up these observations, Blokland (1999) created a set of 16 videotapes with examples of clear positive, clear negative, neutral and ambiguous emotions in 4-month-old infants, and showed them to expectant mothers who later participated in an AAI. As in the IFEEL procedure, mothers were asked to provide a label for each expression and the IFEEL lexicon was used to categorize them. In addition, each response was scored as fully accurate (2 points) if it was in exactly the same category as the normative sample had placed it, partly accurate (1 point) if it was in a related category (e.g. 'caution' for 'fear') and inaccurate (2 points) if it bore no relation to the display (e.g. 'interest' for 'fear'). The mothers were also asked to rate the intensity of each emotion, and were videotaped during the procedure so that their facial expressions could be coded.

As expected, autonomous mothers obtained the highest accuracy scores and were most expressive while viewing the infant videotapes. In fact, they were the only group to show negative expressions in response to negative infant expressions. Dismissing mothers were least accurate and least expressive, and preoccupied mothers were moderately accurate. Unexpectedly, the preoccupied group showed more positive affect than the others, regardless of the stimulus infant's expression. This is consistent with the findings discussed above, showing that in both infants (Tarabulsy *et al.*, 1996) and 3–year-olds (Blokland and Goldberg, 1998) expressions of inappropriate positive affect are associated with resistant attachment.

As in the previous study, Blokland (1999) found that dismissing mothers were likely to use labels of inherently lower intensity and, in particular, they overused labels in the 'interest' category. In addition, autonomous mothers used the widest range of emotion labels and dismissing mothers used the most restricted range. Of specific interest with regard to the formulations of attachment theory, dismissing mothers used 'interest' labels significantly more often than all of the other groups to describe expressions of fear. In contrast, autonomous mothers used 'fear' labels for ambiguous negative emotions more often than did those in the other groups. Although they occurred with extremely low frequency, non-emotion labels (e.g. hungry, cute) were most likely to be used by preoccupied mothers. Thus although we have little information about attachment influences on children's use of emotion language, there is some evidence that adults differ in the use of emotion vocabulary depending on attachment status.

Summary and interpretations

These limited data paint a picture that is consistent with some of the predictions of attachment theorists. First, as expected, secure individuals are more spontaneously expressive and more accurate in reading emotions than those in other attachment categories. Secondly, avoidant/dismissing individuals are minimally expressive, are observed to restrain expression of negative emotions, and appear to underestimate the intensity of negative emotions in others. Although the data are less clear for resistant/ preoccupied individuals, they suggest that there is confusion in both reading and expressing emotions. Several studies have concurred in finding that resistant/preoccupied attachment was associated with predominant expression of positive affect, even in response to negative signals. Furthermore, this group was more likely than the others to label emotions with non-emotion words (Blokland, 1999). Interestingly, the differences in expressing and interpreting negative emotions are generally more consistent than the differences for positive emotions.

What mechanisms could explain these differences? Do individuals in different attachment groups actually experience emotions in themselves and others differently? Or do they have similar experiences but interpret and report them differently? Here considerably more thought and evidence can be marshalled to address the differences between security and avoidance than for any other combination. One important type of evidence comes from the physiological studies discussed in Chapters 5 and 12. On the basis of heart rate and cortisol measurements, avoidant infants appear to experience the same levels of physiological arousal in the strange situation as other infants, even though there is no overt evidence of this distress (Hertsgaard et al., 1995; Spangler and Grossmann, 1993). Similarly, during the Adult Attachment Interview, galvanic skin responses provide evidence of physiological arousal in dismissing adults during emotion-relevant parts of the interview, even though they do not report emotional experiences from childhood (Dozier and Kobak, 1992).

It is data such as these that lead to the conclusion that avoidance entails defensive processes (Bretherton, 1990; Cassidy and Kobak, 1988). A brilliant account of the development of such processes is given by Case (1995). In part, this analysis is based on the observation that certain emotions inhibit each other (e.g. happiness and sadness or curiosity and wariness). Like secure babies, avoidant babies associate proximity to the mother with safety. After all, they receive adequate care, even though their mothers misread or ignore some cues. However, once distressed, the idea of approaching or the act of approach is associated with anger or anxiety about rejection, because avoidant babies are uncertain of the mother's emotional availability. This results in an experience of 'emotional overload' and a need to reduce arousal and conflict rather than deal with the original cause of distress. In other words, they need to use a secondary strategy of deactivation.

Looking away is a behaviour that serves this function from early in infancy, and is thus likely to be used at this point. Looking away and becoming engaged with toys is even more effective, because it engenders interest and curiosity which inhibit the negative affects being experienced. Thus looking away has two desirable outcomes. First, it reduces anger or fear of rejection by turning away from stimuli, such as the mother's face, that could amplify these emotions, and replacing them with stimuli (toys) that arouse an inhibiting affect. Second, it allows the baby to maintain a degree of physical proximity which provides the comfort of knowing that the mother is physically accessible.

Case (1995) argues that this balancing of emotions is automatic rather than conscious, so that the avoidant baby who has been separated from his or her mother subjectively experiences her return as a neutral event even while his or her affective systems are highly activated with conflicting emotions. Thus the infant's subjective experience is distorted. As children mature and develop more complex working models of relationships, the working model of the avoidant child continues to diverge from that of the secure child, particularly with regard to the content of scripts relating to feelings and the nurturance they could elicit. Thus whereas the infant's approach-avoidance conflict is aroused by the need for physical approach, the older avoidant child's conflicts centre on verbal expression of feelings that require comfort or sympathy. Whereas the infant's defensive response is to look away and become engaged in object play, the older child learns to inhibit expression of emotions and use symbolic distractions (e.g. imaginary conversations). At each stage of development, Case (1995) suggests, children add ' a new layer of cognitive and affective structure to the sensorimotor core' of their basic affective style. Thus avoidant individuals achieve a stable affective equilibrium at the expense of 'greater physical distance, and decreased interpersonal intimacy, insight and/or integration.'

One can well imagine that if turning away from intimacy to avoid arousing one's negative feelings is an automatic and characteristic pattern of social interaction, avoidant or dismissing individuals repeatedly restrict their opportunities to register the full impact of the negative emotions of others. This in turn might account for their reports of less intense emotions. In fact, although the difference was not statistically significant, dismissing mothers in Blokland's sample had the shortest latencies to respond to infant emotional stimuli. In other words, they were quickest to look away from the screen.

It is more difficult to tell a coherent story about resistant/preoccupied attachment. Indeed, there are only limited data to support the theoretical notion that these patterns are associated with heightening or exaggeration of emotions. However, these individuals are distinguished from those who are secure in being less appropriately expressive and less accurate in comprehending the emotions of others. It seems likely that one of the distinguishing features of the two main forms of attachment insecurity lies in the strategies of emotion regulation that are used to maintain these forms over the lifespan. If so, only research that keeps these groups distinct can adequately inform us about the role of attachment in emotional development.

Suggested reading

Malatesta, C.Z., Culver, C., Tesman, J.R. and Shepard, B. (1989) The development of emotion expression in the first two years of life. *Monographs of the Society for Research in Child Development*, **54**.
A detailed study of socio-emotional development in the first 2 years of life, with excellent background on different theoretical approaches to the topic.

Case, R. (1995) The role of psychological defenses in the representation and regulation of close personal relationships across the lifespan. In Noam, G. and Fisher, K. (Eds), *Development and vulnerability in close relationships*. Hillsdale, NJ: Erlbaum, 59–88.
A brilliant analysis of the cognitive and affective components of working models of attachment and developmental changes therein.

Cassidy, J. (1994) Emotion regulation: influences of attachment relationships. In Fox, N.A. (Ed.), The development of emotion regulation: biological and behavioral considerations. *Monographs of the Society for Research in Child Development*, **59**, 228–49.
A detailed theoretical discussion of the role of attachment in emotion regulation.

10 Attachment and information-processing

Whereas emotions provide the organizing energy of internal working models, cognitive processes maintain and modify the contents. Bowlby considered cognitive psychology to be one of the fundamental disciplines of attachment theory, and drew upon the cognitive psychology of his time to frame the notion of internal working models. The first volume of the *Attachment and Loss* trilogy focused largely on animal and infant behaviour, but the later volumes were increasingly concerned with mental representations, and Bowlby's original exposition of internal working models appears in the third volume. The idea of internal working models was derived from Craik (1943), who suggested that each organism carries 'a small-scale model of external reality and its own possible actions within its head.' Similarly, Bowlby proposed that from infancy onward we construct models of the world, significant individuals in it, the self, and the relationships between these entities based on actual experiences. In turn, these models guide and focus subsequent experiences. 'Internal working models are best conceived as structured processes serving to obtain or limit access to information' (Main *et al.*, 1985, p.77). The ability to construct such representations evolved because they confer a survival advantage. They allow individuals to selectively attend to information, predict future events and construct plans.

Later theorists, particularly Bretherton (e.g. Bretherton, 1991), Crittenden (e.g. Crittenden, 1995), and Main (e.g. Main, 1991), elaborated Bowlby's ideas by drawing on contemporary advances in cognitive psychology. In this chapter we shall review ideas about the cognitive components of internal working models of attachment and the evidence that supports them. Currently there is considerably more theory available than evidence. Nevertheless, we shall try to answer the question of whether individual differences in information-processing strategies used in the service of attachment are carried over to other domains. As background to this discussion, we shall consider the development of some cognitive skills that are germane to internal working models. Then we shall examine how variation in these skills represents individual differences in attachment across the lifespan. Finally, we shall turn to the limited empirical evidence concerning the generalization of information-processing styles from attachment to other aspects of endeavour.

Salient aspects of cognitive development

Selective attention and memory

Although there has been much controversy over the extent to which experience initially falls upon a 'blank slate' or is deposited into pre-established compartments, there is now evidence that – from the beginning – the human infant is biased to attend to some types of information more than others. In particular, the stimuli provided by other human beings are highly salient for young infants. This is not because they are human but because they exhibit characteristic qualities that readily capture infants' attention.

As we noted in Chapter 2, young infants scan a visual stimulus by attending primarily to areas of high contrast and motion. To complement this bias, both children and adults exaggerate facial expressions and head movements when interacting with an infant. Similarly, infants are biased to attend to sounds that fall within the upper pitch range of the human voice, and to changes in pitch. Correspondingly, individuals 'conversing' with infants typically pitch their voices in the upper register and exaggerate pitch contours. Thus from the very beginning infants engage in selective attention, and those around them behave in a manner that increases the probability of being selected.

As new experiences accrue, information is stored to create memories that guide attention. For example, after repeated presentation of a complex visual or auditory stimulus, an infant – like an older child or adult – 'habituates.' What this means is that he or she attends less and less to each presentation, eventually just enough to confirm that it is indeed 'the same old thing.' However, if the stimulus is modified (i.e. there is new information), attention increases.

Information that is highly salient to personal well-being and safety, such as attachment-relevant information, is not only accorded preferential attention but engenders affective experiences. These, too, are encoded in memory and affect the subsequent deployment of attention as well as the content of internal representations. Initially, infant memories are limited to 'sensorimotor representations' or schemas (Piaget, 1952) that store knowledge of behavioural sequences and their results without consciousness (e.g. reaching for an object and feeling its contours). Although other types of memory soon develop, we rely on procedural memories (Tulving, 1985) throughout our lives to guide activities such as riding a bicycle, playing a musical instrument or taking the bus to work.

Towards the end of the first year, what Tulving (1972) termed 'semantic memories' emerge. This type of memory entails symbolic encoding to summarize generalized events. At first this is evident primarily in gestures (e.g. raising the arms to be picked up). As the child develops, linguistic skills play a growing role in shaping semantic memories. This allows information from sources other than direct experience to be incorporated. Generalized representations of the self, an attachment figure and the relationship between them are of this nature (e.g. 'Daddy likes to read stories to me' can summarize my own observations of Daddy, what Daddy has told me or, more often, both).

In the preschool years, yet another kind of memory appears. Episodic memories (Tulving, 1972) are vivid, detailed, chronologically ordered memories of specific events based on direct experience (e.g. 'One day my mother and I made cookies with raisins, rolled and pressed them into bunnies, and baked them. I tried to eat the raw dough but my mother scolded me. I sneaked some anyway when she wasn't looking. Three cookies burned but we took the rest in a straw basket to a lunchtime picnic in the park with my best friend').

Episodic and semantic memories do not necessarily coincide. As noted above, semantic memories incorporate both an abstraction of one's own experience and information from others. These may not agree (e.g. Daddy may tell me he likes to read to me but may not actually do it very often). My mother may have been generally responsive to my distress and my semantic memory of her may be that she was 'loving,' but in all likelihood there were some times when she was unavailable or preoccupied with other matters and was less responsive. There may have been times when I was being whiny and manipulative and she tried to teach me to present my complaints in a different way by ignoring me when I whined and responding when I expressed myself more directly. I may or may not remember the details of these occasions along with the semantic memory of my mother being responsive. Agreement and disagreement between semantic and episodic memories play an important role in Main's theorizing (e.g. Main, 1991, 1995) about the internal working models underlying different adult attachment patterns.

The ideas of Bretherton (e.g. Bretherton, 1990) and Crittenden (e.g. Crittenden, 1995) concerning internal working models focus less on these distinctions, and rely on Schanks' (1982) notion that memories exist in a complex hierarchy of schemes ranging along a continuum. Some of them are very close to specific experiences and others are quite general. The concept of scripts is particularly important. One way of thinking about scripts is to regard them as the symbolic analogue of procedural memories. Any event which happens frequently and regularly (e.g. bedtime rituals, mealtime) is likely to be encoded in this way, and young children often reveal these memories by enacting them in play (e.g. 'Eat your peas', 'I don't like peas!', 'They're good for you'). Scripts concerning repeated interactions with caregivers are incorporated into internal working models as information about relationships, and thus influence the processing of later experiences.

Beginning in the preschool years and continuing throughout the lifespan, we acquire and develop the ability to recount experiences in narratives. In general, narratives build upon selective attention, integration of memories, and language and communication skills. Thus narrative methods for assessing attachment reflect constructions that are the culmination of the intricate co-ordination of a complex array of skills. Such methods first become possible in the preschool years, and by late adolescence and adulthood are the preferred tools for assessing attachment. Although sensitivity to temporal sequences appears to emerge as early as 20 months of age (Oppenheim and Waters, 1995), it is not until well into the elementary school years that narratives are organized by explicit causal links (Waters and Hou, 1987). Children acquire many of their narrative skills in conversations with attachment figures where shared experiences are 'co-constructed.' If parent–child communication and co-construction processes are disturbed, children are confronted with circumstances that undermine their efforts to make sense of social experiences, and are left without emotional and narrative skills for communicating about salient topics (Oppenheim and Waters, 1995).

Bowlby (1988) cites extreme examples of such disturbances. He describes children who witnessed a parent's suicide but were later repeatedly told (and encouraged to believe) that the death had been caused by an illness or accident. In everyday life, even in well-functioning families, it is natural for parents and children to have different perspectives on shared events. This produces differences in memories of all kinds (scripts, semantic or episodic). The way in which such differences are handled may be important for the child's developing ability to construct a coherent narrative. A fully accurate encoding of differences would retain both the child's and the parent's point of view (e.g. 'I thought I did a good job of cleaning my room but my mother scolded me because it was messy. So I wasn't so eager to do it the next time she asked'). Alternatively, pressure from a parent to accept conflicting information as correct can result in distortion of the conscious memory (e.g. 'I never clean my room'), while the child's original memory is forced into less accessible forms (preconscious or unconscious). It is thought that when such conflicting information is a pervasive feature of attachment experiences, multiple inconsistent internal working models of attachment are retained without conscious awareness of discrepancies (Bowlby, 1988; Main, 1991).

Metacognition and theory of mind

Young children may be particularly vulnerable to such distortions because the ability to retain accurate memories of situations marked by communication and co-construction disturbances requires meta-cognitive skills that are not yet available. Flavell (1979) was the first developmental psychologist to draw attention to the significance of meta-cognition or 'thinking about thinking.' Although children begin to talk about their own feelings and those of others some time in the third year (Bretherton *et al.*, 1981), they are not yet equipped to query their own mental representations or those offered by others. Some time in the fourth year, children manifest a rudimentary ability to step back and consider their own cognitive processes as objects of thought (Oppenheim and Waters, 1995). By the age of 6 years, most children have mastered simple forms of metacognition (Chandler, 1988). For example, most 6-year-olds understand that there is a single world of objects, events, people, etc., which – although experienced and thought about by everyone – is independent of the thoughts of any particular individual. That is, I may know things that others do not, others may know things that I do not, and both my thoughts and those of others may be either true or false. In addition, both my thoughts and those of others can change over time.

Implicit in these notions is an underlying 'theory of mind.' From early childhood we formulate ideas about the mind, its contents and how it works, and eventually recognize that similar thoughts and processes take place in the minds of others. Since attachment figures are the first and initially most salient 'others' that the child encounters, it is plausible that these ideas first develop in the context of attachment relationships, and that children might have a more advanced theory of mind about their primary caregivers than about people in general (Oppenheim and Waters, 1995). In any case, internal working models of attachment come to feature attributions about the contents of the mind of the attachment figure (e.g. 'Daddy likes to read to me'), and differences in metacognitive functioning are thought to distinguish the working models of individuals with different attachment strategies.

Attachment as a theory of information-processing

Against this general background we can now review patterns of attachment through the lifespan and consider how the cognitive processes of working models differ for different attachment patterns.

Infancy

In infancy, as we discovered above, mental representations are almost exclusively procedural and selective attention is a prominent mechanism. Not surprisingly, differences in attentional strategies are the most striking feature of infant attachment patterns. In fact, the patterns of selective attention that are first engaged in infancy characterize attachment patterns throughout the lifespan. Securely attached infants maintain balanced and flexible deployment of attention to both the caregiver and the surrounding environment. In the previous chapter we discussed Kobak's notions concerning deactivation and hyperactivation (e.g. Kobak and Sceery, 1988). Avoidant infants are already using the strategy of deactivation – selectively excluding attachment-relevant information from awareness. Thus they focus on the environment and restrict attention to the caregiver. Resistant infants use a strategy of hyperactivation and are hypervigilant to attachment-relevant information. They maintain a singular focus on the caregiver at the expense of ignoring other environmental information.

While Main (1991) considers both avoidant and resistant infants to have an organized selective attention strategy, Crittenden (1995) points out that both secure and avoidant infants experience predictable caregiver responses, can predict caregiver behaviour, and are confident of the outcome of their strategies. However, she argues, the resistant infant copes with an unpredictable attachment figure, is not able to predict his or her behaviour, and therefore learns to distrust cognition as a reliable source of information. It is not until the preschool years that this latter group discovers a strategy that yields successful prediction of caregiver behaviour, one that entails alternation of angry and coy behaviour (note that it is a strategy based on manipulation of affect).

Disorganized/disoriented infants have either failed to develop a strategy for selective attention in attachment-relevant situations, or are unable to maintain their selected strategy. For example, they may be predominantly avoidant but be unable to contain their distress – evidence that distressing attachment-relevant information continues to intrude despite efforts to ignore or suppress it. In addition, behaviours such as stilling, freezing and stereotyped movements may represent lapses in access to needed information. Crittenden (1995) alternatively suggests that the apparent inactivity of stilling and freezing may reflect heightened monitoring and information-processing that allow the infant subsequently to engage an organized strategy.

Childhood

Selective attention continues to play a role in each of the main attachment categories. At reunions, the securely attached child, like the securely attached infant, is able to integrate smoothly attention to play and attention to the attachment figure by greeting the caregiver casually and involving them in the ongoing activity. Conversation is fluent and ranges over a wide variety of topics, including those that are personal. It often includes shared 'updates' (co-constructions) of what happened during the separation. The child volunteers information about what he or she has done and felt, and may ask about the activities of the adult.

The deactivating strategy of avoidant, defended or dismissing individuals is either to exclude or to minimize attachment-relevant information. Thus the avoidant or defended preschooler or 5 to 7-year-old, like the avoidant infant, gives little evidence that the attachment figure's return is important and becomes 'too busy' with another activity to attend to the caregiver beyond polite conformity with social rules. The child neither volunteers information about what he or she was doing or feeling during the separation nor enquires about the caregiver's activities. If there is conversation, it is about impersonal topics. Often the caregiver tries – without success – to engage the child in conversation.

In contrast, the dependent or coercive child's hyperactivating strategy focuses predominantly on the relationship with the caregiver. Thus the child is less able than either secure or avoidant children to continue organized exploration (processing of environmental information) in the absence of the caregiver, and once the attachment figure has returned, play or exploration is minimal. Often the child and the caregiver 'complain' about each other in subtle and indirect ways without concrete discussion. For example, the child may immediately announce that he or she wishes to go home, and then try to leave the room. The remaining time is taken up with conflict in which the child repeatedly presses to leave while the parent repeatedly insists that they must stay. There is little fluid conversation or exchange of information.

In the patterns that Cassidy, Marvin and the MacArthur Working Group (1987, 1992) described as controlling, children demonstrate an organized behavioural strategy, yet it appears to be based on an inappropriate reading of the situation. That is, the child takes the upper hand in a situation where he or she is actually dependent on the parent. While this may afford the child some sense of control and predictability with an otherwise un-predictable parent, it does so at the expense of ignoring or distorting important information. In fact, Crittenden (1995) characterizes the parallel patterns in her classification scheme as employing false cognitions (defended children) or affects (coercive children).

Main (1991) suggests that from infancy onward throughout life, insecure individuals must deploy some of their limited resources in monitoring the availability of attachment figures and engaging strategies to recruit or main-tain their attention. Because the secure strategy does not require such monitoring, it involves less cognitive activity. Main (1991) argues that a consequence of the relatively low information-processing demands of the secure strategy is that secure individuals can devote more attention and working memory to metacognition. Thus the development of both cogni-tive and metacognitive skills should be advanced in secure compared to insecurely attached children.

When attachment is assessed by narrative methods, secure children con-struct a story in which the child character has appropriate affect and a realistic strategy for coping with the situation, often with the help of responsive adults. Thus the story *is* a story – it has a beginning, a crisis or conflict, and a successful resolution. Although many of the insecure (predominantly avoidant) children attribute appropriate emotions to the story child, they often avoid the key issue of the story (e.g. insisting for a separation story that the parents cannot be going away on holiday). They either cannot imagine what the child could do about the situation, or they invent magical solutions. Thus the story has a beginning but may not have a crisis or conflict, and there is difficulty in bringing it to a plausible resolution (Bretherton *et al.*, 1990; Main *et al.*, 1985). Children who are considered to be controlling or disorganized invent unexpected catastrophes without solution, or are unable to respond at all (Main, 1995). In summary, although there is little explicit information about the narratives of children who are dependent or coercive, securely attached children appear to have better narrative skills than their insecure peers when recounting stories about attachment themes.

Adolescence and adulthood

The interpretation of the Adult Attachment Interview is highly dependent on analysis of cognitive processes in the construction of autobiographical narratives. Hesse (1996) suggests that the subject is presented with two tasks – first, to access, retrieve and reflect on memories of childhood while second, and simultaneously, maintaining coherent collaborative discourse with the interviewer. While the secure/autonomous individual successfully co-ordinates these two tasks, the insecure individual does not. Like the minimally communicative avoidant children, the dismissing adult volunteers little information. The questions of the interview are apparently answered, but with minimal attention to the attachment-relevant information that is requested. Thus dismissing individuals avoid the first of Hesse's tasks while superficially engaging in the second. The striking features of dismissing interviews are repeated inability to access memories, the use of brief, incomplete answers, and conflict between semantic and episodic memories, all of which combine to produce relatively incoherent narratives.

Preoccupied interviews are incoherent in a different way. They are marked by repeated intrusion of episodic memories that are not relevant to the question, difficulty in organizing semantic memories (and hence confusion about past events) and inability to follow the demands of the task. Detailed descriptions of specific incidents readily surface, but the speaker sometimes admits to forgetting what the question was. There is difficulty in staying on topic, handing turns back to the interviewer, and 'moving on' in a timely way from one topic to the next. With such individuals the interviewer struggles to keep track of answers, move on to the next question, and conclude the interview within the allotted time.

Secure/autonomous individuals display an ability to engage in meta-cognitive monitoring during the interview. For example, they may indicate that their memories could be erroneous, that other people might have a different view, or that their current ideas are different to what they thought at the time. Their narratives give the impression that the speaker is reflecting on the information as it is retrieved and organized. They may spontaneously identify contradictions or points that would confuse the interviewer (e.g. using a pet name for a family member and stopping to inform the interviewer 'Oh, sorry, you wouldn't know . . . that was my sister's nickname'). On the other hand, insecure individuals provide inconsistent or incomprehensible information with little awareness that they have done so. An additional scale for measuring 'self-reflection' during the AAI (Fonagy et al., 1991) indicated that autonomous mothers and fathers of infants score highest on this scale, followed by preoccupied and then dismissing parents.

Transcripts are assigned to the unresolved (for loss or trauma) category when they reveal mental disorganization or disorientation during the part of the interview concerned with loss and/or trauma. The primary evidence for such disorganization is a lapse in metacognitive monitoring of reason or discourse. The speaker may show confusion about the date of a loss by placing it at different ages in response to different questions, or they may speak of a dead person as if he or she were still alive. There may be excessive detail when recounting loss or trauma experiences, or unexplained dysfluency in discourse style. Main and Hesse (1992) suggest that these lapses in metacognitive monitoring are mediated by associated lapses in working memory.

In summary, across the lifespan there is evidence that each attachment pattern is associated with a unique style of processing attachment-related information, and these differences are key markers in the schemes we use to classify attachment.

The question of generalization

To what extent are the differences noted thus far in the assessment of attachment evident in other activities? Are there specific activities in which these differences should be most evident? For example, we might expect that attachment-related, information-processing skills are most likely to be transferred to other social relationships such as those with peers. Most of the studies described below focus on processing of either attachment-relevant information or general social cognitions, but some of them have examined more general aspects of information-processing. In fact, the limits of generalization have not yet been well articulated. We shall first consider studies of children and then those of adults. From the above discussion we can make some general predictions. Of course attachment is not the only factor that influences cognitive and metacognitive skills, but the theory predicts that individuals with secure attachments should generally be more competent than insecure individuals. We might also predict that, since avoidant/dismissing strategies focus attention on non-attachment information, individuals who use this strategy should rank next in general competence, with distinct differences in their performance on attachment and non-attachment task content. We would predict that dependent/coercive/ preoccupied individuals would be the least competent of the three organized attachment groups, since they are doubly compromised – they have difficulty in organizing attachment-related information, and their strategy of focusing on attachment relationships is thought to interfere with necessary attention to other activities.

It is not clear what predictions should be made concerning disorganized/ controlling/unresolved attachment and cognitive skills. In infant attachment assessments, these individuals appear to be least able to organize information and make decisions. In contrast, in adulthood, those who are unresolved with regard to loss or trauma experience only occasional lapses of organization during the assessment interview, and only in the context of specific topics. In the years between infancy and adulthood, behavioural patterns of attachment strategies linked with disorganization are organized, but there has been little discussion of explicit information-processing strategies in this group. One prediction is based on the observation of Moss and her colleagues (Moss *et al.*, 1999) that in the preschool and early school years, mother–child problem-solving is related to the child's concurrent attachment classification and is disrupted in disorganized-controlling dyads' dysfunctional communication. This observation suggests that disorganized attachment may be associated with very poor cognitive and metacognitive abilities. An alternative position (e.g. Kirsch and Cassidy, 1997) is that, other than the potential handicaps associated with insecure attachment, disorganization of attachment does not have any specific role in shaping general information-processing.

Childhood

As early as the toddler years, the exploratory play of securely attached children is characterized by longer play bouts, more focused concentration and more cognitively sophisticated exploration than that of insecure children (Belsky *et al.*, 1984; Main 1983). We noted earlier (in Chapter 2) that securely attached infants were advanced with regard to development of object permanence compared to their insecurely attached peers (Bell, 1970). In addition, securely attached toddlers were more likely to use self-directed speech (an early form of metacognition) in problem-solving (Main, 1983), and showed superior problem-solving skills to their insecurely attached peers (Matas *et al.*, 1978). At 3½ years, when mother–child dyads were given a 'grocery-shopping task' requiring both metacognitive skills and collaboration, secure children engaged in more task-relevant activity and more object exploration, and engaged in a higher proportion of metacognitive activity (e.g. monitoring and evaluation) than their insecurely attached counterparts (Moss et al., 1993).

In a study of memory and attention, 3-year-old boys who had been securely attached infants remembered positive events more accurately than negative events, while the reverse was true for those who had been insecure (Belsky et al., 1996b). However, in this same group of children, the expected differences in distractibility during positive and negative events were not found. In contrast, Kirsch and Cassidy (1997) found that 3½-year-olds who had been insecurely attached infants looked away from attachment-relevant pictures more often than did those who had been securely attached infants, with the insecure-avoidant group showing this effect most dramatically. When these same children were presented with stories in which a mother was responsive, rejecting or over-reacting to a child's distress, it was predicted that each attachment group would best remember the story that was most consistent with their own experience (i.e. the secure group would be best at remembering the responsive story, the avoidant group best at remembering the rejecting story, and the resistant group best at remembering the over-reactive story). Instead, the children in the secure group remembered the responsive stories better than did those in the avoidant group, and also remembered the rejecting stories better than did those in the resistant group. Although these studies document differences in attention and memory related to early attachment, in each case some of the expected differences failed to materialize.

One area to which attachment-related cognitive processes may be generalized is that of representations of the family. There has been some concerted effort to analyse family drawings of 5 to 9-year-olds from an attachment perspective. The basic technique of these studies is to provide children with standard materials and ask them to draw a picture of their family. Several early but unpublished studies (Grossmann and Grossman, 1991; Main et al., 1985) suggested that school-age children who had been securely attached infants were distinguished from their insecurely attached peers by drawing more complete and individualized figures (i.e. variations in clothing, hair-style, posture and expression).

The first published study (Fury et al., 1997) was based on elaborating a coding scheme developed by Kaplan and Main (1986) and applying it to drawings of 171 third-graders in the Minnesota longitudinal study. This scheme reflects the concepts discussed above with regard to how children in each attachment group process information about relationships. More specifically, the system includes a list of signs thought to be associated with an early history of insecurity, avoidance, resistance or disorganization (see Table 10.1 and Figure 10.1). With the exception of the signs of resistance,

Table 10.1 Examples of infant attachment markers in children's drawings[a]

Insecurity	Avoidance	Resistance
Absence of background	Lack of individuation	Figures close together
Figures not grounded	Arms downward	Figures separated by barriers
Incomplete figures	Exaggerated heads	Unusually small figures
Omission of mother or child	Lack of colour	Unusually large figures
Mother not feminized	Disguised family members	Figures in corner
Figures not gender-differentiated	Child apart from mother	Exaggerated soft body parts
Neutral or negative affect	Unusual signs or symbols	Exaggerated facial features
		Exaggerated hands and/or arms

[a] Reproduced with permission from Fury et al. (1997).

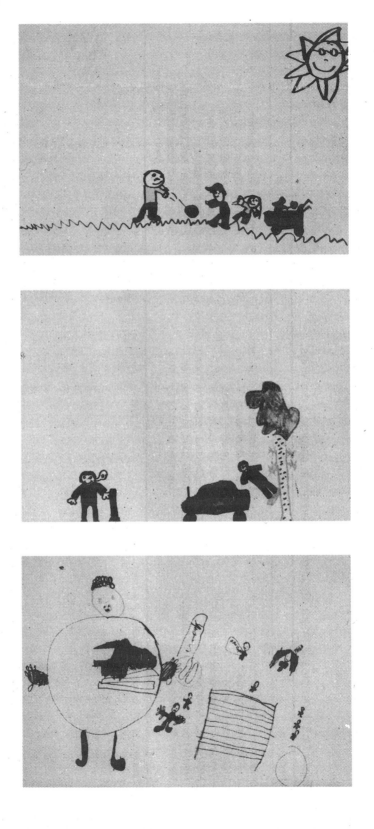

individual signs were not necessarily associated with early attachment history. However, when coders used the full system of signs plus additional qualitative ratings to guess each child's early attachment classification, a significant association was found between classification based on the drawing and prior observations in the strange situation.

Although Fury and her colleagues did not find IQ scores to be associated with the overall score for drawings, a subsequent study of family drawings noted that, among 200 5 to 6-year-olds, secure children demonstrated better fine motor co-ordination and general cognitive ability than did their insecure peers (Pianta *et al.*, in press). Nevertheless, in the Minnesota sample, after IQ and contemporary measures of life stress and emotional functioning had been taken into account, early attachment history still made a significant contribution to the drawing measures.

While the above studies are consistent with general ideas about attachment-group differences in cognitive style, they are rather limited and have not yet been replicated. There is a somewhat larger literature on the relationship between attachment and both general cognitive ability and language skills in childhood. An early narrative review of such studies (Bretherton *et al.*, 1979) indicated that, while many investigators had indeed found positive associations between early attachment quality and broad measures of cognitive function, a substantial number of studies failed to do so. With regard to language development, the evidence seemed to be more consistent but showed no difference in language competence between secure and insecurely attached children.

A more recent meta-analysis reached quite different conclusions (van IJzendoorn *et al.*, 1995). In studies of children ranging from infancy through to age 10 years, although there was an association between attachment and IQ scores, it was relatively small (effect size 0.09). In contrast, although there were fewer studies of language development in the first 4 years, the association between attachment and language was considerably stronger (effect size 0.28), with secure children, as expected, having an advantage. For the most part, both of these reviews concentrated on the differences between secure and insecure children, because the number of

---

Figure 10.1 Examples of drawings with typical characteristics of children who were secure, avoidant or resistant as infants. (a) 'Secure' drawing. The figures are grounded, differ in clothing, hair-style, body position and action, and are oriented towards each other and engaged in joint activity. (b) 'Avoidant' drawing. The mother is 'disguised.' She is in the car. The 'self' figure is climbing the tree and has no hands. Although the figures are coloured differently, their postures are identical and they are facing forward, not engaged in joint activity. (c) 'Resistant' drawing. The entire drawing is brown. The extremely large figure with an exaggerated abdomen is the mother, and all of the extremely small figures were described as 'self' figures jumping over the fence that is a barrier between the self and the mother.

resistant infants in the population is so small. However, in the meta-analysis, on the assumption that those who had been resistant infants should now be particularly disadvantaged, an analysis was performed to see whether the number of resistant cases in the sample was related to effect size. This analysis was only possible for the more numerous studies of general cognitive skill, but it showed that, indeed, the more resistant infants that were included in the sample, the stronger was the effect size. This finding is consistent with the notion that the selective attention pattern associated with resistance and its later analogues may have a persistent negative effect on acquisition of general cognitive skills. The disorganized classification was ignored in these analyses because most of the studies had not used it.

The most ambitious study to explore links between attachment and cognitive skills followed 85 Icelandic children from age 7 to 15 years, and 51 of these to age 17 years (Jacobsen *et al.*, 1994). Attachment was assessed at age 7 years with a narrative method based on a pictured separation story. At 7, 9, 12, 15 and 17 years, the children participated in a battery of Piagetian tasks to assess concrete and formal operations, At 9, 12, 15 and 17 years, additional tasks involving syllogistic reasoning were administered. As control or mediating factors, measures of IQ, self-confidence, and attention deficits were assessed. At all ages and on all tasks children classified as secure at 7 years of age were most competent, and children classified as disorganized encountered the most difficulties. (In this particular study, the 4 children classified as dependent were ignored because they constituted too small a group for analysis.) Although there were corresponding group differences in both IQ and attention deficits, neither of these measures accounted for the effect of attachment. Instead, for the Piagetian tasks, attachment exerted its effects primarily through effects on self-confidence. The authors reasoned that enhanced self-confidence enabled secure children to engage in more intense and sophisticated exploration.

Attachment effects on syllogistic reasoning tasks were not attributable to any of the control variables. Although secure and insecure-avoidant children showed a consistent improvement over time on syllogistic reasoning tasks, this was not true of the insecure-disorganized group. At 17 years of age, their performance was little improved over their initial performance at age 9 years. This study provides clear evidence in support of the notion that secure attachment is associated with cognitive advantages and disorganized attachment may interfere with some aspects of cognitive development. However, in so far as we can tell from these data, the effect of attachment on the Piagetian tasks is exerted primarily through self-confidence (and the more sophisticated exploration it permits), rather than through specific information-processing skills. On the second type of task (syllogistic reasoning) the possible mechanisms involved are less clear.

The findings from a French-Canadian sample were quite similar in pointing out unique difficulties associated with disorganized attachment, but they also found links with both self-esteem and dysfunctional mother–child interaction during problem-solving tasks (Moss *et al.*, 1999). During these tasks, the children in the disorganized group engaged in less metacognitive activity than did those in the other groups. Consistent with the earlier meta-analysis (van IJzendoorn *et al.*, 1995), there were no differences between the attachment groups in language skills, but children with disorganized-controlling attachment patterns were significantly poorer in mathematical skills than those with organized attachment strategies. Both academic self-esteem and mother–child collaborative problem-solving made independent contributions to this outcome. These data point out the importance of attempts to study the mechanisms whereby attachment may affect broader aspects of cognitive development, and the desirability of using tasks that focus on specific processing skills.

Adults

Given the interest in working models of attachment that has characterized attachment work in the 1980s and 1990s, it is somewhat surprising that the examination of adult thought processes in relation to attachment has been fairly limited. You may recall from Chapter 3 that validity data for the AAI suggest that adult attachment patterns are not related to IQ scores or style of discourse in discussing a non-social topic (work history, Crowell *et al.*, 1996). (Note that this contrasts somewhat with the data for children. Possibly the small effect of attachment on IQ scores during childhood is primarily related to developmental aspects of cognitive competence, and is less evident once adult levels are achieved.)

However, there is evidence that discourse regarding other relationships reflects some of the features that characterize attachment styles. For example, Zeanah and his colleagues (Zeanah *et al.*, 1994) designed an AAI-like interview to assess a parent's 'working model of the child.' To date it has been used primarily with parents of infants. In the interview the parent is asked to discuss perceptions and subjective experiences of their infant and their relationship with the infant in a format that follows the AAI. Like the AAI, the interview is recorded, a transcript is constructed, and the transcript is scored for aspects of narrative style and coherence.

Three general styles have been identified, namely 'balanced,' 'disengaged' and 'distorted,' intended to correspond to the autonomous, dismissing and preoccupied categories, respectively. As yet, there is no evidence of specific links between the AAI and Working Model of the Child classifications, but two studies have shown concordance with infant attachment classifications (Benoit *et al.*, 1997; Zeanah *et al.* 1994). However, like AAI/infant attachment concordance, this effect is largely accounted for by matches between balanced representations and secure infant attachment. Thus it is not yet clear whether the narratives produced in the Working Model of the Child Interview satisfactorily demonstrate an extension of information-processing style from the attachment domain to the caregiving domain.

A second attempt of this type involved assessment of a current dating or marital relationship using an interview format and scoring system parallel to those of the AAI (Current Relationship Interview; Crowell, 1990; Owens and Crowell, 1993). The same classification categories (autonomous, dismissing, preoccupied and unresolved) are used. In a study of 45 engaged couples, 64 per cent of individuals were similarly classified as secure or insecure on both interviews (Owens et al., 1995). Again this reflects primarily autonomous–autonomous matches, and the links between specific types of insecurity were weak. However, the coherence scores on the two interviews were significantly correlated.

Although constructing AAI-like measures to assess other social relationships is one way of exploring generalization of attachment-based information-processing, an alternative approach is to examine performance on experimental information-processing tasks with or without an attachment-related content. In one such study, when pictures were presented repeatedly at very brief exposures, psychology students classified as secure on the AAI identified attachment-related threats (e.g. adult anger towards a child) sooner than their insecure peers, but there was no evidence of the expected differences between dismissing and preoccupied students (van Emmichoven, 1998). A similar approach was used to administer a battery of experimental tasks to adult women (Atkinson et al., 1998). Before the information-processing tasks were administered, subjects watched an emotionally disturbing film with attachment content (an edited version of one of the Bowlby and Robertson separation films). When asked 1 week later to recall two attachment-related stories (one positive and one negative), the autonomous women remembered more attachment as well as non-attachment details than did the preoccupied women, who in turn remembered more than the dismissing women.

In a second task, women were shown a list of phrases and instructed to remember or forget them. The list included positive and negative attachment items, positive and negative emotion items (unrelated to attachment) and neutral items. After presentation of all of the phrases, the participants were shown a new list containing both the original phrases and new ones, and were asked whether or not they had seen them earlier. Among the phrases they were asked to remember, insecure women remembered more neutral items than did secure women. The reverse was true for all other types of items – autonomous women remembered both attachment and non-attachment emotion items better than did preoccupied or dismissing women. With regard to the items to be forgotten, insecure women forgot fewer control phrases and more target phrases than did autonomous women. Thus the autonomous women demonstrated better conscious control of memory than did their insecure peers, remembering what they were instructed to remember and forgetting what they were instructed to forget. These few preliminary studies illustrate an area that is ripe for exploration and promises to contribute to our understanding of internal working models in adults.

Overview

In this chapter we have considered the cognitive properties of internal working models of attachment and reviewed the way in which assessments of attachment identify each of the known attachment patterns by unique information-processing and metacognitive skills. We also asked whether the cognitive differences that are considered to characterize different internal working models of attachment are evident in related domains. One of the basic ideas of attachment theory is that internal working models are the mechanism by which early attachment experiences are carried forward and influence other aspects of functioning. Thus Bowlby (1980) argued that one's internal working model of attachment becomes a filter which focuses and organizes subsequent social experiences.

Although there is some evidence to support this premise, it is still sparse (particularly for adults), and the data are not always consistent with predictions. The most consistent evidence supports the prediction that secure or autonomous individuals will have cognitive advantages over those who are insecure. Distinctions between different types of insecurity, with a few exceptions (e.g. Jacobsen *et al.*, 1994; Moss *et al.*, 1999), have either not been made or not been supported. Thus it would be premature to make pronouncements about how broadly attachment-based information strategies influence other aspects of social and/or non-social cognition. However, given the central role that theory attributes to internal working models, it is likely that this will be an important area of future investigations. The most productive approaches are likely to be those that focus on articulating specific predictions for different types of insecurity, rely on tasks that assess specific information-processing skills, and consider mediating factors such as self-esteem, parent–child problem-solving interactions, or school experiences.

Suggested reading

Main, M. (1991) Metacognitive knowledge, metacognitive monitoring, and singular (coherent) vs. multiple (incoherent) model of attachment: findings and directions for future work. In Parkes, C.M., Stevenson-Hinde, J. and Marris P. (Eds), *Attachment across the life cycle*. London: Routledge, 127–59.

Bretherton, I. (1990) Open communication and internal working models: their role in the development of attachment relationships. In Thompson, R. (Ed.), *Socio-*

emotional development. Nebraska Symposium on Motivation No. 36. Lincoln, Nebraska: University of Nebraska Press, 57–113.
Two somewhat different perspectives on internal working models of attachment reflecting contemporary cognitive psychology, each written by a leading figure in the field.

Jacobsen, T., Edelstein, W. and Hofmann, V. (1994) A longitudinal study of the relation between representations of attachment in childhood and cognitive functioning in childhood and adolescence. *Developmental Psychology*, **30**, 112–24.
A solid longitudinal study of attachment and cognitive processes from age 7 to 17 years.

11 Attachment and social competence

Contemporary attachment theory asserts that the processes reviewed in Chapters 9 and 10 and the internal working models that they constitute exert strong (often automatic and unconscious) influences on feelings, thoughts and behaviour. By directing attention to some actions and events instead of others, guiding appraisal of information, and selecting what is and is not remembered, internal working models shape behaviour towards others and hence the reactions that one engenders in others. In other words, internal working models of attachment serve as interpretive lenses that focus new experiences. As we have seen, research to study the components and functioning of internal working models is in its infancy. Yet long before attachment theorists and researchers began serious work on the nature and mechanisms of internal working models, evidence was accumulating that individual differences in early attachment were related to a wide array of subsequent social developmental outcomes. As a result, there are numerous studies reporting successes and failures in linking measures of early attachment to later social development, but only limited data to illuminate the mechanisms by which this happens. Such information would include measures of the intervening and concurrent quality of parent–child interactions or relationships, evidence of mediating emotional or cognitive processes, and indicators of other supportive and/or disruptive events and processes.

Hence, although there are notable exceptions, research exploring the consequences of early attachment for later social development is not well integrated with the proposed explanatory framework. The topics investigated in these studies will almost certainly need to be revisited with an enhanced understanding of how working models function. In this chapter, we shall review the existing studies, beginning with a general consideration of mechanisms proposed to account for the effects of attachment on social development. We shall then review studies of social development during childhood, as well as the growing literature on adult attachment and concurrent social functioning.

Mechanisms of influence

Many suggestions have been made as to how early attachment could influence subsequent development. Some arise from attachment theory itself, while others originate from different theoretical perspectives. The notion that working models of attachment are the route by which early attachment influences later social competence currently provides only a broad framework within which we must search for specific mechanisms. One common view is that early attachments *per se* become the prototype for subsequent relationships. That is, individuals subsequently recreate or attempt to replicate their early attachment relationships. This view is shared by some other theories regarding the importance of early experiences (e.g. psychoanalytical theories). If this view is correct, we should find parallels between features of relationships with caregivers that are thought to give rise to attachment patterns and later relationships with social partners. Owens and colleagues, (1995) examined the similarity between adults' descriptions of their experiences with their parents on the AAI and with their marital partners on the Current Relationship Interview, and found little support for the strong form of the prototype hypothesis. In fact, representations of early attachments were only modestly related to those of current relationships. This suggests that although early relationships with caregivers provide a foundation for later intimate relationships, they do not determine the form of these relationships *per se*.

A strong prototype hypothesis is difficult to reconcile with the diverse nature of later relationships. Whereas early attachments involve an immature and relatively powerless child depending on a wiser and more experienced adult for protection, in some later relationships that child may be the older, wiser protector (e.g. as an older sibling), in others an equally inexperienced peer (e.g. childhood friendships), and in still others an equally experienced peer (e.g. marital relationships). Owens *et al.* (1995) suggest instead that romantic partners co-construct their understanding of present relationships. Thus earlier working models of attachment would influence this co-construction process but could not determine it. A similar process might also occur in constructing representations of other close relationships, and would be consistent with the notion that working models, particularly if secure, are open to alteration in the light of new information and experience.

Sroufe, Egeland and Carlson (in press) suggest five ways in which early relationships with parents influence subsequent social competence. Although they focused on peer relationships, these mechanisms could apply equally well to other social domains.

1. By shaping the child's expectations of relationships and their rewards or problems, early attachments provide the *motivational* base for other relationships.

2. The extent to which a child feels effective in early attachment relationships provides an *attitudinal* base for later social experience by shaping the extent to which the child feels prepared to master the challenges of the larger social world.
3. Attachment relationships provide the *instrumental* basis for other relationships by shaping the development of broadly applicable behavioural skills.
4. The pattern of affect regulation in early attachment relationships establishes the *emotional* base for social competence because it is the prototype for the self-regulation required in the broader social world.
5. The rules and roles of reciprocity learned in attachment relationships provide knowledge to form the *relational* base for other relationships.

In short, early attachments provide a foundation upon which subsequent social encounters build. However, these basic attitudes and skills may well be modified by experiences with peers, teachers and other adults. In the longitudinal study reported by these authors (see below), some of these possibilities are evaluated by assessing proposed attachment group differences in particular skills, knowledge and attitudes at several age points.

Another possibility, often pointed out by critics of attachment theory (e.g. Lamb *et al.*, 1984, 1985; Lewis, 1997), is that early attachment may be linked to later social developmental outcomes not because the child's representation of early attachment is influential, but because parents who support particular patterns of early attachment provide similar conditions through later childhood. Thus, according to this view, concurrent conditions are the primary influence on social behaviour at any given time. Early attachment is simply a marker of the caregiving conditions that are likely to prevail later on. This hypothesis of continuity of care can be tested by including assessments of both intervening and concurrent parent–child relationships in research designs. It would also gain support from evidence of high stability in attachment patterns over the lifespan. We have already noted (in Chapter 3) that the evidence for stability is rather mixed. An alternative position is that concurrent relationships with parents are an important influence on social behaviour, but that parent–child relationships can and do undergo change as each developmental period brings its own challenges for both parents and children. Thus, if buttressed by appropriate empirical data, the impact of concurrent relationships with parents could be interpreted as contributing to both effects of early attachment on later social competence and their absence.

These routes of influence need not be mutually exclusive. Indeed, most theorists have argued for complex multiply determined models of social development. However, if the stance of the theory is that internal working models are the primary route by which early attachments influence later behaviour, then specific aspects of an individual's internal working model of attachment must be related to particular later social cognitions and behaviours, and this pathway should be stronger than that of other proposed influences. At present, the evidence available to test this formulation is limited.

Since most children experience more than one attachment figure, it is assumed that different attachment relationships contribute to the formation of a general internal working model of relationships. It is not yet clear how this happens, or how information from different attachment relationships is weighted or combined to arrive at a general model. Is such a model specific to close relationships? Or is it a model of relationships in general, encompassing those with familiar and unfamiliar peers and adults both within and outside the family? What aspects of development should attachment influence? Indeed, early attachment has been linked to so many different aspects of development (e.g. peer and sibilng relationships, self-concept, problem-solving skills, language abilities) that it is worth speculating whether attachment is 'merely a marker of general adjustment' (Belsky and Cassidy, 1994; Sroufe, 1983). Consequently, some theorists have argued for the importance of discovering what attachment does *not* predict as well as what it does predict (e.g. Belsky and Cassidy, 1994; Sroufe, 1983).

In this text, we have proceeded from the assumption that attachment is a particular aspect of some relationships as experienced by the individual. If, as Bowlby and some subsequent theorists suggest, early attachment experience is the cornerstone of personality development, then its influence should indeed be very broad. However, we then need to construct and evaluate models to explain how this breadth arises. A more circumspect view is that, although it may influence a broad array of social abilities, attitudes and behaviours, it should be more influential in some domains than in others – for example, it should be more influential in close personal relationships than in general sociability.

Evidence

Concepts of self and others

Attachment experiences are thought to result in internal working models that incorporate an appraisal of the self and the self in relationships which shape a general outlook on social experiences. Thus we might begin with the proposition that different attachment patterns shape the view of the self that enters into social relationships. Although self-concepts have not been widely studied in relation to attachment, three kinds of evidence are relevant. First, there are mixed data on attachment and later 'ego resilience' or self-confidence as rated by teachers or observers in children and self-reports in adolescents and adults. For example, children in the Minnesota longitudinal study who had been securely attached received higher scores on both Q-sort and behavioural measures of ego resilience at 5½ years of age (Arend *et al.*, 1979) and were rated as more self-confident in group situations as adolescents (Sroufe, *et al.*, in press). Similarly, two studies (Kobak and Sceery, 1988; Treboux *et al.*, 1992) found secure college students to be more self-confident than those who were insecure on the AAI. However, several studies of children failed to confirm this pattern (e.g. Barnas *et al.*, 1991; Easterbrooks and Goldberg, 1990; Oppenheim *et al.*, 1988), as did some studies of adults using the AAI (see Crowell and Treboux, 1995, for a summary). However, when adults complete attachment questionnaires, self-classified secure subjects consistently report higher self-esteem than insecure subjects (Borman-Spurrell *et al.*, 1994; Collins and Read, 1990; Feeney and Noller, 1990; Feeney *et al.*, 1994).

Secondly, these concepts can be inferred from the narratives told in response to story stems (See Chapter 10). It has been observed that securely attached children tell stories in which the central figure copes well with problems (often with help from others), that avoidant children appear to be at a loss for problem-solving strategies, and that the disorganized group tell of bizarre and random disasters in which they are helpless. From these findings one can infer that children in the secure group are confident about their ability to face problems and enlist the help of others, while those in the avoidant and disorganized groups lack such confidence. One can also infer that secure children regard the social world as a supportive one, avoidant children expect little help from others, and disorganized children perceive the world to be unpredictable and threatening.

Thirdly, we can examine self-reports and behaviour in experimental tasks designed to assess concepts of self and others. Cassidy (1988) used two assessments of self-image with 6–year-olds whose concurrent attachment had also been assessed. One was a story completion task, and the other was a conversation with a puppet about how the child thought he or she was viewed by others. Secure and avoidant children generally differed in how they described themselves, with a significant majority (68 per cent) of secure children describing themselves positively but acknowledging minor flaws, and the majority of avoidant children (88 per cent) claiming to be perfect, even when pressed about their possible limitations. In a second study, responses to this puppet task were linked with attachment classifications derived from a story-completion task (Verscheurren *et al.*, 1996). There is a similar phenomenon in adulthood, with dismissing adults under-reporting symptoms and problems (Dozier *et al.*, 1991).

In general, while suggestive, the data linking attachment to self-concept and social expectations are limited and inconsistent. They are strongest for adult studies using self-report measures of both attachment and self-concept. Such studies must be interpreted cautiously, as the mechanism of linkage may be similar bias across self-reports, rather than attachment *per se*. Clearly this is a domain that requires further exploration if the claims of attachment theory are to be supported.

Continuing relationships in the family

Possibly early attachment would have its strongest effects on the continuance of those relationships that originally fostered it. Several studies have shown that young children with secure histories are more compliant, cooperative and responsive with their mothers than those who were insecure (e.g. Londerville and Main, 1981; Main, 1983), but other researchers failed to find such links (e.g. Takahashi, 1990; Youngblade and Belsky, 1992).

In a German study based in Bielefeld, Grossmann and Grossmann (1991) asked 6–year-olds and their mothers to make a building with blocks. Children with secure histories showed more assertiveness, self-confidence and involvement, but were also more likely to engage in direct conflict – for example, by refusing to co-operate with maternal suggestions – whereas children with avoidant histories were more inhibited.

Although we generally assume that it is 'good' for children to comply with parental suggestions and requests, it has been suggested that there are appropriate times and ways for children to assert their independence (Kuczynski *et al.*, 1987). Recall from Chapter 8 that while compliance can reflect secure co-operation, there is also an insecure attachment pattern in which timid children comply out of fear of provoking the parent's anger (Crittenden, 1988). In fact, Kuczynski and his colleagues (1987) describe non-compliance as an important feature of developing autonomy that follows a clear progression. Very young children simply ignore parental requests. This later gives way to confrontational refusal ('No!') and eventually the ability to negotiate ('Just a minute,' 'Can I finish this tower first?'). Secure attachment is thought to provide better support for the development of autonomy than insecure attachment. If this is the case, we should find that children who were securely attached as infants or toddlers progress more rapidly through this sequence than their insecure peers. So far, this proposition has not been directly tested.

Although Grossmann and Grossmann (1991) found that early attachment predicted emotional rather than intellectual aspects of behaviour in the block-building task and in mother–father–child play with puppets at 6 years of age, children's perception of parental support at 10 years of age was not related to their earlier attachment history. However, when early attachment was influential, attachment to the mother had more powerful effects than attachment to the father. Main, Kaplan and Cassidy (1985) also found stronger continuity for child–mother than for child–father relationships. Evidence that attachment to the mother is more influential in later functioning than is attachment to the father provides at least one clue to the weighting of information from different relationships in constructing a general working model of relationships.

Earlier (in Chapter 6) we examined the few studies of attachment and relationships with siblings which suggested the existence of some association between the older child's attachment and behaviour towards a sibling. In general, studies of attachment and later family relationships are surprisingly rare, particularly after the early years. Studies of stability of attachment fall into this category, and the rather late development of methods for assessing attachment *per se* in older children may be one explanation for the limited study of this area. However, it is also important to know, for example, whether different patterns of early attachment are related to other features of parent–child relationships beyond the preschool years.

One approach to this question is to use retrospective analysis of concurrently collected data. Thus one study used material from the AAI to rate early childhood relationships as either rejecting or not, and a separate questionnaire in which participants reported current relationships with their parents (Pearson, *et al.*, 1993). Approximately half of the participants reported consistent relationships – 15 per cent were consistently poor and 38 per cent were consistently positive. Regardless of the quality of relationships, consistency *per se* was associated with more coherent AAI transcripts than was inconsistency. A second study (Levy *et al.*, 1998) used questionnaire measures of attachment style to assess attachment, together with free-form descriptions of parents written by participants. Those who described themselves as secure provided more differentiation, elaboration and more positive characteristics and fewer negative characteristics in their descriptions of both their mother and their father. Questionnaires that assess attachment style ask individuals to consider their current and previous romantic relationships, rather than their early attachments to caregivers. Hence, in this case, the inference about the effects of early relationships with parents is that those who have well–differentiated and positive memories of their parents are most likely to perceive themselves as currently secure in romantic relationships.

Despite these few attempts, whether in later childhood, adolescence or adulthood, there is a distinct lack of longitudinal data on the possible role of early attachment in later parent–child relationships, and even less information on sibling relationships.

Children's reactions to unfamiliar peers and adults

There is evidence to indicate that securely attached children are more sociable towards both unfamiliar children (Plunkett *et al.*, 1988) and adults (Grossmann and Grossmann, 1991). When German 10–year-olds in a longitudinal study (Grossmann and Grossmann, 1991) were interviewed by an unfamiliar experimenter, children who had been securely attached as infants appeared comfortable with the interviewer and with the personal questions that were asked. Those who had been insecure as infants were likely to be either difficult for the interviewer to engage, or inappropriately intimate (e.g. seeking close physical contact with the interviewer). However, Jacobson and Wille (1986) failed to confirm attachment-based patterns of sociability towards new peers, and although there are few systematic observations of older children with strangers, several studies failed to find effects of atttachment on sociability with adult strangers in infants and toddlers (Frodi, 1983; Lamb et al., 1982; Thompson and Lamb, 1983). Thus inadequate evidence precludes the drawing of conclusions about early attachment and interactions with strangers. Since strangers are by definition individuals with whom we do not have ongoing relationships, it may in fact be the case that attachment does not have any particular impact on initial responses to strangers.

On the other hand, the formation of relationships depends on a process whereby individuals who are strangers to each other become better acquainted. Behaviour with strangers is probably a domain where context is important. For example, in Chapter 8 we noted that indiscriminate sociability with strangers occurs among children reared in institutions or experiencing multiple foster placements. Indeed, if the function of attachment is protection, it is generally not safe for young children to be overly friendly towards strangers, and such behaviour may well reflect a failure of the attachment system. On the other hand, in the presence of an attachment figure who has indicated that it is safe to engage in social interaction with the stranger, we might expect attachment security to play a role in the child's sociability. Later on, we expect individuals to use appraisal of the context to determine the appropriate level of sociability with particular strangers. Differential disclosure and task focus on the AAI could be interpreted as evidence for different reactions to a stranger on the part of adults, but attachment studies of adults have not otherwise examined behaviour with strangers *per se*.

Peer relationships in childhood

As children grow and develop, engagement with peers and peer friendships become an increasingly important aspect of their social world, and eventually most children move away from their families of origin to form pairbonds with peers and begin families of their own. To what extent do early attachments influence success in the world of peers?

The most impressive data on attachment and peer relationships comes from the Minnesota longitudinal study (for a summary see Sroufe et al.,in press). Attachment was assessed at 12 and 18 months in the strange situation. In preschool, middle childhood and adolescence, children were rated by teachers, trained observers and counsellors at camps and special events organized for study participants. When the child was 13 years old, the family was videotaped in a number of tasks from which ratings of security and family support were made, and still later (at age 15 years) adolescents participated in an interview about friendship. Measures of competence with peers were found to be generally stable across this wide age span. At preschool age, children with secure attachment histories were ranked highest in competence by teachers and were observed to be less isolated and more popular than those with insecure histories. They were more likely to respond to a classmate's distress in a helpful way, whereas those who had been avoidant were less empathetic. While 4–year-olds with secure histories were rarely either victims or victimizers in bullying relationships, victimizers most often had avoidant histories and victims were most often in the resistant group (Troy and Sroufe, 1987).

In middle childhood, children with secure histories were twice as likely as the insecure group to form friendships in the day camps, and to spend more time with a particular friend, as well as spending more time with groups engaged in organized activities (e.g. building something, dramatic play). They were also more likely to maintain gender boundaries, girls playing mostly with girls and boys playing mostly with boys, as is usual in this age group. In adolescence, counsellor ratings of global competence as well as competencies that arise in adolescence (e.g. couple relationships, relationships with mixed-sex groups) were significantly higher for those with secure attachment histories. In addition, in a group problem-solving activity, adolescents with secure histories were rated higher in self-confidence and leadership, and were more likely to to be elected spokeperson for their group, than those with insecure histories.

When multiple-regression techniques were used to control factors such as earlier competence with peers and later family relationships, early attachment continued to make a contribution to peer competence at later ages. In addition, maintenance of age-appropriate gender boundaries was less influenced by previous peer competence and more strongly related to attachment and later family support than other measures of peer competence. These data suggested to the research team that attachment and family experience are particularly implicated in aspects of peer competence 'centered on trust, vulnerability, or freedom to experience emotion and emotional closeness' (Sroufe *et al.*, in press, p.257).

Few other studies of attachment and peer relationships are either as long-term or as comprehensive as this one. In one interesting retrospective attempt, Skolnick (1986) used the Attachment Q-sort to rate descriptive reports of parents and children, and correlated the resulting child security scores with relationship measures in adulthood 30–40 years later. The data showed these early security scores to be related to adult sociability and marital satisfaction. In a longitudinal study based in Regensburg, Grossmann and Grossmann (1990) found that in kindergarten, secure children appeared to be relaxed and friendly and 67 per cent of them were rated as socially competent with peers. Children who had been avoidant infants appeared to be less relaxed, engaged in more frequent conflicts with peers and only 27 per cent were rated as socially competent. Others, too, have reported that securely attached children socialize more competently and are more popular with peers than their insecure counterparts (e.g. Vandell, 1988; Waters et al., 1979). Kerns (1994) used the Attachment Q-sort at age 4 years to find that at age 5 years, pairs with two secure children were more positive and harmonious in interactions than those with two insecure children, and Park and Waters (1989) found that 4-year-old 'best friend' pairs with two secure members had more harmonious interactions than those with only one secure partner. In this same age group, Turner (1991) found that contemporary attachment measures were associated with sex-typed peer behaviours. Compared to securely attached boys and girls, insecurely attached boys were more aggressive with their peers, whereas insecure girls were more compliant with them. Securely attached boys and girls did not differ, which suggests that they were more androgynous (i.e. they incorporated the positive features of both masculine and feminine sex roles) than those who were insecure. While these studies are consistent with predictions from attachment theory, an array of other studies have reported weak, mixed or unexpected findings (e.g. Howes et al.,1994; Lewis and Feiring, 1989; Youngblade and Belsky, 1992).

All of these studies compared individuals with secure vs. those with insecure histories, or secure vs. avoidant groups. Thus they shed some light on the potential advantages of secure attachment for later peer relationships, but contribute little to our understanding of those whose early attachments were resistant or dependent.

Dating and marriage in adulthood

To date, there is minimal longitudinal information with regard to intimate relationships of adults based on childhood attachment. Instead, studies have focused on concurrent measures of attachment and other aspects of social functioning. Studies which used attachment questionnaires are more prominent than those which used the AAI. Since these measures often assess different relationships and/or different aspects of relationships, we shall first consider evidence based on the AAI and then studies which used questionnaire measures.

Because the AAI was developed in the context of studying parental behaviour rather than social competence with other adults, studies of adult social relationships using the AAI are relatively rare and the data are mixed. There are three main findings. First, self-reported marital satisfaction is inconsistently related to classifications on the AAI (see Crowell and Treboux, 1995, for a summary). Secondly, there is some evidence from both self-reports and observation that there is more conflict among couples with at least one insecure partner, and that couples with two insecure partners may be most conflictual. For example, among engaged couples, insecure women reported more verbal and physical aggression from partners, and both partners reported heightened jealousy compared to couples in which the women were autonomous. In this same sample, after 15–18 months of marriage, women who were insecure on the AAI were more likely to report marital conflict, physical and verbal aggression and threats of abandonment from spouses than were those who were autonomous (Crowell and Treboux, 1995).

The third type of evidence suggests that, in married couples, the husband's attachment status affects the quality of the marriage more than that of the wifes. Husbands who were autonomous were in better-functioning marriages and had more positive interactions on structured tasks (Cohn et al., 1992; Kobak and Hazan, 1991). In addition, couples with two insecure members showed the most conflict and negative affect (Cohn et al., 1992).

Thus there is some preliminary evidence that there may be AAI-related differences in contemporary adult partner relationships, but this is a very under-studied area.

Questionnaire measures of attachment were developed in the context of research on couple relationships. These measures of attachment style focus on self-perceived security in adult couple relationships, rather than on past or current relationships with parents. Thus, while we may be able to make inferences about earlier relationships with parents by using other measures (e.g. Levy, et al., 1998), for the most part the studies below ask whether individuals who describe themselves as secure with romantic partners experience their intimate relationships differently to those who describe themselves as fitting one of the insecure patterns. Not surprisingly, this body of work tends to be more coherent with regard to adult relationships than is that with the AAI.

The most extensive work on this topic used the Hazan and Shaver (1987) measure (or variants of it), in which the subject reads a description of Ainsworth's basic attachment types and reports which pattern fits them best. In the initial research with this measure, Hazan and Shaver (1987) reported that different attachment styles were associated with different attitudes towards romantic relationships. Individuals who thought of themselves as secure focused on the enduring aspects of relationships, those who were avoidant felt that romantic relationships did not really exist and 'true love' was rare, whereas those who described themselves as ambivalent felt that true love was rare but that one easily falls in love. These findings were largely replicated in subsequent studies (Collins and Read, 1990; Feeney and Noller, 1990).

Furthermore, self-reported attachment classifications in young adults were related to the quality of their current romantic relationship, their propensity to marry, and their reactions to breakups. For example, 4 years after the original assessment of attachment style, those individuals who considered themselves to be secure were likely to be married, whereas those who considered themselves insecure were either unattached or dating more than one person (Kirkpatrick and Hazan, 1994). Secure individuals were more satisfied with their current relationship and both sought and provided more support in stressful situations than those who were insecure (Collins and Read, 1990; Davis *et al.*, 1994, Simpson, 1990; Simpson *et al.*, 1992). However, ambivalent women and avoidant men reported the highest stability in relationships (Davis *et al.*, 1994). When relationships broke up, ambivalent subjects reported most distress, whereas avoidant subjects were more likely to report relief (Feeney and Noller, 1992).

In short, when current relationships are viewed as attachments, individuals who assign themselves to each of Ainsworth's classifications have different attitudes towards relationships as well as different experiences in relationships. Whether the attachment assessment is the AAI or one of the questionnaires on attachment styles, the direction of effects in these studies is difficult to ascertain. Because the AAI focuses on childhood experiences and relationships with parents, studies that use it are exploring the transfer of experience in one kind of relationship to that in another kind (parent–child to couple, or vice versa). In contrast, studies which use assessments of attachment in current relationships are evaluating relationships between different components of similar relationships. These approaches promise to provide complementary information on attachment and social competence.

Parental behaviour

Since the AAI was largely developed to reflect representations of attachment in parents who had been observed to rear secure, avoidant and resistant individuals, AAI classifications have been studied in relation to both parental behaviour and child attachment outcomes. We have reviewed much of this evidence in previous chapters and will not discuss it further here, other than to remind ourselves that while concordance for security/insecurity is relatively high, it is accounted for primarily by matches between autonomous parents and secure infants, and the preoccupied-resistant link is exceedingly weak. Nevertheless, these studies focused on the initial development of attachment, and show some transfer of attachment patterns from one generation to the next. There are other potentially interesting questions concerning the relationship between adult representations of attachment and aspects of caregiving. Thus we might want to know whether adult attachment status is related to timing and/or spacing of pregnancies, number of children, or child-rearing goals and attitudes as well as behaviour in other parental roles (e.g. teaching, discipline) as children mature.

Overview and conclusions

The literature on attachment and social competence is both extensive and inconsistent. Many of the above sections ended with the observation that we could not draw confident conclusions about attachment and social competence. What could explain this inconsistency? Remember that in the first section of this chapter we noted many ways in which early attachment may be linked to later social outcomes. Some of these lent themselves to expecting change as well as expecting continuity. We also noted that most theorists agree that social competence is multiply determined. The most convincing and coherent findings in support of a role for attachment in the development of social competence came from the Minnesota longitudinal study, an in-depth ongoing investigation marked by a well-articulated view of potential mechanisms and outcomes (e.g. Sroufe *et al.*, in press).

We noted at the outset that an adequate framework for integrating these studies is itself in the process of development. Nevertheless, there is an indication that investigators with a relatively comprehensive view of attachment and its role in development were able to provide concrete evidence to document it. For example, what is most convincing about the data from the Minnesota longitudinal sample is the capability of performing analyses to consider multiple influences such as parent–child or peer relationships across childhood, and the demonstration that after consideration of such factors, early attachment is found to make an additional contribution to social developmental outcomes. It is also evident from such analyses that the contribution of early attachment in this context is small to moderate rather than large. This supports the view that social development is multiply determined, with early attachment being one among many influences.

We suggested that attachment may be more relevant to some types of social interaction than to others. However, because the evidence with regard to attachment and family, peer and stranger interactions is either limited or mixed, it is impossible to determine whether attachment is more influential for social competence in some of these contexts than in others. Surprisingly, there are few discursive reviews or meta-analyses of this material. Many of these areas are ripe for such efforts.

Finally, studies of adult attachment and adult peer relationships have focused primarily on couple relationships. Here consistency of evidence is related to the aspect of adult attachment that is being measured. Not surprisingly, when attachment is assessed as a component of couple relationships it is shown to play an integral role in these relationships. When attachment is assessed with the AAI and focuses on parent–child relationships, the evidence regarding couple relationships is more limited. There is ample evidence of performance in parental roles, particularly the capacity to rear children who become securely attached. Because that is what the AAI was originally designed to do, these data are not surprising. However, there is a need to examine the contributions of adult attachment to other aspects of parental behaviour.

Suggested reading

Thompson, R.A. (1999) Early attachment and later development. In Cassidy, J. and Shaver, P.(Eds) *The handbook of attachment*. New York: Guilford, 265–86.
A masterful review of the child development literature on this topic.

Crowell, J. and Treboux, D. (1995) A review of adult attachment measures: implications for theory and research. *Social Development* **4**, 294–327.
Includes a summary by topic of findings relating different measures of adult attachment to social functioning.

Sroufe, L.A., Egeland, B. and Carlson, E.A. (in press) One social world: the integrated development of parent–child and peer relationships. In Collins, W.A. and Lausen, B. (Eds), *The Minnesota Symposium on Child Psychology. Vol. 30*. Relationships as developmental context. Mahwah, NJ: Erlbaum, 241–61.
An overview of an exemplary research project that provides both a clear model and convincing data for the influences of early attachment on later peer relationships.

12 The psychobiology of attachment

In his exploration of attachment as a universal biobehavioural protective system in primates, Bowlby wrote a great deal about protection from predators. However, he was also concerned with other aspects of protection. He considered the attachment behavioural system to constitute an 'outer ring' of life-support mechanisms functioning as an interface between an 'inner ring' of physiological homeostatic systems and the external environment (Bowlby, 1973). Thus he was concerned with the way in which psychological mechanisms influenced biological ones (psychobiology), and particularly those physiological mechanisms concerned with maintaining stable internal conditions (homeostasis). An attachment behavioural system that functions well provides a protective barrier or 'buffer' between the demands of the external environment and the infant's ability to regulate his or her basic physiological functions (see Figure 12.1). A poorly functioning attachment behavioural system increases the pressures on physiological homeostatic systems and compromises survival.

An obvious illustration of this idea is that, by providing shelter, regulating room temperature and using appropriate clothing, an adult caregiver reduces the demand for the infant to regulate body temperature to a manageable range. In addition, the adult caregiver relies on the infant's appearance and behaviour as cues for action to adjust the external conditions that help to maintain a comfortable temperature. Similar processes operate to maintain the infant's fluid balance and nutrition. In these examples it is easy to see how the joint interaction of infant and caregiver can protect the infant from exposure to potentially dangerous conditions, and enhance their health and hence survival.

However, Bowlby's primary focus, like that of most attachment theorists and researchers, is on psychological development and the ways in which the protective nature of an attachment relationship extends beyond meeting basic physiological needs. The primary function of an attachment figure is to provide comfort in times of stress or danger. The presence of this figure initiates processes that reduce and eventually terminate the physiological arousal that occurs in response to stress and danger. In addition, the confidence that an individual develops in the availability and effectiveness of an

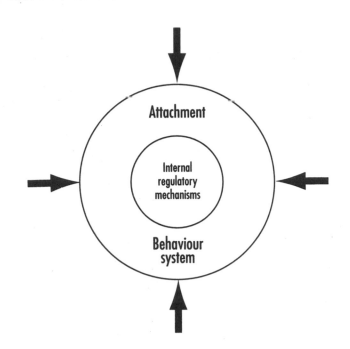

Figure 12.1 The attachment behaviour system as a buffer between external stressors and internal regulatory mechanisms.

attachment figure can modify their perception of stress and hence their stress responses. If help and relief from distress are anticipated as being readily accessible, their initial stress reactions are likely to be contained. This aspect of attachment has been only minimally explored, and much of the experimental research has been conducted in animals other than humans. In this chapter we shall explore the psychobiology of attachment systems and review studies of both animals and humans that begin to elaborate this aspect of the theory.

General theorizing

When concerned with human interactions at the behavioural level, it is easy to gloss over our implicit knowledge that these behaviours – like all behaviour – are organized and initiated within each individual through messages transmitted physiologically primarily by the brain and other parts of the nervous system. However, it is informative to think of behavioural exchanges in terms of the mutual influences of one brain upon another (Schore, 1996). That is, during any social interaction, the brains of the individuals concerned are exchanging information and influencing each other. In addition, the cumulative history of their interactions is stored in the form of temporary or permanent changes in the organization of neurones in each brain. When one of the participants is an infant, one brain is undergoing rapid developmental change, and the nature of these changes will reflect accumulated social interactions.

Current thinking about brain development distinguishes two types of processes whereby the environment influences brain development (Greenough *et al.*, 1987). 'Experience-expectant' processes are related to environmental information that is typical for the organism and often critical for survival and well-being. Since this information is both typical and essential, the brain has evolved to 'expect' it by overproducing synaptic connections between neurones in the areas of the brain that are usually devoted to that information. The eventual 'pruning' and selection of the connections that survive is influenced by experience, with connections that are repeatedly utilized being retained, while those that are not used eventually atrophy. For example, if one eye of a kitten is closed during early development, then representation of that eye is diminished and representation of the open eye is expanded in the visual cortex (Hubel and Wiesel, 1965).

The second type of process is described as 'experience dependent', and is reflected in the generation of new synaptic connections in response to specific events to which the individual is exposed. Since individual differences in specific events cannot be predicted, the brain does not 'anticipate' or prepare for them. Rather, it reacts to these events as they occur, and events that are highly salient or repeated many times are encoded in neural networks that persist.

One recent proposal that attracted a great deal of attention originated with Schore (1996), who focused on experience-dependent processes. He proposed a model of the way in which face-to-face interactions between adult caregivers and infants provide the fundamental context for the postnatal maturation of a system in the prefrontal cortex involved in regulatory, homeostatic and attachment functions. He noted that adults and infants engage in face-to-face games with a great deal of eye contact, smiling and laughter. These periods of mutual delight are linked to internal states in the infant which release neurotransmitters essential to experience-dependent developmental processes. Schore (1996) postulated that this is the primary way in which attachment influences neurobiological development and specifically the neurobiology of emotions and emotion regulation.

The underlying definition of attachment used by Schore (1996) differs from the one we have been developing, although it is consistent with the common trend to combine or confound warmth with the original notion of protection (De Wolff and van IJzendoorn, 1997; MacDonald, 1992). Whereas Bowlby emphasized danger as the context, and fear and distress as the emotions germane to development of attachment, Schore defines attachment in terms of shared positive emotions and mutual visual gaze. Because face-to-face interaction is a relatively infrequent aspect of early infant–caregiver activities, and its occurrence varies considerably across cultures, it seems unlikely to be the 'fundamental context' for normal emotional or neurobiological development. However, although to date the model is only speculative, it may be useful to consider whether any of the concepts Schore (1996) proposed regarding the role of infant–caregiver interactions in brain development are useful for exploring the psychobiology of attachment. The specific structures and processes involved for states of fear, danger and distress undoubtedly have a larger experience-expectant component than those suggested by Schore, because Bowlby was concerned with return to the mother in times of danger, a phenomenon which is universal and related to survival and well-being.

In humans, the primary infant–caregiver relationship is more than the dominant and consistent social relationship that provides stimulation to the developing infant brain. It is a relationship within which the adult provides, shapes and modifies the infant's interactions with the external environment, and thus is a major determinant of the other experiences that the infant encounters. Experiences with both social and non-social stimuli can be growth-enhancing and supportive or growth-inhibiting and adverse. When studying early development in humans, there are obvious limitations on the types of rearing conditions that can be studied to observe effects on physiological organization and regulation. Not surprisingly, the animal literature on this topic is more extensive.

Animal studies

Rat models

The notion of the parent as a regulator of the infant's physiology has been most clearly articulated by Hofer (1995), who serendipitously discovered that rat pups separated from their mothers showed slowed heart rate and decreased temperature and activity. His first assumption, namely that keeping the pups warm in the mother's absence would prevent these changes, proved incorrect. Even with the addition of an artificial heat source, heart rates fell just as low as they did at room temperature, but instead of being less active, the pups were overactive (Hofer, 1973a). This observation suggested that something much more complex was happening, and led to a series of systematic experiments to answer the question 'what is it that is lost when a rat pup is separated from its mother?'.

These studies revealed that different stimuli from the mother rat (e.g. tactile, nutritional and thermal stimuli) regulate different infant behavioural and physiological systems. For example, the decrease in heart rate turned out to be related to loss of the mother's milk. By carefully regulating the rate of milk consumption through a surgically inserted tube, the rat pups could be made to have almost any resting heart rate that the experimenters chose, but this did not affect their activity level (Hofer, 1973b). On the other hand, by providing artificial tactile stimulation on a schedule that resembled that of normal nursing cycles, the experimenters could regulate the rat pups' activity level (Hofer, 1975). Additional studies revealed very specific regulatory links between aspects of maternal stimulation and physiological regulation in the rat pups. The behavioural and physiological changes accompanying separation from the mother were seen as being analogous to what Bowlby had described as the young child's despair at prolonged separations from his or her parents (Hofer, 1995).

Later, with the use of an ultrasound detector, it became evident that separation from both the mother rat and littermates was accompanied by ultrasonic vocalizations that stopped almost immediately if at least one littermate or the mother was returned and provided close physical contact (Hofer and Shair, 1978). These cries, together with the search behaviours that rat pups normally use to locate their mothers, as well as the ways in which rat mothers use these cues to locate their pups, were considered to be similar to human children's separation protests (Hofer, 1995). Thus the repertoire of attachment behaviours that Bowlby had described in humans and other primates could be observed in the interactions of rat pups with their mothers, and the rat afforded a model for studying the underlying physiological mechanisms.

By using clinically effective anti-anxiety drugs, Hofer and his colleagues could begin to elucidate the underlying neural mechanisms for some of these regulatory systems. For example, by administering a drug that blocks receptors in the brain that respond to opium-like chemicals, the comfort that a littermate or mother rat usually provides is rendered ineffective in ending protest vocalizations. This information generates the inference that release of opiates normally mediates the response to comfort in rat pups. Hofer (1995) suggested that the mechanisms he discovered are 'hidden regulators' which are the physiological basis for the affective state of felt security. Eventually, associated mental representations take over to become higher-order regulators of these underlying biological systems. Thus, even in the lowly rat, pups develop expectations regarding comfort and safety that moderate their physiological responses to stress. However, 'even adult humans continue to respond at the sensorimotor-physiological level in some aspects of social interactions, separations and losses, continuing a process begun in infancy.' (Hofer, 1995, p.227).

Much of what Hofer (1995) described is related to the way in which the caregiver of a young infant in any mammalian species initially serves as the regulator of infant physiology. Gradually the infant acquires an increased ability to self-regulate, based on these early experiences with a caregiver. At first, the caregiver is a major component of the regulatory system. As the infant develops, homeostatic mechanisms are increasingly self-regulated, but they continue to reflect what the infant has learned through the caregiver's regulatory contributions.

Non-human primates

Bowlby was very familiar with experimental studies of rearing experience in non-human primates, and some of these were highly influential in his thinking (see Chapter 1). Monkeys have been reared in laboratories under a wide range of conditions that approximate to normal maternal care in different degrees. The more closely the substitute caregiver approximates to the characteristics of another monkey, the more closely the social behaviours of the infant monkey resemble those typical for the species. Thus surrogates that rock back and forth are more effective than those that are stationary (e.g. Mason and Capitano, 1988), a live animal (e.g. a dog) is more effective than an inanimate rocking surrogate (Mason and Capitano, 1988) and peers even exceed the typical monkey mother in eliciting social behaviours (Harlow *et al.*, 1971). However, monkeys raised with peers appear to be more timid when confronted with novelty, less sociable with strangers, and tend to have lower social status in their living groups than mother-reared monkeys (Suomi, 1991).

Different rearing conditions also result in physiological differences that persist into adulthood (Suomi, 1995). Kraemer (1992) summarized the studies that focused on processes affected by neurotransmitters such as the norepinephrine, dopamine and serotonin systems (see Figure 12.2). Under normal rearing conditions, the by-products of norepinephrine, dopamine and serotonin detected in cerebrospinal fluid are stable across time and correlated. These relationships are not as clearly evident in socially deprived monkeys. Furthermore, mother-rearing produces the highest

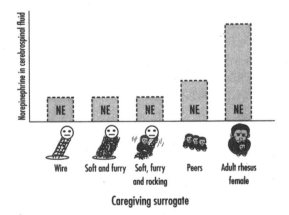

Figure 12.2 Mother vs. surrogate rearing and norepinephrine (NE) levels in monkeys. Bars show that the amount of norepinephrine in the cerebrospinal fluid is substantially increased only for monkeys raised with an adult female. Adapted from Kraemer (1992) with permission of the author.

levels of cerebrospinal norepinephrine. Alternative rearing conditions, including peer-rearing, where the behavioural repertoire is almost intact, are associated with significantly lower cerebrospinal levels of norepinephrine. Thus the brain norepinephrine system is thought to reflect the social history of the infant monkey (Kraemer *et al.*, 1989).

In a landmark article on the psychobiology of attachment, Kraemer (1992) set out to show that the neurobiology of the attachment system in primates constitutes brain 'hardware' rather than 'software.' That is, social attachment is not 'an optional overlay of more basic functions, but is an organizing feature of those functions' (Kraemer, 1992, p.496). Monkeys raised in isolation are characterized by inability to organize their behaviour in response to stress, changes in brain structure reflected in decreased cell connections, and neurochemical dysregulation. Thus, through early interactions with the caregiver, unique neurobiological characteristics are established that constitute a persistent regulatory system which is carried into subsequent environments. The implication is that human attachments are characterized by related processes. Kraemer specifies that this regulatory system does not include cognitive elements, but operates exclusively at the level of homeostatic regulatory processes. However, we may speculate that this regulatory system corresponds to Hofer's (1995) 'hidden regulators' and that working models of attachment are the mental representations that become the higher-order regulators. If this is so, different behavioural patterns of attachment and the working models that they represent should be reflected in different neurobiological organization.

A caution

It is always risky to extrapolate from animal models to human behaviour. In the present case, the analogies to the conditions studied by Hofer and Kraemer have not been measured in human experience. (The studies of institutional care and maltreatment discussed in detail in Chapter 8 may be the closest analogues of the primate studies above.) Generally, animal studies inquire about approximations to the appropriate caregiver in the species. In human studies we are interested in more limited variation in the experience of infants raised by their own parents or by other human caregivers. This narrow range of variation represents only one end of the continuum that is explored in animal studies. We can expect the differences we usually study in humans to be both behaviourally and physiologically more subtle than those described so far.

Human studies

Attachment patterns represent behavioural strategies for managing stress. These strategies are thought to reflect what an individual has learned about the reliability and effectiveness of an attachment figure's behaviour under stressful conditions. Secure/autonomous individuals are confident of the attachment figure's ability and willingness to provide comfort and assistance. They make effective use of an attachment figure to reduce stress. Avoidant/dismissing individuals have learned that attachment figures are unresponsive to their distress and rely on self-regulation. Resistant/ preoccupied individuals have learned that attachment figures are unpredictable but sometimes effective. Therefore they make strong bids for attention by exaggerating their attachment needs – bids which are often ineffective in reducing stress. Those with disorganized attachment lack organized strategies for stress management with regard to an attachment figure. Thus it may be most useful to seek physiological differences in systems related to the physiology of stress. In order to understand the limited data on stress responses and attachment, a brief excursion into the physiology of stress responses is necessary.

The hypothalamic–pituitary–adrenocortical (HPA) system

One biological system that plays a central role in responding to stress is the hypothalamic–pituitary–adrenocortical (HPA) axis, so called because it involves interactions between the hypothalamus and the pituitary and adrenal glands (for a more detailed overview of HPA functioning, see Stansbury and Gunnar, 1994). Its main product in humans is a hormone called cortisol. Cortisol can be detected in blood and urine, but because it can also be measured easily in small samples of saliva, it has become an attractive indicator of stress responses in both adults and children, including infants.

Cortisol has wide-ranging effects on many organs and organ systems. It is thought to have three major functions in reactions to stress. First, it assists in mobilizing energy by influencing metabolism. Secondly, it regulates the activity of other stress-sensitive systems, such as the immune system. Thirdly, it affects cognitive and emotional functions. Its production is influenced by a complex array of physiological and psychological factors. The release of cortisol is stimulated by three types of input, namely internal biochemical processes, physical stressors such as pain and hunger, psychological factors relating to perception of stressors. Two of the psychological factors that are known to influence cortisol production under conditions of stress or challenge are particularly relevant to our thinking about attachment patterns – these are predictability and control.

Studies of both animals and humans show that negative events which are unpredictable and those which are uncontrollable are associated with increased cortisol output (for summaries see Kirschbaum and Helhammer, 1989; Sapolsky, 1992). Secure attachment is thought to derive from the experience of successfully managing aversive experiences by recruiting help from an attachment figure. Thus secure attachment is associated with confidence that one will be able to control negative experiences, in part because the outcome of the preferred (secure) strategy for managing distress is highly predictable. Thus negative events are perceived as less stressful than they would be in the absence of a successful coping strategy.

In contrast, avoidant or dismissive attachment is thought to derive from a history of being unable to recruit assistance from an attachment figure when confronted with stressful experiences. Such individuals develop different coping strategies (e.g. deactivation, as discussed in Chapters 9 and 10) that make greater demands on their internal resources than does the secure strategy. Particularly for the young child, this strategy will be of variable success in managing discomfort, and is thus associated with uncertainty about the outcome of the preferred coping strategy.

Resistance or preoccupation is associated with a history of unpredictability in recruiting assistance in times of stress, but the attachment figure does sometimes respond appropriately. Here the preferred strategy is to direct energy towards producing distress signals (hyperactivation of the attachment system, as discussed in Chapters 9 and 10), which makes demands on internal resources and does not necessarily have a predictable outcome. Although it has been studied less intensively, it seems likely that disorganization is associated with a history characterized by lack of both predictability and control. Thus individuals characterized by insecure attachment use coping strategies that place a heavier load on internal resources, are less predictable in outcome and do not necessarily confer a sense of control.

The cortisol stress response and its development

A certain amount of circulating cortisol is necessary for routine activities. In normal adults, cortisol secretion follows a cycle that is linked to daily activities (e.g. waking, sleeping, elimination) and physiological changes. Activity in the HPA system occurs in pulses, and increases in circulating cortisol levels reflect the accumulation of a series of these pulses. Cortisol levels rise during the last hours of sleep, are highest in the early morning, fall rapidly after awakening and then decline more slowly throughout the day. Human infants begin to develop the adult cycling pattern gradually from birth onwards. The full adult pattern emerges by 2 years of age, but the early-morning peak in cortisol levels usually appears by 3 months of age (Price et al., 1983; Spangler, 1991).

Responses to stressful events are imposed on this pattern of daily variation. When a stressful event occurs, it is 10–15 minutes before increases in cortisol levels occur, and 20–30 minutes before peak concentrations are reached. Then the excess cortisol is gradually cleared from the circulation. Because it is unethical to subject infants to high levels of stress, researchers have had to be resourceful in identifying naturally occurring stresses to study. Mild restraint, routine innoculations and separations are the main stressors that have been studied. In the newborn, significant increases in cortisol levels occur in response to stressors ranging from mild restraint to circumcisions by new residents (summarized in Gunnar, 1992). The cortisol response to routinely scheduled innoculations decreases over the course of the first 15 months as responses are gradually dampened with repetition of the experience (Gunnar et al., 1996; Lewis and Thomas, 1990). During daily activities, non-stressful events such as naps and car trips are associated with decreases in cortisol levels (Larson et al., 1991). Thus the pattern of cortisol secretion both in daily cycles and in reaction to stressful events undergoes developmental changes during infancy, which is the time when the first attachment is taking shape.

Animal studies provide evidence that early caregiving experiences contribute to individual differences in these developmental changes. For example, the amount of licking and grooming that individual rat mothers perform in the first 10 days of the pups' life is negatively correlated with HPA activity after acute stress (Liu et al., 1997). Thus rat pups of mothers who did more licking and grooming showed less increase in HPA activity when stressed. In some species, rat pups that are handled daily for the first 3 weeks of life show reduced HPA responses to a variety of stressors in adulthood (e.g. Levine et al., 1967). In contrast, rat pups that are separated from their mothers in the first 2 weeks of life show larger cortisol responses to the stress of restraint than those which are not separated (Plotsky and Meany, 1993). These data were interpreted as indicating that early maternal behaviour 'programmes' HPA responses to stress in the offspring. In non-human primates, separation from the mother is known to be a potent stimulant of cortisol output (Coe et al., 1983). In response to social separation, peer-reared rhesus monkeys consistently show more extreme cortisol reactions than do mother-reared cohorts (Suomi, 1997). Thus we can predict firstly that human infants will also show cortisol responses to separations such as the strange situation, and secondly that prior history of care will influence these responses.

Attachment and physiology in human infants

Several studies have examined the relationships between caregiving and cortisol secretion during stressful events for human infants. For example, Gunnar and her colleagues (1993) observed that 9-month-old infants showed increases in salivary cortisol levels in response to a 30-minute separation from the mother. However, for half the infants the substitute caregiver was instructed to be responsive during the separation. For the other half the substitute caregiver was told to ignore the baby as much as possible and only to respond to cries. Infants in the 'responsive' condition showed much smaller cortisol increases than those in the 'ignoring condition. These data show that separation does elicit a cortisol stress response in human infants, and that contemporaneous caregiving conditions influence the magnitude of the response.

The interesting question for our purposes is whether differences in physiological reactivity are linked with patterns of attachment. The reasoning above suggested that we should expect the smallest stress response to occur among securely attached infants and the largest stress response to occur among disorganized infants, with the avoidant and resistant groups being somewhere in between.

One approach to studying stress responses is to assess indicators of autonomic nervous system activation, such as heart rate. Early studies in which heart rate was monitored during the strange situation showed that, regardless of attachment classifications, most infants show heart rate acceleration during stranger approach and separations (Donovan and Leavitt, 1985; Spangler and Grossmann, 1993; Sroufe and Waters, 1977b). Furthermore, Spangler and Grossmann (1993) found that in contrast to secure infants, whose heart rate declined during object play, avoidant infants experienced heart rate accelerations when engaged in play. This observation is consistent with the notion that the avoidant infant's use of play when under stress is a defensive strategy rather than true exploration. Clearly, the separations of the strange situation are physiologically arousing for all infants, including those who appear unperturbed and are considered to be avoidant.

Cortisol stress responses have also been studied in the context of the strange situation. Although attachment group differences in cortisol levels were not evident when saliva samples were collected immediately after the strange situation (Gunnar, 1989), subsequent studies sampled at 15 minutes (Hertsgaard et al., 1995) and 30 minutes (Spangler and Grossmann, 1993; Spangler and Schieche, 1998) after the end of the strange situation. The most consistent finding from these studies is that secure infants, as expected, showed no increase in salivary cortisol levels. In two studies, disorganized infants secreted more cortisol than all of the other attachment groups (Hertsgaard et al., 1995; Spangler and Grossmann, 1991), but in the largest such study, involving 106 infants (Spangler and Schieche, 1998), this effect could not be replicated. Instead, resistant infants displayed the largest increase in cortisol levels. Interestingly, in this study avoidant infants only showed increased cortisol levels if they were temperamentally fearful and/or showed negative emotion.

There is evidence that these differences in attachment groups occur in situations other than the strange situation. In the most convincing of these studies (Nachmias et al., 1996), 77 18–month-olds and their mothers participated in a 'coping session' and, on a separate visit, in the strange situation. The coping session included presentation of three novel experiences, namely a mechanical robot, the entrance of a clown who tried to engage the child, and a puppet show. These activities were designed to assess the child's willingness or reluctance to enter into new situations (behavioural inhibition). During each activity, the mother was asked to be involved as little as possible for the first 3 minutes, and then to assist the child in any way that seemed appropriate for the second 3 minutes. Saliva samples were collected at both sessions.

In both sessions, increases in cortisol levels occurred only for children who were both inhibited and insecurely attached to their mothers (this effect was replicated by Spangler and Schieche, 1998). Thus children who were not inhibited during the coping session showed no increase in cortisol levels in either session (see Figure 12.3). Children who were inhibited but secure also showed little or no increase in cortisol levels. Children who were both inhibited and insecure showed significant increases in cortisol levels in both sessions. It was also observed that the mothers of secure and insecure children differed in the strategies that they used to help their children to cope with novel events. For example, the mothers of secure children were more likely to encourage their children to approach the novel stimulus and to offer comfort, whereas the mothers of insecure children were more likely to demand that the child approach without offering any comfort. Children's coping strategies received higher ratings of competence when the mother received lower scores for demanding approach. Both mother and child coping strategies contributed to predicting cortisol responses.

We noted that in monkeys, physiological measures do not necessarily parallel behaviour (Kraemer, 1992; Figure 12.2). Similar observations have also been made for human infants. Most infants show parallel crying and cortisol responses to inoculation, but some show intense crying with a low cortisol response, while others cry very little and display a high cortisol response (Lewis et al., 1993). Although avoidant infants show little distress in the strange situation, their heart rate and cortisol measures indicate that they are physiologically aroused (Donovan and Leavitt, 1985; Hertsgaard et al., 1995; Spangler and Grossmann, 1993; Sroufe and Waters, 1977b). It has been suggested that dissociations of this kind are more common among insecurely attached infants (Gunnar et al., 1996a).

What can we make of such discrepancies? In stressful situations, infants – like adults – are disposed to engage in selected behaviours that are part of their coping repertoire. If these behaviours have reliably resulted in comfort in the past, the expectation of effective coping should reduce the perception of stress and minimize the need to mount a physiological stress response. In contrast, if these behaviours have not been associated with consistent stress reduction in the past, the uncertainty of gaining comfort or the expectation of failing to get it will increase perceived stress and elicit a physiological stress response. Thus it is not the behaviour *per se* that is associated with physiological stress, but the perception of its effectiveness

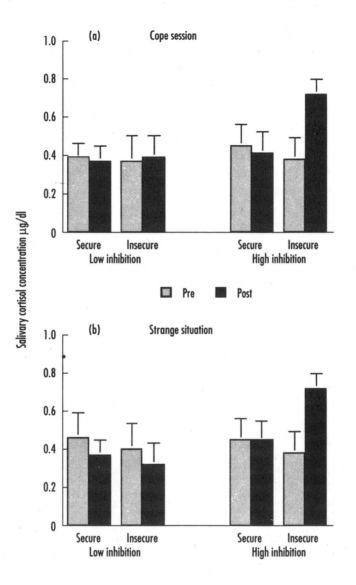

Figure 12.3 Pre- and post-session salivary cortisol levels (in μg/dl) in (a) the cope session and (b) the strange situation as a function of inhibition and attachment security. Bars reflect standard errors of the mean. Reproduced from Nachmias et al. (1996) with permission.

(Gunnar, 1999; Spangler and Schieche, 1998) based on the history of previous coping efforts.

Attachment and physiology in adults

Adult physiological concomitants of attachment have been minimally studied. Comparison of college students who experienced death of a parent before the age of 12 years with those who did not showed that both attachment losses and reports of family conflict in childhood were related to cardiac and cortisol reactivity during two stressful tasks (Luecken, 1998). When maternal and infant heart rate are measured during the strange situation, both mothers and infants in insecure dyads are more likely than those in secure dyads to show acceleration of heart rate at the entrance of a stranger and at impending separations (Donovan and Leavitt, 1985). In one promising investigation, Dozier and Kobak (1992) recorded skin conductance during the AAI. They found that adults who used a 'deactivating strategy' (consistent with dismissing attachment) showed increases in skin conductance (reflecting arousal indicative of conflict or inhibition) during the parts of the interview concerned with emotionally arousing material. More recently, a pilot study showed differences in cortisol reactivity during the AAI for adults with secure vs. insecure attachment strategies when classifications were based on a questionnaire measure (Adam et al., 1996). In addition, further work from the same laboratory suggested that secure/autonomous attachment qualities in the mothers of toddlers were associated with more pronounced daily cycling of maternal cortisol levels – that is, a higher peak in the morning and a more rapid decline in cortisol over the course of the day (Adam, 1998). Thus, although the study of attachment and adult stress responses has barely started, there are already some early data which are consonant with Bowlby's ideas.

Overview

In this chapter we have considered theories of how early experiences with a caregiver can influence fundamental aspects of neurobiological organization. Although there is an intriguing theoretical framework focusing on positive emotions (Schore, 1996), the chapter selectively considered conditions related to negative emotions, as these were considered to be more clearly related to attachment constructs and are more clearly supported by empirical evidence. We used data from animal and human studies to demonstrate preliminary support for the idea that different attachment behavioural patterns in humans would be associated with differences in physiological functioning, particularly in response to stress. Although the evidence is limited, it is consistent with Bowlby's view of the attachment behaviour system as an outer protective container of physiological responses. The data further suggest that insecure attachments may be less effective than secure attachments in fulfilling this role. This area of research will certainly expand as increasingly non-invasive methods of assessing physiological change become available.

Suggested reading

Kraemer, G.W. (1992) A psychobiological theory of attachment. *Behavioral and brain sciences* **15**, 493–541.
A comprehensive review of the primate literature of the time, with a physiological model of the effects of early-rearing experience on brain development.
Hofer, M.A. (1995) Hidden regulators in attachment and loss. In Goldberg, S., Muir, R. and Kerr, J. (Eds), *Attachment theory: social, developmental and clinical perspectives*. Hillsdale, NJ: The Analytic Press, 203–30.
An eminently readable summary of groundbreaking work on the psychobiology of attachment.

Spangler, G. and Schieche, M. (1998) Emotional and adrenocortical responses of infants to the strange situation: the differential function of emotional expression. *International Journal of Behavioural Development* **22**, 681–706.
A comprehensive study of temperament and attachment influences on infant adrenocortical responses.

Stansbury, K. and Gunnar, M. (1994) Adrenocortical activity and emotion regulation. In Fox, N. (Ed.), The development of emotion regulation: biological and behavioral considerations. *Monographs of the Society for Research in Child Development* **59**, 108–43.
An excellent introduction to the HPA system, written for developmental psychologists.

Part IV

Health implications of attachment

13 Attachment and mental health

This chapter begins a section focused on the health implications of attachment. The data on attachment and mental health are far more extensive than those on physical health, in part because the basic ideas of the theory first arose in mental health settings. Therefore we shall first consider mental health, and then turn to physical health in Chapter 14. In Chapter 11 we examined the notion that secure attachment confers specific advantages in the development of social competence. An extension of this assertion is that insecure attachment entails specific handicaps or threats to mental well-being. The strongest form of this position is that insecure attachment has a causal role in the development of psychological disturbance (psychopathology). As we shall see, the empirical data show this position to be untenable. The more commonly accepted view is that early attachment is one factor among many that either add protection or increase vulnerability to subsequent disorders. However, the notion that early parent–child relationships are an essential ingredient in the origins of psychopathology is not unique to attachment theory, and has been widely endorsed in both popular and professional literature even in the absence of empirical evidence. The development of procedures for assessing attachment provided important tools for generating empirical evidence on this topic, and gave rise to attempts to link patterns of attachment to problem behaviour, deviant behaviour or diagnosed disorder.

Attachment theory has its roots in clinical observations, and studies of attachment in clinical populations played an important role in shaping the theory and assessment of attachment. In Chapter 8, we considered the effects of maternal disorder on the development of early attachment. In the present chapter we are concerned with the effects of attachment on later disorders, and the use of attachment theories and methods in clinical practice.

The availability of methods to assess attachment allowed empirical tests of the relationship between one aspect of parent–child relationships and psychopathology. However, concurrent with the advent of this technology, our perspectives on the origins of psychopathology became more complex. For example, one framework for understanding the development of

aggressive disorders considers family stressors, discipline and child characteristics (e.g. temperament or neurobiological problems) in addition to attachment (Greenberg et al., 1993). The development of a suitably complex
model for understanding the roots of psychopathology is an enterprise
beyond the scope of this text. In this chapter we shall review the evidence
for links between attachment and psychopathology as one component in
the origins of disturbance. We shall also consider possible applications of
attachment theory to clinical practice.

Research strategies and limitations

There are two basic strategies for evaluating the proposition that attachment plays a role in the origins of psychopathology. The first is to conduct
prospective longitudinal studies beginning early in life that follow individuals as they mature. While this provides direct measures of childhood
attachment, only a small number of clinical cases emerge. The study of
populations at high risk for psychopathology can substantially increase the
size of the diagnosable group, but this remains a strategy which invests
valuable resources in studying individuals who, for the most part, do *not*
develop psychopathology. As a result, studies of this type often look not at
disorders *per se* as outcomes, but at individual differences in problem
behaviours such as aggression or social withdrawal. However, understanding variation in problem behaviour within the normal range may or may not
be useful for understanding frank psychopathology.

An alternative strategy is to study concurrent attachment in clinical
samples. This approach ensures an adequate number of clinical cases, but
we cannot necessarily infer the nature of prior attachment. First, as noted
in Chapter 3, changes in attachment can occur during the lifespan. Even if
the highest stability estimates are assumed (80 per cent), at least 1 in 5 individuals undergo changes in attachment at some time. In all likelihood the
figure is considerably higher than this. Secondly, the presenting psychopathology may alter or obscure some aspects of prior attachments. Not surprisingly, although there are notable exceptions (Allen et al., 1996; Carlson,
1998), the propective longitudinal strategy has been used primarily in the
study of childhood behaviour disorders, and the concurrent strategy pre-
dominates in studies of adult disturbance.

A variant of these methods, common in clinical studies, is retrospective.
In this strategy, information regarding early experiences is retrieved either
from objective sources (e.g. medical records) or on the basis of self-report,
after specific outcomes (clinical diagnoses) have been identified. Thus a
relatively common finding is that many individuals who experience depression also report death of a parent early in childhood (e.g. Harris and
Bifulco, 1991). Such information provides what we call a 'backward' prediction because the outcome is identified first. It is possible to use data

from prospective longitudinal studies in this fashion by selecting subjects with different outcomes and comparing them on earlier measures. In one such attempt, Lyons-Ruth, Alpern and Repacholi (1993) were able to demonstrate the different results of backward and forward prediction of hostile aggressive behaviour from early attachment. Backward prediction invariably yields stronger effects than forward prediction. In other words, the ability to predict backwards (depression in adulthood predicts early loss of a parent) does not necessarily allow us to make successful forward predictions (death of a parent in childhood does not predict depression in adulthood).

Hypotheses

Whether in childhood or adulthood, hypotheses regarding the possible links between attachment and psychiatric disturbance vary in specificity. Before examining the data, it is useful to outline these possibilities.

Insecure attachment increases vulnerability to behaviour problems

This is the broadest and most general hypothesis. It makes no distinction between different forms of insecurity or different types of disturbance. This hypothesis has been widely investigated partly because, as noted in many previous chapters, investigators gain flexibility for statistical analysis by 'lumping' insecure groups together. However, this prediction is not unique to attachment theory. It would also be made by most other theories of psychological development – early disadvantage persists or lays the groundwork for later disadvantage.

Different insecure attachment patterns increase vulnerability to different disorders

Major attachment strategies and internalizing and externalizing disorders

Attachment theory offers a typology of non-optimal early relationships, and it is expected that these are associated with different outcomes. The predominant theoretical reasoning (e.g. Cassidy and Kobak, 1988; Dozier *et al.*, 1999; Renken *et al.*, 1989) links avoidant attachment with externalizing problems – that is, those in which behaviour causes disruption and inconvenience for others (e.g. aggression, conduct disorder, criminal behaviour). It is argued that children engaged in an early avoidant relationship learn through the caregiver's lack of response firstly to ignore their own feelings of distress and secondly that 'you cannot count on or trust others.' As they grow to maturity, they assume that others are uncaring and act accordingly, in a manner that may imitate or exaggerate the way in which they perceive themselves to have been treated. In addition, the frustration of unmet attachment needs gives rise to anger which is not expressed towards the parents but is displaced towards others.

You may find this formulation counter-intuitive from what you know of different attachment patterns. After all, is it not avoidant and dismissing individuals who 'cover up' their feelings and needs by using a deactivating strategy? Why would this not lead to 'internalizing' problems (those in which the child or adult experiences internal pain and misery but does not inflict it on others, e.g. depression, social withdrawal)? Such a script also seems to be consistent with the information summarized in Chapter 9 linking avoidant, defended or dismissing attachment with a style of emotional expression that inhibits or restrains emotions, particularly those that are negative.

Traditional theorizing links resistant, dependent or preoccupied attachment with internalizing disorders (e.g. Dozier *et al.*, 1999; Erickson *et al.*, 1985; Renken *et al.*, 1989). It is argued that because the caregiver responds inconsistently, the child becomes preoccupied with maintaining the caregiver's attention at the expense of exploring the larger world. Consequently, the child – and later the adult – is fearful of undertaking new endeavours and remains enmeshed in family issues, and otherwise isolated and withdrawn.

Again this formulation may seem to conflict with the observation that the pouty or frankly tantrum-like behaviour of resistant babies and dependent preschoolers in the strange situation shares behavioural similarities with externalizing problems. In addition, we also found in Chapter 9 that resistant, dependent or preoccupied individuals are thought to use a hyperactivating attachment strategy associated with exaggerated emotional expression, which may also seem to be more consistent with externalizing disorders.

In short, there may be two different views regarding the relationships between different forms of insecure attachment and internalizing vs. externalizing psychiatric disorders. Each of these approaches predicts very different kinds of disorders to be associated with different forms of insecure attachment.

Disorganization is linked with dissociative disorders

The most specific hypothesis regarding attachment-disorder links suggests that behaviours which mark disorganized attachment in infancy (e.g. stilling, freezing, stereotyped movements) parallel features of dissociative states, reflect moments of dissociation in infancy and/or establish the pathway to later dissociative disorders (Liotti, 1995).

Disorganized (or unresolved) attachment is linked with
psychopathology
A more general hypothesis regarding disorganization is that the attachment
strategy *per se* is less important for the development of psychopathology
than is the absence of an organized strategy. While this hypothesis is
specific with regard to type of attachment, it is not specific with respect to
type of disorder. Many of the earlier studies were unable to make use of the
criteria for disorganization, but since disorganization was first identified in
high-risk or clinical samples, it has been frequently associated with both
psychological disturbance and its predisposing risk factors.

Disorganization in conjunction with an alternative insecure
classification is associated with disturbance
Increasingly, attempts have been made to distinguish between disorganization of attachment that reflects persistent and extreme examples of inappropriate care and that which may reflect transient difficulties. For
example, as we pointed out in Chapter 3 when we discussed lack of
resolution of mourning, disorganization is a normal reaction to important
attachment-related losses. This type of disorganization is usually transient
as the bereaved individual gradually comes to terms with the loss and re-
organizes his or her life. Nevertheless, we also found that this type of disorganization or lack of resolution with respect to loss (or trauma) is
associated with disorganized attachment in infants. However, we might
expect that this kind of disorganization of attachment in the infant will, like
the parent's disorganization, be transient rather than long term.
    The hypothesis that disorganization is related to psychopathology only
when it is also paired with an alternative insecure classification posits that
an infant whose attachment is disorganized as a result of his or her (otherwise autonomous) mother's loss of a parent close to or during a pregnancy
experiences very different care to one who is disorganized as a result of
ongoing inappropriate care by a disturbed or severely overburdened
mother. The first is likely to be disorganized-secure, while the second is
likely to be disorganized-insecure. The difference in experiences marked by
these different forms of disorganization should be associated with differential vulnerability to disturbance.
    In the sections below, we shall consider the extent to which there is
evidence to support each of the above hypotheses.

Attachment and behaviour problems in childhood

Attachment disorders

This is probably a good place to emphasize that insecure attachment *per se* is
not a disorder. Ainsworth's original descriptions of attachment strategies in

infancy distinguished three patterns within the normal range of functioning. The choice of the labels 'secure' and 'insecure', although descriptive, may have been unfortunate because it is not uncommon to find discussions which imply that insecure attachment is a disturbance. This is not the case.

If we use Crittenden's (1995) notion that attachment patterns reflect a dynamic balance between reliance on affective and cognitive information and processes, avoidant (or dismissing) individuals are those who direct minimal attention and energy towards emotion-laden activities and invest heavily in cognitive activities. It is worth noting that this pattern is consistent with stereotyped expectations for male behaviour. Furthermore, it is likely that individuals recognized for their high achievement are characterized by this pattern. Indeed, Bowlby's official biographer, Jeremy Holmes (1993), suggested that Bowlby himself was dismissing. By way of contrast, individuals who are resistant, dependent or preoccupied are focused on socio-emotional relationships to the exclusion of intellectual activities. This pattern overlaps with stereotyped prescriptions for female behaviour. It is possible that such individuals are drawn to 'people-oriented' professions and may have advantages in artistic endeavours such as acting or creative writing.

A further qualification is that, although secure attachment has typically been considered optimal in middle-class North American society, theorists agree that different patterns of parental behaviour and accompanying patterns of organized attachment can be optimal under other cultural conditions. In Chapter 7 we noted cultural differences in the distribution of attachment patterns that were related to cultural beliefs, expectations and values that shape parental behaviour and child-care arrangements and hence infant patterns of attachment.

However, in the early years of life there are disturbances in attachment that are qualitatively different to these normal variations. The early categorization of attachment disorders in young children was based on behavioural observations (discussed in Chapter 8) of children who had either been maltreated in their families or reared in institutions (Zeanah, 1996). Current diagnostic manuals (the *Diagnostic and Statistical Manual*, fourth edition, and the *International Classification of Diseases*, tenth edition) include 'reactive attachment disorder' as one of the few disorders diagnosable in children under 3 years of age, and indicate that this may be either inhibited (characterized by a withdrawn unresponsive child who seeks comfort in deviant ways) or disinhibited (indiscriminately social). The first you may recognize as based on the behaviour of children in maltreatment samples, and the second as based on children reared in institutions.

Zeanah (1996) suggested that a more useful view of attachment disorders should be less concerned with purported causes of disturbed behaviour and more concerned with child behaviour itself. He suggested three types of disorder:

1. non-attachment, in which there is no evidence of a preferred caregiver and the child is either withdrawn or indiscriminately friendly;
2. disordered attachment, in which the child clearly has a preferred caregiver, but uses that caregiver in distorted ways by being either extremely clingy or engaging in reckless and dangerous behaviour (Lieberman and Pawl, 1988);
3. disrupted attachment, which describes the grief response of children who have lost a caregiver.

Any one of these may be characterized by inhibited or disinhibited behaviour. These diagnostic categories, as well as those suggested earlier, lack empirical evidence to validate their clinical usefulness. Nevertheless, we note here that while children who fit any of these descriptions would clearly be insecurely attached, not all insecurely attached children are disordered – indeed, most are not.

Attachment as a risk factor for childhood disorders

There have been very few studies of children with clinically diagnosed psychiatric disorders. Two related studies (Greenberg et al., 1991; Speltz et al., 1990) concurred in showing that preschool boys with disruptive (externalizing) behaviour disorders were more likely than their non-disturbed peers to be insecurely attached. Furthermore, the most frequent attachment pattern was controlling. In one other study (Birkenfield-Adams, 1999), concurrent attachment was assessed for boys with gender-identity disorder, a comparison group with 'other psychiatric diagnoses' and normal controls. In the group with mixed psychiatric diagnoses, avoidant and controlling attachment accounted for all but 15 per cent of the cases. In contrast, attachment in the group with gender-identity disorder was equally distributed across avoidant, secure and dependent categories.

More commonly, the participants in studies of childhood behaviour problems have been followed prospectively and are not clinically disturbed. A full psychiatric work-up is not cost-effective in these studies, as only a very small number of clinical cases are likely to be found. Instead, questionnaire measures that serve as screening tools for behaviour problems are completed by parents and/or teachers. These indicate the frequency with which problematic behaviours occur, and often divide behaviour problems into internalizing and externalizing subtypes. Alternatively, the problem behaviour outcomes may be based on ratings of trained observers in classroom or laboratory settings.

There are numerous studies of this type in the literature, and the outcomes are not always consistent. Some studies have found more problems in preschool and early-school-age children who had been insecure as infants than in those who had been secure (e.g. Erickson et al., 1985; Lewis et al., 1984; Renken et al., 1989), but others failed to find such connections (e.g. Bates *et al.*, 1985; Goldberg *et al.*, 1990). In most of these studies, the number of resistant infants was small and they were either dropped from the analysis or avoidant/resistant comparisons were not pursued. Thus it is possible that reported secure/insecure differences are linked to avoidance rather than to insecurity *per se* (Goldberg *et al.*, 1995).

The predicted links between avoidance and externalizing problems have indeed been found (e.g. Erickson *et al.*, 1985; Lewis *et al.*, 1984; Renken *et al.*, 1989). In contrast, links between resistance and internalizing problems have only been reported occasionally (Lewis *et al.*, 1984; Warren *et al.*, 1997). This absence of effects may reflect both the rarity of resistant attachment and the relative invisibility of internalizing disorders in children. Children who do not disturb others can readily be ignored and are not likely to be referred for treatment unless their symptoms are extremely deviant.

More recently, with the availability of the disorganized classification, Lyons-Ruth, Alpern and Repacholi (1993) found that infant disorganized attachment was the best predictor of teacher ratings of hostile behaviour in 5-year-olds. However, a high percentage of this group were judged to have an underlying avoidant strategy. In an overview of Canadian studies of attachment and behaviour problems in normal, risk and diagnosed groups, I found that as children were more definitely disturbed, secure attachment decreased in frequency and disorganized attachment increased, but there were no obvious patterns for avoidant or resistant attachment and no evidence that avoidance or resistance was linked with particular disorders (Goldberg, 1997).

Despite a substantial number of studies investigating early attachment and behaviour problems, there have been surprisingly few attempts to summarize these data, no published meta-analyses and only a few discursive reviews. A recent meta-analytical attempt to summarize studies of children up to age 6 years that assessed attachment and behaviour problems either prospectively or concurrently (Atkinson *et al.*, 1999) revealed one of the reasons for this. A total of 18 studies with 1351 participants were located, but because many of them did not use the full 4-category classification scheme for attachment and/or combined all insecure groups, the number of studies available to test most of the above hypotheses was small, and there was minimal opportunity to examine the effects of other variables on attachment-behaviour problem associations. Thus for the most part these meta-analyses are very preliminary. Nevertheless, they offer an overview of what conclusions can be drawn from the mixed findings of the available studies.

There were a number of small but significant effects which supported the first hypothesis (that insecure attachment would be associated with more behaviour problems than secure attachment) and partially supported the second hypothesis, namely that avoidant children were more likely to have externalizing behaviour problems than secure or resistant/dependent children, but avoidant children also had more internalizing problems than resistant/dependent children.

The effect sizes for disorganization were somewhat larger. Disorganized children had more externalizing behaviour problems as reported by teachers than the secure (effect size 0.31) and avoidant children (effect size 0.21), but did not differ from the other groups on parent reports. Finally, there was some evidence that effect sizes increased as the time interval between attachment and behaviour problem assessment decreased. Thus some of the largest effects were for studies using the concurrent strategy.

In a review of the role of attachment in origins of aggressive disorders in children (Lyons-Ruth, 1996), there were distinct differences in findings from studies of high- and low-risk samples. In the latter, disorganization was most often linked with an alternative classification of security, and appeared to have little significance for later disturbance. In the former, disorganization was most often linked with avoidance and was strongly associated with later externalizing problems. This led to the suggestion that it is the combination of disorganization and avoidance, rather than disorganization alone, that contributes to later disturbance, particularly disturbances associated with hostile-aggressive behaviour.

In summary, there is some evidence to link both organized insecure and disorganized attachment with behaviour problems. The former effect is very small, and the latter moderate. Although children who were avoidant infants do seem, as predicted by traditional theorizing, to have more externalizing problems than those who have been secure or resistant, contrary to prediction they also have more internalizing problems. The prediction that resistant or dependent attachment would be associated with internalizing problems was not supported. However, there is evidence that the combination of disorganization and avoidance predicts externalizing disorders.

Attachment and psychopathology in adolescents and adults

Because many fully fledged psychiatric disorders first make their appearance in adolescence, studies of adolescents are included here with disorders of adulthood, rather than in the previous section. As indicated above, most of these studies involve assessments of attachment that are concurrent with assessment of pathology or clinical diagnosis.

Insecure attachment and psychiatric disturbance

A very common finding is that the history of psychiatric patients is riddled with negative attachment-related experiences such as loss, abuse or conflict. Not surprisingly, most empirical studies of adolescent and adult psychiatric populations are marked by a very low incidence of autonomous attachment. For example, on the basis of the AAI administered to 13- to 19-year-old psychiatric patients with a mixture of disorders, only 21 of 133 (16 per cent) were judged to be autonomous, compared to 50 per cent in normative samples (Adam et al., 1995). Similarly, among mentally disturbed criminal offenders in two Dutch forensic hospitals, only 5 per cent were found to be autonomous (van IJzendoorn et al., 1997). A meta-analysis of studies of clinical populations (van IJzendoorn and Bakermans-Kranenburg, 1996) confirmed this impression, insecure attachment patterns being strongly over-represented in adult clinical samples, with only 12–14 per cent being autonomous.

Although autonomous or secure attachment is relatively rare in clinical populations, it is not absent, and therefore secure attachment is not a guarantee of mental health. In one study comparing autonomous women with many negative childhood experiences (i.e. those who would be considered 'earned secure') with those who were continuously secure, the earned secure group were found to be more vulnerable to depressive symptoms (Pearson et al., 1994).

It seems likely that the importance of attachment in the development of a disorder is likely to be diminished when genetic or other constitutional factors are known to be more central (Dozier et al., 1999). As an example, we can consider different forms of depression. There is some evidence that major depression (severe and acute) is more often associated with autonomous attachment than is dysthymia, a disorder with less severe but more chronic depressed mood (Fonagy et al., 1996; Tyrell et al., 1999). One interpretation of this finding is that major depression has a stronger biological component than does dysthymia. However, when we consider that the direction of effects is unclear when assessments of attachment and disorder co-occur, another interpretation is that a chronic condition may disrupt internal working models of attachment more than a severe but acute disorder.

Links with specific disorders

Most psychiatric disorders are relatively heterogeneous. Thus depression varies in severity, chronicity (frequency of episodes), and presence or absence of swings to mania. It may occur with both internalizing and externalizing symptoms. Disorders often occur together, in which case we describe them as 'comorbid.' Thus a person can be diagnosed with depression and comorbid anxiety or comorbid eating disorder. The fact that some studies report depression to be associated with preoccupied attachment (Cole-Detke and Kobak, 1996; Rosenstein and Horowitz, 1996), whereas others link it to dismissing attachment (Patrick et al., 1994) may reflect predominance of different depressive disorders in different samples and/or different rates of comorbid disorders. Thus one difficulty in linking particular patterns of attachment to specific disorders arises from the mixed and overlapping diagnoses that are characteristic of current diagnostic practices.

Another difficulty may be the confounding of attachment with proclivity to report symptoms or seek treatment. Kobak, Sudler and Gamble (1991) postulated that preoccupation would be linked to depressive symptoms in adolescents. Among adolescents selected on the basis of high self-reported levels of depression, both secure and preoccupied strategies were associated with increased reports of symptoms, but the effect of security/insecurity was more consistent than that for preoccupation (Kobak et al., 1991). However, other evidence indicates that although dismissing and preoccupied individuals differ in reporting symptoms of all kinds, these self-reports do not necessarily correspond to other measures of disturbance.

In a sample consisting of 40 mental health clients with at least two psychiatric hospitalizations, 21 individuals fulfilled the criteria for diagnosis of schizophrenia, and 19 individuals met the criteria for affective disorder (Dozier et al., 1991). Individuals with schizophrenia were rated as more dismissing than those with affective disorder, but regardless of diagnosis, individuals who were more dismissing reported fewer symptoms on a self-report instrument than did those who were more preoccupied. In another sample of 76 seriously disturbed adults who completed a self-report symptom inventory, dismissing individuals reported fewer symptoms than those in the preoccupied group, but clinicians and AAI interviewers rated dismissing individuals as more disturbed (Dozier and Lee, 1995). Thus dismissing individuals may report fewer symptoms than those who are preoccupied, but be equally disturbed, if not more so.

In several reports, ordinarily rare forms of insecure attachment occur with significantly higher frequencies in clinical samples. For example, two studies found a particular variant of preoccupied attachment characterized by fearful preoccupation with traumatic events to be common in patients with borderline personality disorder, with 47 per cent showing this attachment pattern in one study (Fonagy et al., 1996) and 83 per cent in another (Patrick et al., 1994). Similarly, among adolescents, a rare form of dismissing attachment in which the individual derogates attachment figures or experiences was predictive of later criminal behaviour (Allen et al., 1996). Thus rather than dismissing or preoccupied attachment per se being related to psychiatric disturbance, it may be particular and unusual forms of insecurity that provide the linkage.

Although a meta-analysis (van IJzendoorn and Bakermans-Kranenburg, 1996) provided little evidence to suggest that either dismissing or preoccupied attachment is associated with specific disorders, a more recent discursive review which included a number of new studies that were not available for the meta-analysis (Dozier et al., 1999) concluded that the adult evidence does support a link between dismissing attachment and externalizing disorders, as well as one between preoccupation and internalizing disorders. Further work with more carefully delineated psychiatric samples, as well as examination of unusual patterns of insecurity, may be fruitful directions of further investigation.

Disorganization (unresolved mourning/trauma) and psychopathology

Clinical samples of adolescents and adults are also characterized by a high frequency of unresolved attachment. Indeed, unresolved attachment is the most common non-autonomous classification in most psychiatric samples. For example, in one small study of 20 anxiety-disordered mothers, all of these women were found to have insecure attachments, and 14 (70 per cent) were unresolved for loss or trauma. Among 13- to 19-year-old psychiatric patients, Adam, Sheldon-Keller and West (1995) found 52 per cent to be unresolved. In many cases this classification was based on severe separation experiences in which the adolescent was unwillingly ejected from his or her home or placed in residential or foster care. Patients with borderline personality disorder appear to be marked by a combination of high prevalence of experiencing sexual abuse and high scores for lack of resolution of abuse (Fonagy et al., 1996; Patrick et al., 1994). Some studies further suggest that the unresolved classification in these clinical samples is particularly associated with preoccupation (Adam et al., 1995; Fonagy et al., 1995, 1996, 1997; Patrick et al., 1994). In one study of adolescent psychiatric patients, 77 per cent of those who were both unresolved and preoccupied had made suicide attempts or reported intense suicidal ideas (Adam et al., 1996). Other studies indicate that antisocial personality and criminality are linked to a combination of unresolved and dismissing working models of attachment (Allen et al., 1996; Rosenstein and Horowitz, 1996).

'Cannot classify' and disorder

In the above study of mentally disturbed criminals (van IJzendoorn et al., 1997), dismissing, preoccupied and unresolved attachments were equally represented together with a relatively new and usually rare classification – 'cannot classify.' This latter classification is assigned when an individual shows clear evidence of contradictory patterns of attachment. For example, someone who was clearly dismissing towards their father and clearly preoccupied with regard to their mother would qualify for this classification. It would also be used for someone whose transcript was very low on coherence but did not reflect enough dismissing or preoccupied characteristics to be given either of the standard insecure classifications. Hesse (1996) suggests that whereas the unresolved classification is marked by brief and transitory collapse of an underlying attachment strategy, 'cannot classify' reflects a more global collapse or breakdown of strategy. If so, then this category should be over-represented in clinical samples. Indeed, there are several reports to suggest that this is the case, with one study reporting 'cannot classify' as the assigned classification for 25.8 per cent of previously hospitalized vs. 6.6 per cent of similar non-hospitalized students (Allen *et al.*, 1996), a second reporting that 37 per cent of maritally violent men vs. 10 per cent of non-violent men were placed in this category (Holtzworth-Munroe *et al.*, 1992), and a third (Adam *et al.*, 1995) finding a high incidence of the 'cannot classify' category in a mixed adolescent patient sample.

Disorganization and dissociative disorders

The most compelling evidence for a link between a specific form of attachment and a specific disorder is that for early disorganization and dissociation. First, there is the observed similarity in the behavioural indices of both disorganized attachment in infancy and dissociative states in adolescence and adulthood. Secondly, there is retrospective case material to support the hypothesis linking disorganization and dissociation (Liotti, 1995). However, the best evidence comes from the only published long-term prospective study of early attachment and later disturbance. Carlson (1998) analysed data for 157 participants in the Minnesota longitudinal study who had been followed from infancy to age 19 years in order to examine the long-term effects of disorganized attachment in infancy. Neither resistance nor overall insecure attachment were related to measures of psychopathology based on teacher and self-report measures through childhood and adolescence. At 19 years of age, each adolescent completed a self-report instrument that assessed dissociative experiences such as disturbances in memory, identity, awareness and cognition (e.g. lack of memory for significant events). Avoidant attachment, disorganization, behaviour problems in elementary school, and the quality of parent–child relationships at 13 years predicted psychopathology outcomes at 17½ years. Furthermore, disorganization made a significant contribution to psychopathology outcomes even after all other contributing factors had been controlled.

The most striking finding was that disorganized attachment in infancy was consistently and significantly related to specific items tapping dissociative experiences on both general psychopathology assessments and self-reports of dissociative experiences at 19 years of age. The predictors of dissociative experiences also included childhood behaviour problems and disturbances of parent–child relationships in later years, but disorganized attachment made a significant contribution after these other predictors had been controlled. The data from this study are among the first to test the specific hypothesis that early disorganized attachment is linked with later dissociative states. Although they show that both adolescent psycho-pathology in general and dissociative experiences in particular are best predicted by a combination of factors, early disorganized attachment was shown to make a significant contribution on its own.

Overview: attachment and psychiatric disturbance

Studies of children, adolescents and adults concur in finding associations between psychological disturbance and attachment. In non-diagnosed populations studied prospectively, although insecure attachment *per se* does have an effect on behaviour problems, it is only a very small one. Clearly, insecure attachment cannot be a primary cause of psychological disturbance on its own. Rather, insecure attachment is a risk factor that operates in concert with other coexisting conditions to increase or decrease vulnerability to disorder. Interestingly, whereas prospective studies of children suggest that avoidance is implicated in both internalizing and externalizing behaviour problems, both preoccupied and dismissing adults are over-represented in clinical populations.

The strongest associations generally come from studies of concurrent attachment in clinical populations, and must be qualified by the fact that the direction of effects is unclear. On the one hand, there is evidence that psychiatric patients often have highly traumatic attachment experiences that exceed the normal range in community samples. The high frequency of extreme and unusual forms of attachment, such as disorganization, lack of resolution of abuse or separation, derogation of attachment, preoccupation with traumatic events and 'cannot classify' may reflect these experiences. Such evidence, even in the absence of prospective studies, implicates early caregiving experiences in later disorder. However, the lack of adequate prospective data and the possibility that psychiatric disturbance may disrupt internal working models of attachment prevents us from making clear causal attributions. The exceptions are two cases where we do have prospective data – one where dismissing and unresolved adolescent attachment predicted later criminal behaviour (Allen *et al.*, 1996) and a second linking early disorganization to later dissociative experiences (Carlson, 1998).

The study of the possible role of attachment in psychiatric disorders is one of the most rapidly growing areas of attachment research. Detailed study of attachment in clinical samples may result in further distinctions within attachment categories, such as unresolved and 'cannot classify,' or the discovery of patterns that are not seen at all in normative groups. Improvements in psychiatric diagnosis will also be important in this endeavour. Better nosology of heterogeneous disorders and understanding of the nature of comorbid disorders will also set the stage for exploring more precise relationships between attachment and psychiatric disorders.

Clinical applications

The high proportion of clinical cases marked by unusual attachment patterns suggests that whether disturbance of attachment is a contributing or resulting factor, there may be a role for attachment theory and research in diagnosing, treating and preventing psychiatric disorders.

A caution: attachment assessments as clinical tools?

Despite the clinical roots of attachment theory and the major contributions that study of clinical populations has made, the most common measures of attachment were designed as research methods to examine group data, rather than as clinical tools to assess individuals. Psychometric data for evaluating attachment data on a case-by-case basis are not currently available. By far the greatest drawback to clinical use of most attachment measures is that they are inordinately time-consuming and cannot be used in a cost-effective manner in the typical clinical practice. For example, the strange situation requires a space with appropriate video equipment and someone to run it, a 'stranger' to participate in the assessment, and a trained scorer who can spend up to 2 hours to code each 30-minute tape. The Attachment Q-sort appears to be most valid when completed by trained observers who spend one or more half-day sessions observing in the home in addition to sorting time. The AAI in and of itself might be completed and recorded in a normal clinical session, but proper transcription takes 8–12 hours, and a highly trained coder may take 4–6 hours to arrive at a classification.

Many of the studies described above were conducted by clinician researchers who are able to support the use of these procedures through research grants. While there are less time-consuming measures of attachment (see Chapter 3), these also seem to tap somewhat different aspects of relationships that apparently have less in common with a clinical orientation. Thus, while attachment measures may have some clinical utility, they are not yet available in forms that have proven clinical validity or cost-effectiveness.

Applications in diagnosis

Despite these limitations, attachment theory and research may still have important applications to clinical practice. Some of the techniques developed by attachment researchers can be incorporated in diagnostic procedures (see Zeanah *et al.*, 1997, for a detailed case illustration). For example, although transcribing and scoring the AAI may not be clinically feasible, the interview itself may provide an effective format to elicit important material. In addition, even without the use of the AAI, familiarity with its orientation and focus on narratives provide a framework for listening and generating hypotheses about the implications of attachment problems in particular cases.

Similarly, while it may not be cost-effective to use the strange situation for the purpose of classifying attachment, the observation of separation and reunion of young children and their caregivers/parents may contribute useful information without derivation of an attachment classification. An important lesson from strange-situation research is that reunions can be more telling than separations when evaluating individual differences. In the past, clinicians have focused on how children separate from parents when they arrive for assessments. Attachment research suggests that what happens when the child returns to his or her parents is at least as important.

Applications in treatment

An increasing number of clinicians have given thoughtful attention to the ways in which attachment concepts may enrich psychotherapy (e.g. Holmes, 1993; Lieberman, 1997, Rutter, 1997; Slade, 1999). Such contributions apply not only to case formulation and remediation of disturbance, but also to an understanding of the nature of the therapeutic relationship (Byng-Hall, 1990; Holmes, 1993). One approach is to conceive of the therapeutic process as one in which the therapist attempts to provide a corrective emotional experience by serving as a secure base for exploration of difficulties. Another is to view the task of therapy as one in which the therapist supports the patient in constructing a coherent narrative of previously confusing and damaging experiences.

Aspects of attachment may also be relevant to the choice of treatment or effectiveness of treatment. For example, preliminary data in one study indicated that in a highly disturbed group of adult patients, individuals judged as dismissing on the AAI were more likely than others to show improvements during psychotherapy (Fonagy et al., 1996). One possible implication of such findings is that a different form of psychotherapy or approaches other than psychotherapy may be more effective with pre-occupied patients. Patients with different internal working models of attachment are likely to make different demands on a therapist (Dozier et al., 1994), in return making the latter's task different. Whereas the task of a therapist with dismissing patients is to increase awareness of emotional experiences, that of a therapist with preoccupied patients is to co-construct a framework for organizing and reflecting on emotions (Slade, 1999). In one study, therapists who were themselves autonomous were found to be better able to implement these different approaches (Dozier et al., 1994).

Applications in prevention

Perhaps most important of all, attachment theory and research have alerted us to the importance of stable dependable protective care for developing children, and have taught us to appreciate and consider the experience of young children when making decisions about foster care, adoption, divorce and custody (Rutter, 1997). Moreover, it has become increasingly clear that although loss of a parent through death or divorce has a significant impact on young children, and implications for subsequent development, the quality of ongoing and subsequent relationships are crucial to the way in which such losses are absorbed and resolved (e.g. Bretherton *et al.*, 1997; Harris *et al.*, 1986). Furthermore, an understanding of how attachment develops and may go awry has informed a number of early interventions to prevent the formation of insecure attachment.

Given that insecure attachment *per se* is not a disorder but rather a risk factor that increases vulnerability to disorder when accompanied by other risk factors, early interventions have been directed primarily towards high-risk infants and their families. Thus the target populations have been those characterized by a mixture of risk factors such as low income, lack of social support, parental depression, difficult infant temperament and/or infant medical problems. On the basis of the theory concerning transmission of attachment (see Chapter 4), these attempts have taken one of two routes. The first is based on altering maternal behaviour, particularly enhancing maternal responsiveness, while the second focuses on altering maternal representations through therapy and support for the mother.

A successful example of the former is a study in which Anisfeld and her colleagues (1990) provided one group of low-income mothers of preterm infants with a cloth baby carrier and a second group with a plastic baby seat. The use of the cloth carrier was expected to increase mother–infant physical contact, augment the impact of infant cues, and thus enhance the likelihood that the mother would respond to the latter. This increased responsiveness was expected to produce an increase in secure attachment. The plastic baby seat was considered to constitute a control condition. In fact, at least half of the mothers in the experimental group reported daily use of the carrier. In this study, although the group difference in sensitivity (in favour of the experimental mothers) was not significant, the difference in infant attachment was significant – 83 per cent in the experimental group were securely attached at 13 months, compared to 38 per cent in the control group.

An example of the second type of intervention was one in which Lieberman, Weston and Pawl (1991) randomly assigned insecurely attached infant–mother dyads among recent low-socioeconomic status Hispanic immigrants to either a therapeutic intervention or a control group. The intervention consisted of unstructured home visits over the course of a year to provide a 'corrective attachment experience' to the mother. Observation of mother–infant interactions at the end of the year indicated that experimental mothers were more empathically responsive to their toddlers, but there were no differences in attachment as measured by the intervenor's Attachment Q-sort for the toddler.

These two examples illustrate the variety of possible outcomes in these theoretically based interventions. It is assumed that maternal representations influence maternal responsiveness, which in turn influences infant attachment. However, interventions may successfully change one maternal component with or without a corresponding change in the other, and infant attachment may or may not be affected. Although neither of the above studies assessed maternal representations directly, in the first example infant attachment was affected in the absence of effects on maternal behaviour, and in the second, maternal behaviour was influenced without a corresponding influence on child attachment.

A meta-analysis of 12 attachment-based intervention studies (van IJzendoorn *et al.*, 1995) showed that the effects on maternal sensitivity (mean effect size = 0.58) were generally larger and more consistent than the effects on infant attachment (mean effect size = 0.17). Enhancing maternal sensitivity and/or infant attachment did not necessarily involve a change in maternal representations. In addition to their clinical implications, these findings also direct us to reconsider the underlying transmission model.

A striking finding of this meta-analysis was that short-term interventions with a specific focus were more effective than long-term comprehensive interventions. Because none of the studies had a long-term follow-up, the interpretation of this finding is unclear. It may be that a direct focus on specific aspects of mother–infant relationships brings about more rapid but possibly shorter-lasting changes, while long-term interventions are slower to change specific behaviours, but are longer-lasting and more general in their effects.

This type of preventive work is in its infancy, and will undoubtedly continue to expand in the future, with new insights and applications to clinical practice. At the same time, it is necessary to delineate the limits of attachment theory and research in the clinical domain. It is unlikely that attachment and attachment-based interventions are relevant to every disorder. Thus an important future task is to distinguish disorders in which attachment constructs are useful and appropriate from those in which they are not.

Suggested reading

Atkinson, L. and Zucker, K. (1997) *Attachment and psychopathology*. New York: Guilford Press.
An edited volume of theoretical, empirical and clinical papers on the topic.

Dozier, M., Stovall, K.C. and Albus, K. (1999) Attachment and psychopathology in adulthood. In Cassidy, J. and Shaver, P.R. (Eds), *Handbook of attachment theory and research*. New York: Guilford Press, 497–519.
A comprehensive review of what is known about attachment and adult psychiatric disorders.

Zeanah, C.H. (1996) Beyond insecurity: a reconceptualization of attachment disorders of infancy. *Journal of Consulting and Clinical Psychology*, **64**, 42–52.
A critical review of attachment disorders in infancy.

Greenberg, M.T., Speltz, M.L. and DeKlyen, M. (1993) The role of attachment in the early development of disruptive behavior problems. *Development and Psychopathology*, **5**, 191–213.
This article develops a relatively complex model for understanding the role of attachment in the development of externalizing behaviour problems.

Slade, A. (1999) Individual psychotherapy: an attachment perspective. In Cassidy, J. and Shaver, P.R. (Eds), *Handbook of attachment theory and research*. New York: Guilford Press, 575–94.
A thoughtful discussion of the applications of attachment constructs in the therapeutic process.

14 Attachment and physical health

Because attachment theory originated in the experiences of a clinician with an interest in mental health, it is not surprising that the literature on attachment and mental health is far more extensive that that on attachment and physical health. Nevertheless, there is growing evidence that attachment constructs have the potential to add immeasurably to our understanding of physical health as well. Certainly the concept of attachment as a protective system includes the notion of protection from illness. Illness is repeatedly mentioned as one of the conditions that normally activates attachment behaviour, yet this is a neglected aspect of attachment theory and research. Behaviour during illness and the responses that it elicits are thought to play a role in the development of attachment. Thus when illness occurs, both past and present attachment experiences influence help-seeking behaviour. Furthermore, the information we reviewed in Chapter 11 suggests that attachment influences the type of support system in which individuals are embedded, as well as the ability to use it effectively. Some but not all professional caregivers are potential attachment figures, and attachment history could also influence an individual's attitude and behaviour towards such figures, and hence aspects of treatment.

Secondly, behaviour patterns linked to attachment may expose or shelter the individual from psychological and physical stressors. For example, we noted in Chapter 13 that insecure attachment, when it coexists with other disadvantages, predicts health-risk behaviours such as drug use. In recent years there has been an increasing emphasis on the psychology of health behaviours – that is, behaviours concerned with maintaining physical health (e.g. diet, exercise, strategies for coping with stress), preventing disease (e.g. check-ups, non-smoking, use of sunscreen) and managing disease so as to promote recovery and minimize damage (e.g. adherence to treatment, relationships with professional caregivers). It seems likely that attachment experiences and their concomitants play a role in these behaviours.

In Chapter 12, we discussed ways in which early attachment experiences and the expectations of care that they engender organize aspects of neurobiological development. Armed with this information, it is not an impossible leap to speculate that features of this early-established physiological organization increase or decrease vulnerability to particular diseases. In this chapter we shall speculate on all of these possibilities and integrate empirical information where it is available. This discussion is not intended to suggest that attachment supplants other routes to health and disease. Attachment is considered here as one of the many factors (genetic, constitutional and environmental, for example) that interact to promote health and disease.

Illness as an attachment situation

Bowlby's original formulation of attachment included illness as one of the conditions in which protection of an attachment figure was important. In fact, you will recall that separations during hospitalization were one focus of the early work that Bowlby and Robertson undertook at the Tavistock Clinic (Chapter 1). The basic structure of the AAI repeatedly asks adults to review their experience of parental behaviour when they were ill, hurt or emotionally upset. Thus it is well accepted that illness is one of the key conditions that activates attachment behaviour. Although there has been some research on the development of attachment in children with specific early-identified chronic health problems (see van IJzendoorn *et al.*, 1992), other than the retrospective memories elicited on the AAI, there has been virtually no attention paid to attachment behaviour during childhood illnesses. One study examined parent and child behaviour during emergency hospitalization in relation to attachment security (Posada and Jacobs, 1999), and a second study explored the effects of attachment-based interventions to support parent–child relationships during hospitalization (Fahrenfort, 1993). Although hospitalization exacerbates attachment needs and raises barriers to meeting them, it is not a universal experience of childhood. However, all children experience at least some routine childhood illnesses during which they are cared for at home by their parents. We know very little about the role that such experience may have in the formation and maintenance of attachment strategies or health/illness behaviour.

It seems likely that early experiences with parents during routine illnesses are influential in the development of later illness behaviours, including the readiness with which an individual turns to attachment figures when ill. How quickly and comfortably do children report symptoms of illness to their parents? How comfortable are adults in seeking medical help for complaints? If one has had a history of sympathetic attention and appropriate care during past illnesses (conditions theoretically germane to secure attachment), the likelihood of promptly and confidently seeking care should be increased. Individuals who experienced scepticism about the seriousness of symptoms, or who were encouraged (or perhaps even forced on occasion) to carry on and 'keep a stiff upper lip' (a likely scenario for avoidant or dismissing attachment), may be more likely to delay help-seeking and perhaps belittle the usefulness of seeking help. We might also speculate that those whose history of parental response to illness was inconsistent or unpredictable (i.e. the conditions thought to generate resistant/preoccupied attachment) would be disposed to exaggerate complaints in an attempt to elicit and maintain the attention needed.

There is now a vast and growing literature documenting the importance of social relationships for health. Associations between social support and physical health have been found in a diverse array of medical conditions, including heart disease, cancer and infectious diseases (Uchino *et al.*, 1996). Whereas much of the literature on social support focuses simply on its presence or absence, it is also known that individuals differ in the social networks they develop and the ways in which they use them. Hence social support may be best conceptualized as an individual-differences variable rather than a situational variable. Much of the material discussed in Chapter 11 suggests that secure or autonomous individuals are more likely than their insecure counterparts to develop and maintain accessible social networks that will be used in times of stress, including illness.

A further question is whether relationships with health-care providers are attachment relationships and, if so, whether individual differences that parallel attachment classifications can be observed. A health-care provider could easily fit the description of a 'stronger, wiser' figure to whom one turns for help when distressed. I would speculate that the best candidate for filling this role would be either a primary-care physician with whom one has a relatively long history of sharing health and personal information, or a specialist who is instrumental in the prolonged care of a chronic illness. To my knowledge, there has been no research on this topic, but it offers intriguing possibilities for investigation. This domain represents only one small part of the broader area of health behaviour to which we shall now turn.

Attachment and health behaviour

In most of the industrialized world, the prevalence of acute infectious disorders has steadily declined as a result of improved sanitation, immunization programmes, and the development of new drugs. Whereas most of these changes benefit entire populations, individuals can further protect themselves from infectious disease by engaging in practices that reduce their own exposure or vulnerability (e.g. handwashing and innoculations). During the time period when acute infectious disorders declined, there was a corresponding increase in the prevalence of chronic conditions such as cardiovascular disease, cancers, and conditions resulting from accidental injuries. The role of behavioural factors in preventing these conditions is increasingly evident. For example, it has been estimated that a reduction in smoking could avoid 25 per cent of cancer deaths as well as 350,000 premature deaths from heart attack. Similarly dramatic effects on heart disease, diabetes, gastrointestinal cancer and stroke could be achieved with weight reduction and increased exercise levels among potentially vulnerable adults (Taylor, 1990). Why do some people regularly engage in health-promoting behaviours, while others persist in behaviour that is known to cause physical damage even after the symptoms have appeared? Why do some people react to signs of illness by seeking and following treatment, while others delay in obtaining medical assistance or fail to adhere to treatment? Individual differences in personality are thought to give rise to these different approaches to health and illness.

One personality factor that has been implicated in health and illness behaviours is that of coping style – a characteristic way of reacting to problematic or stressful situations (Lazarus and Folkman, 1984). We have already identified attachment strategies as general approaches to managing stress. Thus attachment strategies are in fact coping strategies. However, there are other complex and varied ways of describing coping style that do not invoke attachment constructs *per se*. At least some of these characterizations exhibit considerable overlap with the classic descriptions of attachment patterns.

One general feature of coping strategies describes the focus of effort. A distinction is made between strategies that focus on solving the problem and those aimed at regulating emotional distress (Lazarus and Folkman, 1984). A second important dimension concerns the choice between approaching and engaging in active efforts vs. avoiding by diverting attention away from the problem (Holahan and Moos, 1987). A tripartite classification scheme that incorporates both of these dimensions and has a great deal in common with primary attachment strategies arose from observations of children coping with cancer (Phipps et al., 1995). Some children avoid acknowledging the significance of their illness – they minimize its importance, underestimate its severity and ignore salient information. This strategy, described as 'denial,' is both emotion-focused and avoidant, and shares features with avoidant or dismissing attachment. Individuals who take this approach disconnect themselves from experiencing emotional distress, or 'blunt' its impact. Just as dismissing or avoidant individuals do not seek direct comfort from an attachment figure when they are distressed, for fear of experiencing rejection, these individuals turn away from potentially useful information or supports in order to avoid negative emotions associated with illness. Such individuals shut out information, underestimate the consequences of failing to adhere to treatment, and exhibit low treatment compliance.

A study which corroborates possible links between avoidant attachment and poor adherence was conducted among patients with diabetes (Ciechanowski et al., 1999). Control of diabetes is routinely assessed objectively by a haemoglobin marker in the blood. Patients who were avoidant in attachment style were found to be less successful than others in adhering to treatment as indicated by both objective haemoglobin assays and ratings from health-care providers.

In contrast to with 'deniers,' some individuals are 'sensitizers.' Given the same objective conditions, they exaggerate rather than minimize the significance or risks of illness. They perceive their illness as more serious than is warranted, they unnecessarily give up enjoyable activities out of a preoccupation with avoiding danger, and they behave as if they are more helpless than is in fact the case. This coping pattern is emotion-focused but approaching, and shares features with resistant or preoccupied attachment. Just as the resistant or preoccupied individual exaggerates emotions, clings to conflictual attachments and is unable to explore autonomously, the sensitizer exaggerates distress and helplessness, depends on others to take responsibility for his or her treatment, and is unable to explore or attend to care of the illness. Since such individuals abrogate responsibility for treatment, they are only likely to adhere to treatment to the extent that someone else supervises or implements it. Because they exaggerate negative emotions, they are also likely to be pessimistic and are predicted to have poor psychosocial outcomes as well as poor compliance with treatment.

The third strategy characterized children who focused away from aversive aspects of illness (blunting responses), but still sought information about the illness and its treatments. This strategy protects against emotional turmoil but involves active coping with illness. Thus it combines both emotion-focused and problem-focused coping, and shares features with secure or autonomous attachment. In the same way that secure attachment represents an integrated and flexible approach which allows for full exploration with use of an attachment figure as needed, adaptive blunting integrates emotional and cognitive responses in a way that facilitates exploration of possible solutions. Adaptive blunting is expected to be associated with high levels of optimism and flexibility, good treatment compliance, and good psychosocial adaptation.

Although these descriptions emerged from the study of children with cancer, they can be regarded as more general coping strategies. Because they overlap with descriptions of the primary attachment strategies, it is tempting to speculate that individuals who are secure are predisposed to approach problems, including those of health and illness, with the strategy of adaptive blunting, that those who are dismissing or avoidant are inclined to use strategies of denial, and those who are preoccupied or resistant are likely to adopt sensitizing strategies. I am not aware of any research that empirically documents such links, but this would seem to be another likely route for demonstrating relationships between attachment and health/illness behaviour.

Most of the health psychology research in these domains has been conducted with adults. In the case of young children, parental dispositions toward health and illness behaviour largely determine the manner in which the child's health is maintained and illnesses are treated. However, as children grow older, they are first expected to co-operate with these regimes and then to take increasing responsibility for activities such as nutritional intake, toothbrushing, handwashing, getting adequate sleep, recognizing symptoms of illness and attending regular medical check-ups. How this transition from parental to child responsibility occurs is undoubtedly shaped by the nature of parent–child relationships. One might predict that the secure parent–child relationships that are thought to support child autonomy would be associated with more effective transfer of health-care responsibility to children.

Furthermore, since protection from illness is implicitly included in the concept of attachment, the parental behaviour that supports secure attachment should be associated with more effective health care. In one large paediatric practice, there was an association between infant attachment status and use of health-care services up to age 3 years. Secure infants were most likely to have completed routine paediatric visits on time than those in other attachment groups. Insecurely attached infants, particularly those who were avoidant, made more acute visits for illnesses of low severity than secure infants (Berger and Damberg, 1997). These findings may reflect differential parent care and management of health-related issues, differential infant vulnerability, or a combination of these two factors.

This discussion has focused on coping strategies because, we suggested, attachment *is* a coping strategy. Attachment may also affect health and illness behaviours indirectly by influencing the development of traits, attitudes or abilities thought to be important in personal health care. For example, one model represents health habits as involving appropriate self-regulatory goals, and the ability to monitor outcomes and to make behavioural adjustments to meet those goals (Ewart,1991). This self-regulatory system is seen as interwoven with close social relationships in which individuals jointly facilitate or impede each other's regulation. Previously (in Chapters 9, 10 and 12), we considered the extent to which attachment is implicated in self-regulation. Whether individual differences in self-regulation in other domains can be extended to health habits has yet to be examined. However, the nature of close relationships *is* what attachment is about. Thus attachments would be expected to play a role in theorized joint regulation in the above model. Because these are secondary effects of attachment on health, it is probably more useful at this stage to pursue the study of attachment effects on personality traits *per se* than to integrate attachment directly into such models. However, there is the possibility that individual differences in vulnerability to disease are affected by attachment history.

Vulnerability to illness

Stress and disease

Theories about links between stress and illness have a long and venerable history (see Chrousos and Gold, 1992, for a review) with Selye (1946) being credited with the first general statement of our current formulation. Briefly, Selye postulated that a constellation of psychological and physiological symptoms occurring in some seriously ill patients could best be understood as the consequence of severe and prolonged adaptations to stress. The normal response to stress includes an intricate cascade of physiological changes, including increases in heart rate, respiration, glucose levels and blood pressure, activation of the immune system and inhibition of functions associated with growth (Chrousus and Gold, 1992). If these changes persist indefinitely, they lead to physiological damage. Normally, built-in regulatory feedback loops serve as 'brakes' on the stress response and ensure that it will be of limited duration. For example, in addition to its other effects, cortisol, which is produced by the HPA axis in response to stress (see Chapter 12), serves to 'turn off' the immune system (Maier et al., 1994). If the 'brakes' should fail or operate inefficiently, the stress response is prolonged and/or may become dysregulated (i.e. either overactive or underactive). Thus, to follow our example, if cortisol was to be chronically overproduced, the immune system would be persistently suppressed and impaired in its ability to repel infectious disease. Alternatively, if cortisol was to be chronically underproduced, the immune system would become overactive with a resulting increase in vulnerability to conditions such as asthma, ulcers and cardiovascular disease.

Social support and physiological processes

Although exposure to environmental stressors has a documented influence on the occurrence of illness in both adults and children, the magnitude of this relationship is modest, and there are subsets of individuals with 'extraordinary resilience and exaggerated susceptibility' (Boyce and Jemerin, 1990). Thus individual differences in emotional, behavioural and biological response to stress are thought to mediate the stress–illness relationship. A number of studies have examined possible physiological mechanisms to explain this link. A critical evaluation of this body of work, based almost exclusively on studies with adults, reached the conclusion that both naturalistic studies and those that manipulated social support in the laboratory concur in showing the following.

1. Social support has specific effects on cardiovascular, endocrine and immune functioning after controlling for personality traits and other confounding variables.

2. Although they influence health outcomes in their own right, health-related behaviours do not account for these effects.
3. Family support is more important for optimum physiological functioning than social support from other sources.
4. The emotional component of social support makes a significant contribution to these effects (Uchino *et al.*, 1996). The authors suggest that the most promising explanatory mechanism is that social support buffers the effects of stress.

Although attachment concepts have not been integrated into this body of work until very recently, attachment fits the specified criteria of being firstly a family-based source of support and secondly a source of emotional support. Furthermore, we have already noted in Chapter 12 that there is evidence to support Bowlby's notion that buffering of stress responses is a key function of the attachment behavioural system. Such buffering can occur in several ways. First, an effective attachment figure anticipates and avoids danger for his or her dependent charge. As a result, fewer situations that engender a stress response are encountered. Secondly, once an attachment is formed, the perception that comfort is available in times of stress serves to modify perceived stress and its associated physiological components. Thirdly, we considered evidence that early attachment influences the organization of some physiological stress responses. Individuals in different attachment groups may show different patterns of daily cortisol cycling (Adam, 1998) and differing parameters of cortisol stress response (Hertsgaard *et al.*, 1996; Spangler and Grossmann, 1993; Spangler and Schieche, 1998). Although the full implications of these differences have yet to be developed, these observations suggest that secure attachment is a more effective stress buffer than insecure attachment. The implication of this assertion is that secure attachment should serve to promote health. Likewise, insecure attachment is a less effective stress buffer and could therefore be associated with increased physiological vulnerability to illness. Is there any evidence that this is the case?

Evidence

Animal studies indicate that disruption of attachment is associated with vulnerability to disease (Reite and Boccia, 1994). When laboratory rats were separated from their mothers at different times during development and periodically subjected to conditions known to generate gastric ulcers (food deprivation plus restraint), time of separation was found to be related to the likelihood and severity of ulcers (Ackerman *et al.*, 1975). During the first 3 weeks of life, when all rat pups were with their mothers, they were resistant to gastric ulcers. If they remained with the mother until 21 or 25 days of age, they continued to be resistant until sexual maturity (62 days of age). Thereafter, their susceptibility gradually increased. However, if the mother was removed from the litter on day 15, pups tested 1 or 2 weeks later invariably developed ulcers, although their susceptibility then gradually declined until adulthood. In addition, the early-separated rats showed more severe lesions than the other groups, and were the only group that developed ulcers in reaction to food deprivation alone (without restraint).

There is compelling evidence that brief maternal separations in non-human primates affect immune regulation. However, among bonnet monkeys whose mothers are removed from the natal troop, these changes are reduced for those who spend their separation time with an alternative attachment figure compared to those who lack such a figure (Boccia *et al.*, 1993). Furthermore, there is ample evidence in both animals and humans of changes in immune and endocrine functioning related to morbidity and mortality following bereavement (Stroebe *et al.*, 1993).

The studies which led me to consider the role of attachment in disease involved following infants with chronic health problems through the first 7 years of their lives. The original purpose was to examine the effects of illness on the formation of attachments and later social development, but as the work progressed, we saw that attachment might also influence health. One group of infants had been diagnosed with cystic fibrosis during the first year of life, a second group had been diagnosed with congenital heart disease, and a third was a comparison group of healthy infants. All of the children participated in the strange situation at 1 year of age. In addition to behavioural observations and questionnaires, we obtained specific health information from medical records.

We found evidence that secure attachment is advantageous for the child's health, as well as indications that avoidant attachment specifically compromises physical well-being. First, among infants with congenital heart disease, those who were securely attached at 1 year were initially rated by the cardiologist as more severely ill at diagnosis than those who were insecure, but the secure group experienced significantly more improvement in health over the first year than their insecurely attached peers (Goldberg *et al.*, 1991).

Second, we found that among infants diagnosed with cystic fibrosis, those who showed avoidant attachment at 1 year did not differ from the others on any medical measures at the time of diagnosis. However, unlike the others, they showed no improvement in nutritional status after diagnosis, and had consistently lower weight for their height than any other group up to 4 years of age (Fischer-Fay *et al.*, 1988; Simmons *et al.*, 1995). Not surprisingly, they were more likely than the others to be treated with specific nutritional interventions such as nutritional supplements and/or surgical insertion of a feeding tube. By the age of 7 years they also showed poorer general health (Goldberg, Washington, Simmons and MacLusky, unpublished data).

Several other studies of infants and toddlers have shown links between attachment and physical growth. In a study of toddlers with and without eating disorders (Chatoor *et al.*, 1998) a continuous rating of security based on strange-situation observations was correlated with weight for height. Chronic malnutrition in an impoverished Chilean sample was associated with high rates of disorganized attachment (Valenzuela, 1990), and insecure attachment has been observed in 49–92 per cent of children with non-organic failure to thrive (Brinich *et al.*, 1989; Crittenden, 1987; Gordon and Jameson, 1979; Ward *et al.*, 1993). These associations are in sharp contrast to the meta-analytical finding that medical problems are generally not related to infant attachment (van IJzendoorn *et al.*, 1992).

Because feeding is a joint activity of infant and caregiver, it is impossible to distinguish the direction of effects in associations between attachment and nutritional status. It may be that parent–child behavioural problems that interfere with feeding also contribute to the formation of an insecure attachment. In some failure-to-thrive samples, other conditions detrimental to attachment (e.g. maltreatment) are present, and insecure attachment is over-represented among mothers of infants with non-organic failure to thrive (Benoit *et al.*, 1989). Another possible explanation is that poor nutrition gives rise to infant behaviours that make it more difficult for the caregiver to provide the sensitive care necessary for secure attachment (Valenzuela, 1990). However, in the light of our previous discussion, it is also appropriate to consider the possibility that the development of insecure attachment patterns interferes with physiological processes essential to growth. We noted above that the stress response includes inhibition of growth-promoting processes. Prolonged stress is associated with suppression of growth-hormone secretion and a decrease in its effect on target tissues (Chrousos and Gold, 1992). When the attachment behavioural system is not effective in buffering stress (i.e. it is insecure), the resulting increase in exposure to stress may actually inhibit growth.

Although these studies could not be considered conclusive, they present an intriguing picture and indicate that further investigation of the relationship between attachment and physical growth patterns is warranted. Although traditionally biology is thought to influence psychology, we now know that such effects are more likely to be bidirectional.

When children in all three groups in our chronic illness study were scored on a general severity of illness scale that included parent reports of everyday illnesses such as colds and earaches, as well as standard scores assigned by physicians, securely attached children in each diagnostic group consistently had the lowest scores and avoidant children had the highest. This was especially marked among the healthy group. Furthermore, in the healthy group this pattern became stronger over the first 3 years of life (Janus and Goldberg, 1997).

In these studies, unlike the rat and monkey studies described above, we cannot rule out confounding factors. However, we are not alone in identifying a potential link between insecure attachment and increased physical symptoms. Among preschool children with asthma, 42 per cent were insecurely attached, compared to 16 per cent in a comparison group (Mrazek et al., 1987). Boys who were insecure at 12 months of age were characterized by more somatic complaints at 6 years than their secure counterparts (Lewis et al., 1984). Among adults who experienced bombing raids in Israel during the Gulf War, those with insecure attachment styles reported more physical distress symptoms than those who were secure (Mikulincer et al., 1993). Similarly, adults who identified themselves as non-secure in couple relationships reported more psychosomatic illnesses than those who considered themselves to be secure (Hazan and Shaver, 1987, 1990), and a high rate of physical symptoms was characteristic of first-year psychology students who considered themselves to be avoidant in attachment style (Kotler et al., 1994).

Two studies of physically ill patients have linked attachment status to physiological markers. In the first study of patients with chronic hepatitis C, those who were preoccupied (using Bartholomew's four-category model) had a greater number of unexplained somatic symptoms than those who were secure or avoidant (Ciechanowski et al., 1998). In the second study, patients with ulcerative colitis who were identified as dismissing on the Reciprocal Attachment Questionaire (West et al., 1987) were more likely to be characterized by a physiological marker of disturbance in immune functioning than were those in other attachment groups (Maunder et al., 1999).

In short, while the evidence is not conclusive, there is growing support for the notion that attachment patterns may be differentially associated with vulnerability and resistance to disease, and that security is more advantageous for physical health than insecurity. Although several studies showed avoidant attachment to be associated with a greater propensity to physical symptoms than other forms of insecurity, many studies did not differentiate between insecure forms of attachment, and this pattern was not consistent across studies that did so.

Overview

This chapter has been largely speculative because, despite a long and compelling history in animal research and extensive data on the role of social support in adult illnesses, attachment constructs have only recently been introduced into the health psychology of humans. This is somewhat surprising given the original formulation of attachment as a protective system that includes protection from illness.

The speculation and evidence we have discussed may be summarized in the model depicted in Figure 14.1. Attachment may be implicated in physical health through direct influences on physiological organization and health

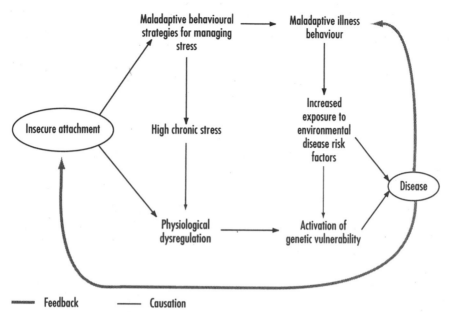

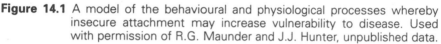

Figure 14.1 A model of the behavioural and physiological processes whereby insecure attachment may increase vulnerability to disease. Used with permission of R.G. Maunder and J.J. Hunter, unpublished data.

behaviour, as well as through indirect effects on personality traits, attitudes and competencies that play a role in health behaviour. Both speculation and evidence suggest that secure attachment is beneficial to health, whereas insecure attachment is likely to increase the risk of disease. Thus insecure attachment contributes to physiological dysregulation both directly and via poor behavioural stragies for managing stress. In turn, each of these factors increases vulnerability to disease. Physiological dysregulation does so more or less directly by activating genetic vulnerabilities, whereas poor stress management does so via maladaptive health/ illness behaviours that increase exposure to disease risk factors. Disease, in turn, has effects on both attachment and health/illness behaviours. Although there is some evidence that avoidant attachment may predispose individuals to these processes more than other forms of insecurity, it is as yet insufficient to allow firm conclusions to be drawn.

Suggested reading

Maier, S.F., Watkins, L.R. and Fleshner, M. (1994) Psychoneuroimmunology: the interface between behavior, brain, and immunity. *American Psychologist* **49**, 1004–17.

An excellent discussion of the immune system and the role of stress in disease written explicitly for a psychological audience.

Uchino, B.N., Cacioppo, J.T. and Kiecolt-Glaser, J.K. (1996) The relationship between social support and physiological processes: a review with emphasis on

underlying mechanisms and implications for health. *Psychological Bulletin* **119**, 488–531.
A comprehensive and detailed review of the literature on social support, with specific attention to social support as a buffer for stress.

Taylor, S.E. (1990) Health psychology: the science and the field. *American Psychologist* **45**, 40–50.
An overview of the field of health psychology.

Part V

Evaluation of attachment theory and research

15 Attachment theory and research: an appraisal

The purpose of this chapter is to undertake a critical evaluation of what attachment theory and research have accomplished, to highlight continuing controversies, and to identify issues for future research. This is the chapter I found most difficult to write and to complete. It is not that there is any lack of material or ideas concerning the status of attachment theory and research. Rather, my own thinking (and probably that of other attachment researchers) is constantly undergoing revision as new data and ideas emerge. I cannot imagine a conclusive appraisal of which I will not want to rescind or revise some portion in the next week, month or year! So this chapter will remain forever a 'work in progress' which should encourage students to undertake similar appraisals. In undertaking this task, we shall be referring to many of the previous chapters as reminders of earlier discussions or data summaries. Thus this chapter can also serve as a review of where we have been.

'Attachment' is the most recent and current label for the emotional bonds between children and parents. Its immediate predecessors, 'dependency' and 'object relations', each represented a distinct theoretical approach that enjoyed a period of enthusiastic reception, research and exploration. Is attachment something more than the latest 'buzzword' for the same old thing? When the next burst of enthusiasm for a different approach comes along, what will be the legacy of attachment theory and research? What, if anything, does it add to our understanding of close relationships and development? These questions focus on contributions and accomplishments. There have also been – and continue to be – many controversies and criticisms.

The history of attachment theory and research is marked by assaults from eager critics. Indeed, as we noted in Chapter 1, Bowlby's original ideas were summarily rejected by his psychoanalytical colleagues, and he was more or less ostracized from their company for many years. Ainsworth's work was also subjected to heated criticism and, until the publication of Sroufe and Waters' (1977a) paper on 'Attachment as an organizational construct,' and the emergence of supporting data from other laboratories, it was neither understood nor accepted by the larger community of developmental psychologists. In addition to negative criticism from those antagonistic to the theory (e.g. Kagan, 1998; Lamb *et al.*, 1984; Lewis, 1997), there have been constructive critical assessments of the field by those within it (e.g. Belsky and Cassidy, 1994), as well as debates regarding particular issues, (such as the exchange between van IJzendoorn (1995) and Fox (1995). This chapter draws on some of this material and is divided into two main sections. The first section considers the achievements of attachment theory and research, and the second is devoted to controversies and challenges.

Accomplishments

Changing our view of close relationships

In one of her early papers on attachment theory, Ainsworth (1969) summarized the ways in which it differed from the psychoanalytical and learning theories that prevailed at the time. We reviewed these differences in Chapter 1. Most recently, Michael Rutter (1997), who has provided several constructive critical reviews of attachment constructs and research, suggested that Bowlby's original formulation advanced our understanding of intimate relationships in the following ways. First, it clearly differentiated attachment from other aspects of close relationships. Secondly, it envisioned attachment as a phenomenon that normally extends over the lifespan instead of being a childish preoccupation to be outgrown. Thirdly, it placed attachment within an appropriate biological context. Fourthly, it introduced a mental mechanism whereby early experiences could be carried forward as well as altered. Finally, it suggested ways in which early insecure attachments could be linked to later psychopathology. Today we can see that Bowlby's monumental work provided the bare bones of a general framework which inspired subsequent workers to engage in creative interpretation and further development. Many details of the original theory have yet to be elaborated. Thanks to the inspired efforts of Mary Ainsworth, Bowlby's basic ideas about the nature of attachment were translated into a paradigm for assessing infant attachment that made many of the propositions eminently testable. Although we shall argue below that some important constructs have not been tested, or have been inadequately tested, the translation from speculation to testability was the crucial catalyst that sparked the explosion of research and ideas for the remainder of the twentieth century.

Generating a coherent and growing body of data

One of the key functions of a theory is to provide a road map that entices researchers to embark on the journey of discovery. From this perspective, 'correctness' of the theory is less important than its intuitive appeal and testability. In this role, attachment theory has served remarkably well, capturing the imagination of several generations of prolific researchers. Historically, we can identify several phases in attachment research. These phases overlap in the sense that each new phase did not replace the previous one, but rather layered new perspectives over the existing foundation. In the first phase, research focused on identifying predictors of infant behaviour in the strange situation and outcomes attributable to the resulting attachment classifications. The second phase was marked by two parallel developments, namely the extension of methods for assessing attachment beyond infancy, and the identification of disorganized attachment and its clinical implications. As attachment assessment moved beyond infancy, it also moved, as Main and her colleagues (Main *et al.*, 1985) suggested, 'to the level of representation.' This led to a third phase focused on exploration of attachment representations (internal working models) and their emotional and cognitive components. In each phase there have been both theoretical and empirical developments contributing to a growing body of coherent work.

What do I mean by 'coherent'? After all, many of the previous chapters are marked by comments regarding the inconsistency or incompleteness of the data. What I mean is that attachment theory acted as a 'lightning rod' to energize a dynamic centre of activity focused on developing and telling a 'story' about parent–child relationships and their role in development. Innovative methods were generated to conduct this work. Although many parts of the narrative are unclear, or even unformed, the ideas and data provoked enthusiastic debate and activated a significant number of researchers and theorists to pursue its promise, and others to argue vehemently that the story is all wrong. All this, I would suggest, has been good for the science of child development. It has forced all of the protagonists to think deeply and critically about both the theory and the phenomena it purports to explain. It has sent them back to the drawing-board, back to the laboratory and back to the home in search of better ideas and better data. It has brought public attention to the emotional needs of young children in domains relevant to public policy (e.g. allowing parents to stay in hospital with their children, phasing out large orphanages in most countries, and examining day care critically). In the preface to the *Handbook of Attachment* (Cassidy and Shaver, 1999), the editors note that anyone who does a literature search on the topic of attachment will find well over 2000 entries ranging across many different disciplines and covering every age period from infancy to old age. All of these phenomena testify to the generative power of attachment theory.

Giving credibility to an organizational approach to behaviour

Bowlby's ideas about control systems and Ainsworth's incorporation of them into the strange situation marked a shift towards examining and assessing organization of behaviour rather than behaviour *per se*, which was originally not well understood. Thinking about the organization of the attachment system has changed over time, and will probably continue to change. Bowlby first described the attachment behavioural system as one activated by signs of danger and 'turned off' by contact with an attachment figure. This notion was soon modified to one in which the attachment system is continually active in monitoring the environment and it is attachment behaviour that is turned on or off, a modification which Bowlby accepted (Main, 1999).

However, it is easy now to forget that when the strange situation was first introduced, researchers in the field were accustomed to measuring infant–adult relationships by recording the frequency and duration of discrete behaviours. The notion of examining behavioural organization was difficult to integrate into this approach. Thus it was natural for some researchers to adopt the strange situation primarily as another opportunity to 'count and measure' (see, for example, the description of Kotelchuck's study of fathers in Chapter 6 and of Fox's study of kibbutzim infants, in Chapter 7). When the duration or frequency of infant behaviours did not differ between adult figures, or when infant behaviours (e.g. vocalizing, locomotion, looks, cries) were uncorrelated, they concluded that the attachment constructs were erroneous.

Attachment researchers retorted that such correlations were not relevant to the construct (Sroufe and Waters, 1977b). When behaviours serve the same function, they can replace each other and thus would not yield high correlations (e.g. an infant who crawls directly to his or her mother and is picked up may not need to cry for attention; interaction at a distance such as looking and vocalizing may preclude the need for physical contact). Furthermore, the durations and frequencies of behaviour and even sequential analyses do not necessarily capture the general organization of behavioural systems.

In current developmental thinking, systemic approaches are common and well accepted. Indeed, a current criticism of attachment work is that it focuses on only a limited portion of the child's social system (Lewis, 1997). Attachment theory and methodology contributed to moving the field in this direction.

Bridging the gap between researchers and clinicians

Although Bowlby's original ideas were provoked by his own clinical experience, initially they were not incorporated into the clinical practice of his colleagues. The development of the strange situation and its potential for testing some of Bowlby's propositions appealed primarily to students of developmental psychology, but two emerging phenomena were important in bringing attachment theory and research back to their clinical origins.

The first was the interest in studying special populations of infants as 'natural experiments' that might alter parent–infant relationships. These studies contributed to the discovery of atypical attachment patterns and their over-representation in clinical populations. In order to pursue this theme, developmental researchers had to form collaborations with clinicians in psychology as well as other disciplines (e.g. medicine, social work, physiotherapy). These clinicians were eager to join such collaborations as they grasped the implications of atypical attachment patterns.

The second significant move occurred with the development of the AAI. The content of this interview was familiar to clinicians who were accustomed to exploring family experiences with adult patients. The discovery that there was a systematic way to codify the resulting narrative, and that the classifications obtained were related to phenomena such as infant attachment and parent and/or child clinical status was naturally appealing. Consequently, a cohort of clinicians was among the first to undertake the AAI training and to use the AAI in research as well as in clinical practice. Some of these clinicians, as well as some from subsequent training cohorts, have become prominent contributors to the field of attachment theory and research. The result of these changes is an ongoing dialogue between clinicians and researchers that has already enriched the field, and promises to continue doing so in years to come.

Controversies and challenges

The following points are listed in no particular order as issues which provoke controversy or warrant further thought and investigation.

But sabre-toothed tigers are extinct! Broad vs. narrow definitions of attachment

Bowlby's original description of a 'safety-regulating' system placed a heavy emphasis on protection from predators. As one of my colleagues likes to remind me, sabre-toothed tigers are extinct. The kind of protection that Bowlby considered in his original reasoning is no longer necessary. Therefore there must be other ways in which attachment is adaptive, and the current meaning of attachment requires broader interpretation. To this argument I usually reply that even in the absence of sabre-toothed tigers, there are more than enough dangers from which young children need protection, including the predations of disease, injury and ill-intentioned or disturbed conspecifics. Despite the absence of predators, infants are not likely to survive for very long without the presence of a caring adult. Thus even in the present supposedly gentler conditions, it is adaptive for infants to become fearful at the prospect of separation from a familiar caregiver. In fact, Main (1999, p.853) argues that because of the importance of its tie to survival, the attachment behavioural system should be conceived as 'standing first in the hierarchy of infants' behavioral repertoire.'

In fact, although most attachment researchers begin their discourse with a nod to attachment as a protective phenomenon, a wide range of implicit definitions are in use, ranging from one extreme with those which insist on illness, injury and emotional upset as the unique domain of attachment to definitions at the other extreme which use the term to mean everything about early parent–child relationships. Although Bowlby was very emphatic about the difference between attachment interactions and other aspects of infant–parent relationships, he himself implicitly broadened the definition when he endorsed Ainsworth's notion that attachment in humans develops as a function of a caregiver's general sensitivity to infant signals (Goldberg et al., 1999). Thus, he suggested, an infant learns about the caregiver's physical and emotional availability in a general sense and comes to expect comfort and safety from danger as a special case of general availability. In fact, this is the approach that most studies of the precursors of attachment have taken. In retrospect, in view of the theoretical emphasis on protection, it is rather surprising that so few of the many existing studies looked specifically at parental protective behaviour and its role in the development of the behaviour patterns observed in the strange situation.

While general sensitivity to infant signals does make a small to moderate significant contribution to the development of attachment (see Chapter 4), it also influences other important developmental phenomena. For example, a sense of self-efficacy – children's belief that they have control over life events – is also thought to arise from caregiver sensitivity. While feelings of self-efficacy are arguably important in personality development, they are not the same as feeling safe. Similarly, children with generally responsive parents come to expect that people will be co-operative rather than conflictual. Again, while important, this is different to an expectation of safety and protection. During early infancy, protective issues may indeed intrude into all aspects of infant–caregiver relationships because the infant's physiological vulnerability is relatively pervasive. However, other systems soon begin to develop, become differentiated and function in their own right. While we have learned a great deal about precursors and outcomes of behaviour in the strange situation, it is not clear that what we have learned explicitly speaks to Bowlby's ideas about protection and its role in development. In fact, as we noted in Chapter 1, the introduction of the strange situation and identification of individual differences in attachment patterns diverted the field away from Bowlby's original preoccupation with normative development of attachment and its functions, and into a focus on individual differences.

As the definition of attachment is broadened, it overlaps with other constructs and behavioural systems relevant to parent–child relationships, loses its unique features, and is potentially indistinguishable from other theoretical approaches (Goldberg *et al.*, 1999). These are the primary arguments for maintaining a narrow definition.

What are some of the arguments for adopting a broader definition? We have already noted that in infancy – the period where attachment has its origins – protective issues may in fact pervade all aspects of care. Even beyond infancy, it may be appropriate to interpret protection rather broadly, going beyond the confines of illness, injury and emotional upset. However, it would also be appropriate to delineate its limits before attachment becomes a general term for child–parent relationships. Secondly, for practical reasons it may not be feasible specifically to parse out different functions of relationships, particularly when evaluating caregiver sensitivity. Although it may well be the case that some caregivers are enchanting playmates but unreliable attachment figures, that some are solid attachment figures but inept teachers, and so on, we may also find that sensitivity across these different domains is highly correlated. If so, it would be impossible to extricate sensitivity to protective needs from general sensitivity. This would have important implications for the 'attachment as protection' construct. It would render it an intuitively appealing construct, but one that could not be operationally defined. Attempts to build a broad and differentiated model of parent–child relationships are germane to deciding how feasible and useful it is to limit or extend the attachment construct.

Other boundaries

A second way in which attachment theories may be broad or narrow refers to the range of phenomena affected by attachment. Are its influences limited specifically to close social relationships, to all social behaviours and relationships, or to a wide range of outcomes including achievements beyond the social domain? It is possible that the above confusions about the origins of attachment patterns contribute to an inappropriately broad interpretation of outcomes. As we broaden the definition of attachment, it is natural to expect a broader range of relevant outcomes. We pointed out in Chapter 11 that several attachment researchers have expressed concern that attachment has been linked to such a wide array of developmental phenomena that its original meaning is in danger of becoming diffuse and indistinguishable from that of an indicator of general adjustment (Belsky and Cassidy, 1994; Sroufe, 1983). Belsky and Cassidy (1994) proposed several possible models for the origins and influences of attachment security that vary in the scope of outcomes attributed to attachment. Unfortunately, they note, we do not have enough evidence to choose between them.

A quick review of the previous chapter topics indicates that attachment is thought to play a role in remarkably diverse areas of development. We have discussed relationships within and beyond the family, social competence, emotional and cognitive development, psychopathology and physical health. You may find yourself asking, 'Does attachment organize every-thing? Where are the boundaries of attachment?' Rutter (1997) raised this same question as one that is important for future work on attachment. Lewis (1997), too, has criticized attachment theory as one which 'tries to explain too much and, in doing so, explains little' (p.162). It is unlikely that all of the complexity of social relationships or individual functioning can be reduced to the single concept of attachment. Bowlby himself took great pains to differentiate attachment from other aspects of relationships. Yet he thought of it as the cornerstone of personality development, and hence as relatively broad in its impact. It is natural for a powerful and successful theory to push its borders outward in attempts to discover its limits. However, in the glow of attachment theory's initial successes, other relationships and other aspects of relationships have fallen into the shadows and been neglected. There is much to be gained by efforts to restore the balance.

To consider one example, the AAI has been validated primarily by show-ing that it predicts infant attachment patterns (see Chapter 3). Although we discussed some early threads of evidence that could point to a genetic mode of transmission (see Chapter 5), the general assumption is that the link between adult state of mind with respect to attachment and infant behaviour in the strange situation is via behavioural aspects of caregiving. Reliance on corresponding infant attachment to validate AAI classifications thus suggests that the AAI is actually a marker of caregiving behaviour, rather than an index of adult attachment *per se*. Caregiving, although related to attachment, is an organized behavioural system that merits atten-tion in its own right (George and Solomon, 1999). The appropriate bound-ary between attachment and caregiving could be delineated via two potential lines of work – first, detailed study of the caregiving system and how it is linked to and distinguished from attachment, and secondly, further work on the role of attachment in close relationships in adulthood. Establishing such a boundary promises to enhance our understanding of both constructs.

Confounding methods and constructs

A continuing problem in attachment theory and research lies in the confu-sion of methods and constructs. Most of those planted firmly in attachment research are well aware of the limits of the available methodology. However, as the strange situation gained increasingly wider use and became the 'gold standard' for development of other measures both in infancy and beyond, 'attachment' for many implicitly came to mean 'what the strange situation measures.' Similarly, adult attachment has come to mean 'what the AAI assesses.' The way in which we label individuals 'autonomous' or 'avoidant' very much parallels the way in which we say someone has 'an IQ of 105.'

The original IQ tests were designed to predict ability to succeed in the school system. They did not assess a particular trait, but acquired this implicit definition with usage. Of course, there is nothing inside the person that can be labelled 'IQ', and in the same way there is nothing specific in the person that can be labelled 'secure' or 'dismissing.' The behaviours that lead us to classify a particular attachment pattern are 'markers' that we take to reflect features of a complexly organized system operating in the natural environment.

Some of the negative criticisms directed towards attachment theory are primarily criticisms of the methods, particularly the strange situation (e.g. Lamb *et al.*, 1984). Thus in Chapter 5 we considered the views of those who believe that the strange situation reflects temperamental differences rather than functioning as an indicator of infant–caregiver relationships. In general, these critics do not argue that infant–parent relationships are irrelevant to development. They argue that they are less important than temperamental dispositions, but generally concede a role for caregiving influences in development. However, they argue that the strange situation does not assess either caregiving influences or infant–caregiver relationships. Given that the strange situation has been so central to the development of attachment theory and research, this is potentially a very damaging blow. In fact, behind these criticisms is the implicit suggestion that a theory built on such a shaky foundation must itself be at fault.

Because methods for assessing attachment at later ages are more diverse, and there is less agreement about the 'gold standard' for 3- to 5-year-olds or 7- to 11-year-olds, there is a greater likelihood of relying on multiple measures. Yet the validation of most of these measures continues to depend on concordance with infant attachment assessed in the strange situation. As we pointed out in Chapter 3, this approach to developing new measures assumes that attachment patterns remain stable, an assumption that may not be justified (see below). In fact, while the strange situation has done yeoman service in the initiation of empirical attachment research, there is an inherent danger in basing an entire theoretical edifice on any one assessment procedure. Happily, there have been recent attempts to move the focus of research efforts back to direct observation of attachment phenomena in naturalistic settings (e.g. Waters *et al.*, 1995).

Development of attachment itself (stability and instability of patterns)

Bowlby, and later Ainsworth, described the development of attachment as occurring in four stages which were completed in the preschool years. Thus these early formulations suggested that significant developmental changes were restricted to the first few years of life. Furthermore, as noted in Chapter 3, the capacity to observe patterns of attachment beyond infancy was relatively late to develop. It is not surprising, therefore, that the early wave of empirical enthusiasm was devoted to predicting behaviour in the strange situation and prediction of later competencies from it. Both theoretically and empirically there was an implicit assumption that attachment patterns were not likely to change beyond the early years. Thus there was a wide gap between the theoretical notion of attachment as a lifespan construct and the actual understanding of what happens to attachments beyond the early years.

Two aspects of development can be considered – first, universal developmental changes in attachment behaviour and representations, and secondly, stability/change in individual attachment strategies over time. There is a suggested framework for the former (Waters et al., 1991), but the limited empirical data are primarily relevant to the latter. Although attachment theory acknowledges the possibility that attachment strategies change with changes in circumstances, there has been a greater focus on the propensity of attachment strategies to persist over time. In Chapter 3, we reviewed the evidence regarding stability of attachment and found that it was in fact mixed both for short-term and for long-term studies. Some studies have been able to show relatively high long-term attachment stability under very stable conditions (e.g. Waters et al., 1995). Others have shown that the presence of significant disruptive events predicts attachment instability (Beckwith et al., 1995; Lewis, 1997; Zimmerman, 1994).

It is the old story of the glass that can be half empty or half full. Attachment proponents interpret the data as evidence of stability, while attachment antagonists interpret the data as evidence of instability. However, these findings together with the evidence that 40–70 per cent of adults who are secure on the AAI fall into the 'earned secure' classification and were most probably insecure in childhood (Pearson et al., 1994; Phelps et al., 1998), indicate that – except under very stable life conditions – there is probably considerable change in attachment strategies over the lifespan. The notion that infant attachment initiates a specific developmental line in which strategies are stable for life is theoretically elegant, but no longer seems realistic. Such an acknowledgement suggests that the study of stability and change in attachment strategies over the lifespan is an area that merits attention, and one that has until now been neglected.

In 1991, Grossmann and Grossmann outlined a four-point agenda for attachment research. They included our needs to understand the following processes: (1) the caregiving patterns and caregiver–infant interactions that culminate in individual differences in attachment patterns assessed at 12–18 months in the strange situation; (2) the transformation of these from concrete dyadic interaction patterns to their representations within the individual; (3) stability and change in attachment strategies across the lifespan; and (4) the transmission of attachment patterns from parents to children. Tasks 1 and 4 have been the primary focus of endeavours thus far, with tasks 2 and 3 only recently gaining attention.

A further issue concerns the formation of new attachments beyond infancy. Although a fair amount of effort has been invested in attempts to understand factors that influence the formation of early attachments, there is a paucity of information regarding the initiation of new attachments later on. Yet it is evident that such attachments are formed and play an important role for their participants. Particularly in adulthood, when partners who are similar in experience and knowledge may serve as reciprocal attachment figures, it is not clear what factors are important in establishing and maintaining attachments.

Forms of insecurity

Ainsworth's identification of two different forms of insecure attachment has been described as a true discovery, one that could not have been predicted, for in her early observations the home behaviour of infants who were later found to be avoidant did not differ from that of those later identified as resistant in the strange situation. Once the strange situation revealed differences, Ainsworth and her team could show that the differences observed in the laboratory did have home correlates in both infant and maternal behaviour (see Chapters 4 and 5, respectively). Much of the theorizing about individual differences invokes these two patterns, whether in infancy or in later years, and in fact there is considerable intuitive appeal to these theoretical ideas which we have exploited throughout the previous chapters. The discovery of the disorganized pattern of infant attachment and its later analogues further enriched theorizing about the origins and effects of individual differences in attachment.

However, much of the existing research suffers from an inability to exploit fully the richness of these theoretical ideas. A theme that has been woven into many of the earlier chapters is that the uneven distribution of these patterns has led researchers either to 'lump' insecure cases together or to discard data from the smaller groups, usually the resistant/preoccupied group. Both strategies cast aside valuable information. Although Cassidy and Berlin (1994) devoted a full paper to describing what was known about resistant/preoccupied attachment, our understanding of this type of attachment is still limited. However, it is also the case that studies which retain these distinctions often produce data that do not show the expected differences (see Chapter 13; also Thompson, 1999). Are these failures attributable to lack of power resulting from small group size, inadequate measurement, failure to attend to mediating variables, or unique sample characteristics? Or do we need to reconsider the theoretical predictions? These are important questions for the field.

The reduction of comparisons to those between secure and insecure attachment groups results in simple 'good vs. bad' comparisons and findings that would be predicted by many other theoretical approaches, thus losing much that is unique and appealing about attachment theory. In practice, there is probably no danger of losing the distinctions between different forms of insecure attachment. The less common forms become more prominent in clinical populations, and there are some meaningful links between disorder and specific forms of attachment in these populations (see Chapter 13). Even in community samples there are sometimes surprisingly consistent findings about resistant infants or dependent children (see, for example, the discussion regarding cultural differences in Chapter 7). The focus on secure vs. insecure attachment was a first useful step in many domains, but a broader appreciation of different forms of insecurity is necessary for future endeavours.

Infant determinism

Emphasis on stability has earned attachment theory and research a reputation for focusing on 'infant determinism,' the notion that phenomena occurring in infancy wield a special power over later events (Kagan, 1998; Lewis, 1997). Attachment theory is not alone in emphasizing the importance of the early years. Nevertheless, its critics often attack this premise as one which is unique to attachment theory. Having already established the fact that attachment theory allows for change in attachment strategies *per se* (although proponents have been loath to study these), there are two issues concerning infant determinism – one is whether a first attachment can be formed beyond the normal window of opportunity, and the second issue is how influential this first attachment is in subsequent development.

With regard to the first point, data from both early and recent studies of children reared in harshly depriving conditions have shown us that there is both good news and bad news. The good news is that there is considerable potential for subsequent formation of attachments. The bad news is that a disproportionate number of them are insecure and atypical (see Chapter 8). Thus there is evidence to suggest that it is desirable for the first attachment to be formed in an early developmental period, although the precise limits of this period are not really known. It is also clear from the pioneering work of Dozier and her students (see Chapter 8) that even in infancy, those subjected to grossly inadequate care quickly develop behaviour patterns that present obstacles to sensitive care from normally sensitive parents. Because this work focuses on how attachments are formed after a period of deprivation, they may hold the key to an all-important question, namely why it is that some children are apparently able to recover fully from early deprivation while others do not. Can we identify specific early experiences as positive or negative influences? What are the physiological manifestations or markers of these experiences? What aspects of subsequent care make a difference?

The second issue is the extent to which early attachment 'determines' subsequent development. Most of the research we have reviewed (see Chapters 9 to 13) suggests that the effects of early attachment on later development are reliable but small to moderate. As Thompson (1999) notes, 'The outcomes of attachment security appear to be more contingent and provisional than earlier expected.' Thus early attachment does not by any means 'determine' later development, but rather it makes a unique contribution along with other influences. Proponents of attachment examine these findings and argue that this is consistent with theoretical predictions. Critics of attachment argue that this undermines the theory – attachment is far less important than Bowlby and his early followers thought. Bowlby himself argued both for and against determinism – change is always possible, but change is also constrained by prior adaptation. A favourite analogy reflecting this position (e.g. Sroufe, 1997) is that of the branches of a tree. One may arrive at many different end points from a given starting point, and there are opportunities to cross from one main limb to another via smaller branches. However, the further out one moves on a particular limb, the less likelihood there is of crossing over to other limbs. Thus a particular infant attachment pattern does not determine the end point but weights the likelihood of reaching one end point compared to another.

'Mother blaming'

A common complaint regarding attachment theory is that it unfairly continues a tradition of blaming mothers unduly for their children's successes and failures (e.g. Chess and Thomas, 1982). Bowlby himself sometimes spoke broadly, referring to a 'principal attachment figure,' and other times more narrowly of the 'mother', but in fact, as we noted in Chapter 6, most of the research has been done with mothers. The 'over-representation of mothers' in research and theory reflects the fact that, despite an increasing emphasis on shared parenting, mothers are still 'over-represented' among the primary caregivers of young children. As a result, however, much of the literature repeatedly refers to mothers when the concepts and ideas could also apply to other attachment figures.

Nevertheless, since mothers *are* the primary caregivers of infants in most families, the care they provide for infants and young children *is* important for development. Such an assertion does not necessarily 'blame' mothers. Most parents want the best for their children and make every effort to do the best job they can under the conditions that they face. Through studies of adult attachment and attachment under adversity, we have started to appreciate how the experiences, context, and resources of some mothers compromise their ability to be the parents they would like to be. Research on attachment as well as related domains in child development has enabled us to appreciate the complexity and power of the factors that impinge on parents' abilities to care for young children. We have considered some of these in Chapter 8. What is perhaps most remarkable about the findings of the research reviewed there is that the majority of mothers rise to meet the challenges of infant illness, infant prior deprivation and poverty.

Nevertheless, Bowlby did emphasize the importance of a consistent care-giver over the first few years of life, and although he conceded that this person did not have to be the mother, popular interpretation has placed this burden squarely on the shoulders of mothers. In part this reflects not only the findings or teachings of attachment theory, but also popular attitudes in most cultures (see Chapter 7).

Thus, the idea that early day care could result in an increase in avoidant attachment (Chapter 7) did in fact make some mothers feel guilty, and led some researchers to express concerns about generating such guilt. Although more recent careful research suggests that much of this guilt was unnecessary, it is likely to persist despite newer findings, in part because most cultures continue to believe that young children should be at home with their mothers.

To muddy the issue further, some of the popular literature confuses the notion of 'bonding' introduced by Klaus and Kennell (1976) with that of attachment. The concept of bonding was introduced to describe the development of parents' emotional ties to their children, and attention was focused on ways in which opportunities for close contact in the immediate postpartum period benefited the bonding process. These ideas, like the early Bowlby–Robertson work on hospitalization, brought about some positive changes in hospital practices at deliveries, and produced a highly controversial literature. It is not unusual to find magazine or newspaper headlines using the term 'bonding' to refer to attachment. Such confusions do a disservice to both constructs, but they also highlight the value of having those based in the research community speaking directly to the public as well as to their colleagues. Many attachment researchers (myself included) have been reluctant to take on this responsibility.

The nature of internal working models

For much of the early history of attachment theory, the notion of internal working models, although attractive as a mechanism for carrying early experiences forward, provided not much more than a 'black box' that explained little. In recent years theorists have started to peer into the black box in order to discern what might be inside. A 1999 summary of what is known about internal working models of attachment (Bretherton and Munholland, 1999) still leaves many questions unanswered, and suggests that the following five areas concerned with development, integration and operation of working models need attention: (1) developmental changes in child–parent relationships as a function of the child's acquisition of attribution-making and perspective-taking skills; (2) development/integration of the self where early attachment classifications with the two parents are discordant; (3) the mutual negotiation/construction of adult attachment relationships, particularly between partners with discordant attachment status; (4) the development of a coherent attachment biography among those with in-secure childhoods; and (5) the regulatory role of representation in attach-ment relationships. Clearly, there is much to learn about what internal working models of attachment are, how they preserve attachment-related information, and how this information is organized and functions to regu-late new experiences.

It is not difficult to add to this list. For example, we can point to the repeated assertion that, in infancy, attachment relationships with different caregivers are distinct. Yet in adulthood, the AAI, an interview which covers childhood experiences with both parents (and other significant caregivers), is thought to reflect a 'state of mind' with respect to attachment not ordi-narily differentiated by relationship. How this integration occurs remains a largely unstudied puzzle.

A central question is that of the status of internal working models. Because we cannot observe working models directly and must make infer-ences from their 'products' (e.g. drawings, narratives, social behaviour and self-reports), we need to consider the nature of their existence. To what extent do such models exist beyond serving as a useful explanatory con-struct? Are there physiologically identifiable structures or processes for the cognitive and emotional components of internal working models of attach-ment? Recent developments in neuroscience do indeed suggest that some such structures and processes exist. We briefly introduced some of this information in Chapter 12, and Main (1999) has suggested potential experiments in the neuroscience and physiology of attachment that could prove illuminating. What we described above as the 'third phase' of theorizing and empirical research focused on internal working models is well under way. Will the 'fourth phase' involve the psychophysiology of attachment? A considerable amount of hard work lies ahead if the construct of internal working models is to fulfil its promise as an explana-tory construct.

In retrospect

At the start of this volume we referred to the popular notion that parent–child relationships play a central role in children's psychological develop-ment. We noted that prior to the development of attachment theory it had been difficult to support this common belief with empirical evidence. The evidence we have reviewed here indicates that the effects of attachment *per se* are highly reliable, but that they are small to moderate rather than large. Early attachment is less influential and also more modifiable than we once thought. Does this amount to a central role in development? This is probably the place to remind ourselves that attachment is only part of the parent–child relationship. We have not concerned ourselves with parents as playmates, disciplinarians, teachers, role models or sources of stimulation, among others. Attachment theory and research advances, but does not exhaust, our understanding of the place of parent–child relationships in development.

John Bowlby died in 1990 and Mary Ainsworth in 1999. In their lifetimes they revolutionized the way in which we think about and observe young children and their parents. They transformed the passive infant who was either a 'blank slate' to be written on or a seething mass of uncontrollable drives to be contained, into a creature who is biased to become sociable and will readily do so when given sensitive care. They transformed early attachment from a child-like preoccupation that impeded autonomous exploration into a source of confidence (a secure base) that provided the very foundation of autonomous exploration. In the new millennium, their intellectual children, grandchildren and great-grandchildren will carry on a respected tradition. They inherit a legacy of many accomplishments, some early promises yet to be fulfilled, and some formidable challenges.

Suggested reading

Lamb, M.E., Thompson, R.A., Gardner, W.P., Charnov, E.L. and Estes, D. (1984) Security of infantile attachment as assessed in the 'strange situation': its study and biological interpretation. *Behavioral and Brain Sciences*, 7, 127–72.
An early critique of the strange situation followed by commentaries. Interestingly, of the major attachment researchers of the time, only Klaus and Karin Grossmann responded with comments.

Main, M. (1999) Epilogue: attachment theory: eighteen points with suggestions for future studies. In Cassidy, J. and Shaver, P.R. (Eds), *Handbook of attachment*. New York: Guilford Press, 845–88.
A look at emerging issues in the field, written by one of its leading theorists.

Rutter, M. (1997) Clinical implications of attachment constructs: retrospect and prospect. In Atkinson, L. and Zucker, K.J. (Eds), *Attachment and psychopathology*. New York: Guilford Press, 17–46.
A critical evaluation of attachment theory and research, written by an eminent clinician-researcher.

References

Ackerman, S.H., Hofer, M.A. and Wiener, H. (1975) Age at separation and gastric erosion in the rat. *Psychosomatic Medicine* **37**, 180–84.

Adam, E.K. (1998) Emotional and physiological stress in mothers of toddlers: an adult attachment model. Unpublished doctoral dissertation, University of Minnesota, Minneapolis, MN.

Adam, E.K. Pierce, S.L., Holland, J.F, Desmond, E. and Gunnar, M.R. (1996) Cognitive and physiological correlates of internal working models. Presented at the International Society for the Study of Behavioral Development, Quebec City, Canada, August 1996.

Adam, K., Sheldon-Keller, A.E. and West, M. (1995) Attachment organization and vulnerability to loss, separation, and abuse in disturbed adolescents. In Goldberg, S., Muir, R. and Kerr, J. (Eds), *Attachment theory: social developmental and clinical perspectives*. Hillsdale, NJ: The Analytic Press, 309–43.

Adam, K., Sheldon-Keller, A.E. and West, M. (1996) Attachment organization and history of suicidal behavior in adolescents. *Journal of Consulting and Clinical Psychology* **64**, 264–92.

Ainsworth, M.D.S. (1967) Infancy in Uganda: child care and the growth of love. Baltimore, MD: Johns Hopkins University Press.

Ainsworth, M.D.S. (1969) Object relations, dependency, and attachment: A theoretical review of the infant–mother relationship. *Child Development* **40**, 969–1026.

Ainsworth, M.D.S. (1973) The development of infant–mother attachment. In Caldwell, B.M. and Ricciuti, H.N. (Eds), *Review of child development research. Vol. 3. Child development and social policy*. Chicago: University of Chicago Press, 21–94.

Ainsworth, M.D.S. (1977) Infant development and mother–infant interaction among Ganda and American families. In Leiderman, P.H., Tulkin, S.R. and Rosenfield, A. (Eds), *Culture and infancy*. New York: Academic Press, 119–50.

Ainsworth, M.D.S. and Bell, S.M. (1977) Infant crying and maternal responsiveness: a rejoinder to Gewirtz and Boyd. *Child Development* **48**, 1208–16.

Ainsworth, M.D.S., Blehar, M.C., Waters, E. and Wall, S. (1978) *Patterns of attachment*. Hillsdale, NJ: Lawrence Erlbaum.

Ainsworth, M.D.S. and Eichberg, C. (1991) Effects on infant–mother attachment of mother's unresolved loss of an attachment figure or other traumatic experience. In Parkes, C.M., Stevenson-Hinde, J. and Marris, P. (Eds), *Attachment across the life cycle*. London: Routledge, 160–83.

Ainsworth, M.D.S. and Marvin, R.S. (1995) On the shaping of attachment theory and research: an interview with Mary D.S. Ainsworth (Fall 1994). In Waters, E., Vaughn, B.E., Posada, G. and Kondo-Ikemura, K. (Eds), Caregiving, cultural and cognitive perspectives on secure-base behavior and working models. *Monographs of the Society for Research in Child Development* **60**, 3–24.

Ainsworth, M.D.S. and Wittig, B.A. (1969) Attachment and exploratory behavior of one-year-olds in a strange situation. In Foss, B.M. (Ed.), *Determinants of infant behaviour. IV.* London: Methuen, 113–36.

Alfasi, A., Schwartz, F.A., Brake, S.C., Fifer, W.P., Fleischman, A.R. and Hofer, M. (1985) Mother–infant feeding interaction in preterm and full-term infants. *Infant Behavior and Development* **8**, 167–80.

Allen, J.P., Hauser, S.T. and Borman-Spurrell, E. (1996) Attachment theory as a framework for understanding sequelae of severe adolescent psychopathology: an 11-year follow-up study. *Journal of Clinical and Consulting Psychology* **64**, 254–63.

Anisfeld, E., Casper, V., Nozyce, M. and Cunningham, N. (1990) Does infant-carrying promote attachment? An experimental study of the effects of increased physical contact on the development of attachment. *Child Development* **61**, 1617–27.

Arend, R., Gove, F. and Sroufe, L.A. (1979) Continuity of individual adaptation from infancy to kindergarten: a predictive study of ego resiliency and curiosity in preschoolers. *Child Development* **50**, 950–59.

Atkinson, L., Chisholm, V.C., Scott, B. *et al.* (1999a) Maternal sensitivity, child functional level and attachment in Down syndrome. In Vondra, J. and Barnett, D. (Eds), Atypical attachment in infancy and early childhood. *Monographs of the Society for Research in Child Development* **64** (258), 45–66.

Atkinson, L., Goldberg, S. and Gotowiec, A. (1999) Attachment and behaviour problems in early childhood: a meta-analysis. Unpublished manuscript, Center for Mental Health and Addiction, Toronto, ON.

Atkinson, L., Kerr, S., Benoit, D. and Poulton, L. (1998) Adult attachment and information-processing. Paper presented at the Waterloo Conference on Child Development, Waterloo, ON, May 1998.

Atkinson, L., and Zucker, K. (1997) *Attachment and psychopathology.* New York: Guilford Press.

Bakermans-Kranenburg, M.J. and van IJzendoorn, M.H. (1993) A psychometric study of the Adult Attachment Interview: reliability and discriminant validity. *Developmental Psychology* **29**, 870–79.

Barnard, K.E., Bee, H.L. and Hammond, M.A. (1984) Development of changes in maternal interaction with term and preterm infants. *Infant Behavior and Development* **7**, 101–13.

Barnas, M.V., Pollina, L. and Cummings, E.M. (1991) Lifespan attachment: relations between attachment and socioemotional functioning in adult women. *Genetic, Social and General Psychology Monographs* **11**, 177–202.

Barnett, D., Ganiban, J. and Cicchetti, D. (1992) Temperament and behavior of youngsters with disorganized attachments: a longitudinal study. Presented at the International Conference on Infant Studies, Miami, FL, April 1992.

Bartholomew, K. and Horowitz, L. (1991) Attachment styles among young adults: a test of a four-category model. *Journal of Personality and Social Psychology* **61**, 226–44.

Bates, J.E. (1980) The concept of difficult temperament. *Merrill-Palmer Quarterly* **26**, 111–30.

Bates, J.E. (1987) Temperament in infancy. In Osofsky, J.D. (Ed.), *Handbook of infant development*, 2nd edn. New York: John Wiley, 1101–49.

Bates, J.E., Maslin, C.A. and Frankel, K.A. (1985) Attachment and the development of behavior problems. In Bretherton, I. and E. Waters, E. (Eds), Growing points of attachment theory and research. *Monographs of the Society for Research in Child Development* **50**, 167–93.

Bateson, P.P.G. (1966) The characteristics and context of imprinting. *Biological Review* **41**, 177–220.

Beckwith, L., Cohen, S.E. and Hamilton, C.E. (1995) Mother–infant interaction and divorce predict attachment representation at late adolescence. Presented at the Meeting of the Society for Research in Child Development, Indianapolis, IN, March 1995.

Beckwith, L. and Rodning, C. (1991) Stability in attachment from 13 to 36 months. Paper presented at Meeting of the Society for Research in Child Development, Seattle, WA.

Bell, S.M.V. (1970) The development of the concept of the object as related to infant–mother attachment. *Child Development* **40**, 291–311.

Bell, S.M.V. and Ainsworth, M.D.S. (1972) Infant crying and maternal responsiveness. *Child Development* **43**, 1171–90.

Belsky, J. (1986) Infant day care: a cause for concern? *Zero to Three* **6**, 1–7.

Belsky, J. (1988) The effects of infant day care reconsidered. *Early Childhood Research Quarterly* **3**, 235–72.

Belsky, J. (1996) Parent, infant and social-contextual antecedents of father–son attachment security. *Developmental Psychology* **32**, 905–13.

Belsky, J. (1997) Variation in susceptibility to environmental influence: an evolutionary argument. *Psychological Inquiry* **8**, 82–186.

Belsky, J. and Braungart, J. (1991) Are insecure-avoidant infants with extensive day care experience less stressed by and more independent in the strange situation? *Child Development* **62**, 567–71.

Belsky, J., Campbell, S.B., Cohn, J.F. and Moore, G. (1996a) Instability of infant–parent attachment security. *Developmental Psychology* **32**, 921–4.

Belsky, J. and Cassidy, J. (1994) Attachment: theory and evidence. In Rutter, M. and Hay, D. (Eds), *Development through life*. London: Blackwell Science, 373–402.

Belsky, J., Garduque, L. and Hrncir, E. (1984) Assessing performance, competence and executive capacity in infant play: relations to home environment and security of attachment. *Developmental Psychology* **21**, 406–17.

Belsky, J., Gilstrap, B. and Rovine, M.J. (1984) The Pennsylvania Infant and Family Development Project. I. Stability and change in mother–infant and father–infant interaction in a family setting at one, three and nine months. *Child Development* **55**, 692–705.

Belsky, J. and Isabella, R. (1988) Maternal, infant and social contextual determinants of attachment security. In Belsky, J. and Nezworksi, T. (Eds), *Clinical implications of attachment*. Hillsdale, NJ: Erlbaum, 41–94.

Belsky, J. and Nezworski, T. (1988) *Clinical implications of attachment*. Hillsdale, NJ: Erlbaum.

Belsky, J., Rosenberger, K. and Crnic, K. (1995) The origins of attachment security: 'classical' and 'contextual' determinants. In Goldberg, S., Muir, R. and Kerr, J. (Eds), *Attachment theory: social, developmental and clinical perspectives*. Hillsdale, NJ: The Analytic Press, 153–84.

Belsky, J. and Rovine, M.J. (1987) Temperament and attachment security in the strange situation: an empirical *rapprochement*. *Child Development* **58**, 787–95.

Belsky, J. and Rovine, M.J. (1988) Nonmaternal care in the first year of life and the security of infant–parent attachment. *Child Development* **59**, 157–67.

Belsky, J., Rovine, M.J. and Taylor, D.G. (1984) The Pennsylvania Infant and Family Project. III. The origins of individual differences in infant–mother attachment: maternal and infant contributions. *Child Development* **55**, 718–28.

Belsky, J., Spritz, B. and Crnic, K. (1996b) Infant attachment security and affective-cognitive information processing at age 3. *Psychological Science* **7**, 111–14.

Belsky, J. and Steinberg, L. (1978) The effects of day care: a critical review. *Child Development* **49**, 929–49.

Belsky, J., Steinberg, L. and Draper, P. (1991) Childhood experience, interpersonal development and reproductive strategy: an evolutionary theory of socialization. *Child Development* **62**, 647–70.

Belsky, J. and Volling, B.L. (1986) Mothering, fathering and marital interactions in the family triad: exploring family systems processes. In Berman, P. and Pedersen, F. (Eds), *Mens' transition to parenthood: longitudinal studies of early family experience.* Hillsdale, NJ: Erlbaum, 37–63.

Bender, L. and Yarnell, H. (1941). An observation nursery (a study of 250 children on the Psychiatric Division of Bellevue Hospital). *Proceedings of the 96th Annual Meeting of the American Psychiatric Association.* Washington, DC: American Psychiatric Association, 1158–74.

Benoit, D. and Parker, K.C.H. (1994) Stability and transmission of attachment across three generations. *Child Development* **65**, 1444–56.

Benoit, D., Parker, K.C.H. and Zeanah, C.H. (1997) Mothers' representation of their infants assessed prenatally: stability and association with infants' attachment classifications. *Journal of Child Psychiatry and Psychology* **38**, 307–13.

Benoit, D., Zeanah, C. and Barton, M. (1989) Maternal attachment disturbances in failure to thrive. *Infant Mental Health Journal* **10**, 185–202.

Berger, S.P. and Damberg, K.R. (1997) Research, clinical practice, behavioural pediatrics and developmental psychology: interlocking the pieces of the puzzle. Presented at the Symposium on Interdisciplinary Reciprocity: Behavioural Pediatrics and Developmental Psychology at the Biennial Meeting of the Society for Research in Child Development, Washington, DC, April 1997.

Berlin, L. and Cassidy, J. (1996) Mothers' self-reported control of their preschool children's emotional expressiveness: associations with infant–mother attachment and children's emotion regulation. Unpublished manuscript, Columbia University.

Bijou, S.W. and Baer, D.M. (1965) *Child development. Vol. 2.* New York: Appleton-Century-Crofts, 1965.

Birkenfield-Adams, A. (1999) Quality of attachment in young boys with gender identity disorder: a comparison to clinic and non-referred control boys. Unpublished doctoral dissertation, York University, Toronto, ON.

Blokland, K. (1993) Infant attachment and three-year emotional expression. Unpublished Masters Thesis, University of Toronto, ON.

Blokland, K. (1999) Maternal attachment and response to infant affect. Unpublished doctoral dissertation, University of Toronto.

Blokland, K. and Goldberg, S. (1998) Attachment and expectant mothers' perceptions of emotion. In *Symposium on Emotional Development: perspectives on the role of maternal perceptions of emotion and internal working models of attachment.* International Conference on Infant Studies, Atlanta, GA, April 1998.

Boccia, M.L., Laudenslager, M.L. and Reite, M.L. (1994) Intrinsic and extrinsic factors affect infant responses to separation. *Psychiatry: Interpersonal and Biological Processes* **57**, 123–30.

Borman-Spurrell, E. Allen, J., Häuser, S., Carter, A. and Cole-Detke, H. (1994) Attachment in young adulthood: how different measures of adult attachment relate to adjustment. Unpublished manuscript, Harvard University.

Bosso, O.R. (1985) Attachment quality and sibling relations: responses of anxiously attached/avoidant and securely attached 18- to 32-month-old firstborns toward their second-born siblings. Unpublished doctoral dissertation, Psychology Department, University of Toronto, Toronto, ON.

Bower, T.G.R. (1975) The object in the world of the infant. In Atkinson, R.C. (Ed.), *Psychology in progress.* San Francisco, CA: W.H. Freeman, 42–50.

Bowlby, J. (1944) Forty-four juvenile thieves: their characters and home lives. *International Journal of Psychoanalysis* **25**, 19–52.

Bowlby, J. (1951) *Maternal care and mental health*. Geneva: World Health Organization.

Bowlby, J. (1953) *Child care and the growth of maternal love*. Harmondsworth: Penguin Books.

Bowlby, J. (1958) The nature of the child's tie to his mother. *International Journal of Psychoanalysis* **3**, 1–23.

Bowlby, J. (1959) Separation anxiety. *International Journal of Psychoanalysis* **41**, 1–25.

Bowlby, J. (1960) Grief and mourning in infancy and early childhood. *The Psychoanalytic Study of the Child* **15**, 3–39.

Bowlby, J. (1969) *Attachment and loss. Vol. 1. Attachment*. New York: Basic Books.

Bowlby, J. (1973) *Attachment and loss. Vol. 2. Separation, anxiety and anger*. New York: Basic Books.

Bowlby, J. (1980) *Attachment and loss. Vol. 3. Loss, sadness and depression*. New York: Basic Books.

Bowlby, J. (1988) *A secure base*. New York: Basic Books.

Boyce, W.T. and Jemerin, J.J. (1990) Psychobiological differences in childhood stress response. 1. Patterns of illness and susceptibility. *Journal of Developmental and Behavioral Pediatrics* **11**, 86–94.

Brachfeld, S., Goldberg, S. and Sloman, J. (1980) Prematurity and immaturity as influences on parent–infant interaction at 8 and 12 months. *Infant Behavior and Development* **3**, 289–306.

Brazelton, T.B. (1973) *Neonatal behavioural assessment scale. Clinics in developmental medicine. No. 50*. Philadelphia, PA: J.B. Lippincott Co. and Spastics International Medical Publications.

Bretherton, I. (1985) Attachment theory: retrospect and prospect. In Bretherton, I. and Waters, E. (Eds), Growing points of attachment theory and research. *Monographs of the Society for Research in Child Development* **50**, 3–38.

Bretherton, I. (1990) Open communication and internal working models: Their role in attachment relationships. In Thompson, R. (Ed.), *Socioemotional development. Nebraska Symposium on Motivation. Vol. 36*. Lincoln, NB: University of Nebraska Press, 57–113.

Bretherton, I. (1991) Pouring new wine into old bottles: the social self as internal working model. In Gunnar, M.R. and Sroufe, L.A. (Eds), *Minnesota Symposium on Child Psychology. Vol. 23. Self-processes in development*. Hillsdale, NJ: Erlbaum, 1–41.

Bretherton, I. (1992) The origins of attachment theory: John Bowlby and Mary Ainsworth. *Developmental Psychology* **28**, 759–75.

Bretherton, I., Bates, E., Benigni, L., Camaioni, L. and Volterra, V. (1979) Relationships between cognition, communication and quality of attachment. In Bates, E. (Ed.), *The emergence of symbols: validity of a social construction orientation*. New York: Academic Press, 223–69.

Bretherton, I., Fritz, J., Zahn-Waxler, C. and Ridgeway, D. (1986) Learning to talk about emotion: a functionalist perspective. *Child Development* **56**, 530–48.

Bretherton, I., McNew, S. and Beeghly-Smith, M. (1981) Early person knowledge as expressed in gestural and verbal communication: when do infants acquire a 'theory of mind?' In Lamb, M.E. and Sherrod, L.R. (Eds), Infant social cognition. Hillsdale, NJ: Erlbaum, 126–54.

Bretherton, I. and Munholland, K.A. (1999) Internal working models in attachment relationships. In Cassidy, J. and Shaver, P.R. (Eds), *Handbook of attachment*. New York: Guilford Press, 89–114.

Bretherton, I., Ridgeway, D. and Cassidy, J. (1990) Assessing internal working models of the attachment relationship: an attachment story completion task for 3-year-olds. In Greenberg, M.T., Cicchetti, D. and Cummings, E.M. (Eds), *Attachment in the preschool years*. Chicago: University of Chicago Press, 273–310.

Bretherton, I., Walsh, R., Lependorf, M. and Georgeson, H. (1997) Attachment networks in post-divorce families: the maternal perspective. In Atkinson, L. and Zucker, K. (Eds), *Attachment and psychopathology*. New York: Guildford Press, 97–134.

Bridges, L.J., Connell, J.P. and Belsky, J. (1988) Similarities and differences in infant–mother and infant–father interaction in the strange situation: a component analysis. *Developmental Psychology* **24**, 92–100.

Brinich, E., Drotar, D. and Brinich, P. (1989) Security of attachment and outcome of preschoolers with history of nonorganic failure to thrive. *Journal of Clinical Psychology* **18**, 142–52.

Byng-Hall, J. (1990) Attachment theory and family therapy: a clinical view. *Infant Mental Health Journal* **11**, 228–36.

Byng-Hall, J. and Stevenson-Hinde, J. (1991) Attachment relationships within a family system. *Infant Mental Health Journal* **12**, 187–200.

Caldera, Y., Huston, A. and O'Brien, M. (1995) Antecedents of father–infant attachment: a longitudinal study. Paper presented at the Meeting of the Society for Research in Child Development, Indianapolis, IN, April 1995.

Calkins, S.D. (1994) Origins and outcomes of individual differences in emotion regulation. In Fox, N.A. (Ed.), The development of emotion regulation: biological and behavioral considerations. *Monographs of the Society for Research in Child Development* **59**, 53–72.

Calkins, S.D. and Fox, N. A. (1992) The relations among infant temperament, security of attachment, and behavioral inhibition at twenty-four months. *Child Development* **63**, 1456–72.

Carey, W.B. and McDevitt, S.C. (1978) Revision of the infant temperament questionnaire. *Pediatrics* **61**, 735–9.

Carlson, E.A. (1998) A prospective longitudinal study of attachment disorganization/disorientation. *Child Development* **69**, 1107–29.

Carlson, V., Cicchetti, D., Barnett, D. and Braunwald, K. (1989) Disorganized/disoriented attachment relationships in maltreated infants. *Developmental Psychology* **25**, 525–31.

Case, R. (1995) The role of psychological defenses in the representation and regulation of close personal relationships across the lifespan. In Noam, G. and Fisher, K. (Eds), *Development and vulnerability in close relationships*. Hillsdale, NJ: Erlbaum, 59–88.

Cassidy, J. (1988) Child–mother attachment and the self in six-year-olds. *Child Development* **59**, 121–34.

Cassidy, J. (1994) Emotion regulation: influences of attachment relationships. In Fox, N.A. (Ed.), The development of emotion regulation: biological and behavioral considerations. *Monographs of the Society for Research in Child Development* **59**, 228–49.

Cassidy, J. and Berlin, L.J. (1994) The insecure/ambivalent pattern of attachment: theory and research. *Child Development* **65**, 971–91.

Cassidy, J. and Kobak, R.R. (1988) Avoidance and its relation to other defensive processes. In Belsky, J. and Nezworski, T. (Eds), *Clinical implications of attachment*. Hillsdale, NJ: Erlbaum, 300–326.

Cassidy, J., Marvin, R.S. and the MacArthur Working Group (1987, 1992) *Attachment organization in preschool children: procedures and coding manual*. Unpublished document, University of Virginia.

Cassidy, J. and Shaver, P.R. (1999) Preface. In Cassidy, J. and Shaver, P.R. (Eds), *Handbook of attachment*. New York: Guildford Press, x–xiv.

Chandler, M. (1988) Doubt and developing theories of mind. In Astington, J.W., Harris, P.L. and Olsson, D. (Eds.), *Developing theories of mind*. Cambridge: Cambridge University Press, 387–413.

Chase-Lansdale, P.L. and Owen, M.T. (1987) Maternal employment in a family context: effects on infant–mother and infant–father attachments. *Child Development* **58**, 1505–12.

Chatoor, I., Ganiban, J., Colin, V., Plummer, N. and Harmon, R.J. (1998) Attachment and feeding problems: a re-examination of non-organic failure to thrive and attachment security. *Journal of the American Academy of Child and Adolescent Psychiatry* **37**, 1217–24.

Chess, S. and Thomas, A. (1982) Infant bonding: mystique and reality. *American Journal of Orthopsychiatry* **52**, 213–22.

Chisholm, K. (1998) A three-year follow-up of attachment and indiscriminate friendliness in children adopted from Romanian orphanages. *Child Development* **69**, 1092–106.

Chisholm, K., Carter, M., Ames, E.W., and Morison, S.J. (1995) Attachment security and indiscriminately friendly behavior in children adopted from Romanian orphanages. *Development and Psychopathology* **7**, 283–94.

Chrousos, G.P. and Gold, P.W. (1992) The concepts of stress and stress system disorders. Overview of physical and behavioural homeostasis. *Journal of the American Medical Association* **267**, 1244–52.

Cicchetti, D. and Barnett, D. (1991) Attachment organization in maltreated preschoolers. *Development and Psychopathology* **4**, 397–411.

Cicchetti, D. and Beeghly, M. (1990) An organizational approach to the study of Down syndrome: contributions to an integrative theory of development. In Cicchetti, D. and Beeghly, M. (Eds), *Children with Down syndrome: a developmental perspective*. New York: Cambridge University Press, 29–62.

Cicchetti, D., Rogosch, F.A. and Toth, S. (1998) Maternal depressive disorder and contextual risk: contributions to the development of attachment insecurity and behavior problems in toddlerhood. *Development and Psychopathology* **10**, 283–300.

Cicchetti, D. and Serafica, F. (1981) Interplay among behavioral systems: Illustrations from the study of attachment, affiliation and wariness in young children with Down's syndrome. *Developmental Psychology* **17**, 36–49.

Cicchetti, D. and Sroufe, L.A. (1978) An organizational view of affect. In Lewis, M. and Rosenblum, L.A. (Eds), *The development of affect*. London: Plenum, 309–50.

Ciechanowski, P., Dwight, M., Katon, W. and Rivera-Ball, D. (1998) Attachment classifications associated with unexplained medical symptoms in patients with chronic hepatitis C. Paper presented at the Second International Conference on Attachment and Psychopathology, Toronto, ON, October 1998.

Ciechanowski, P., Katon, W. and Hirsch, I. (1999) Attachment style and adherence in the diabetic patient. *Psychosomatic Medicine* **61**, 110.

Clarke-Stewart, K.A. (1978) And Daddy makes three: the father's impact on the mother and young child. *Child Development* **49**, 466–79.

Clarke-Stewart, K.A. (1988) The effects of day care reconsidered. *Early Childhood Research Quarterly* **3**, 293–318.

Clarke-Stewart, K.A. (1989) Infant day care: maligned or malignant? *American Psychologist* **44**, 266–73.

Clarke-Stewart, K.A. and Fein, G. (1983) Early childhood programs. In Haith, M.M. and Campos, J.J. (Eds), *Handbook of child psychology. Vol. 2. Infancy and developmental psychobiology.* New York: John Wiley, 917–99.

Coe, C.L., Glass, J.C., Wiener, S.G. and Levine, S. (1983) Behavioral but not physiological adaptation to repeated separation in mother and infant primates. *Psychoneuroendocrinology* **8**, 401–9.

Cohen, J. (1992) A power primer. *Psychological Bulletin* **112**, 155–9.

Cohen, L. and Campos, J. (1974) Father, mother and stranger as elicitors of attachment behaviours in infancy. *Developmental Psychology* **10**, 146–54.

Cohn, D. (1990) Mother–child attachment of six-year-olds and social competence at school. *Child Development* **61**, 152–62.

Cohn, D., Silver, D., Cowan, P., Cowan, C. and Pearson, J. (1992) Working models of attachment and couples relationships. *Journal of Family Issues* **13**, 432–99.

Cole, P.M. (1985) Display rules and the socialization of affective displays. In Zivin, G. (Ed.), *The development of expressive behavior: biology environment interactions.* New York: Academic Press, 269–90.

Cole-Detke, H. and Kobak, R. (1996) Attachment processes in eating disorder and depression. *Journal of Clinical and Consulting Psychology* **64**, 282–90.

Colin, V.L. (1987) Infants' preferences between parents before and after moderate stress activates attachment behaviour. Paper presented at the Meeting of the Society for Research in Child Development, Baltimore, MD, April 1987.

Collins, N.L. and Read, S.J. (1990) Adult attachment, working models, and relationship quality in dating couples. *Journal of Personality and Social Psychology* **58**, 644–63.

Cowan, C., Cowan, P., Coie, L. and Coie, J. (1978) Becoming a family: the impact of the first child's birth on the couple's relationship. In Miller, W. and Newman, L. (Eds), *The first child and family formation.* Chapel Hill, NC: Carolina Population Center, 295–324.

Cox, M.J., Owen, M.T., Henderson, V.K. and Margand, N.A. (1992) Prediction of infant–father and infant–mother attachment. *Developmental Psychology* **28**, 474–83.

Craik, K. (1943) *The nature of explanation.* Cambridge: Cambridge University Press.

Crawford, J.W. (1982) Mother–infant interaction in premature and full-term infants. *Child Development* **53**, 957–62.

Crittenden, P.M. (1985) Social networks, quality of parenting, and child development. *Child Development* **56**, 1299–313.

Crittenden, P.M. (1987) Nonorganic failure to thrive: deprivation or distortion? *Infant Mental Health Journal* **8**, 51–64.

Crittenden, P.M. (1988) Relationships at risk. In Belsky, J. and Nezworski, T. (Eds), *Clinical implications of attachment.* Hillsdale, NJ: Erlbaum, 136–74.

Crittenden, P.M. (1992) Quality of attachment in the preschool years. *Development and Psychopathology* **4**, 209–41.

Crittenden, P.M. (1995) Attachment and psychopathology. In Goldberg, S. Muir, R. and Kerr, J. (Eds), *Attachment theory: social, developmental, and clinical perspectives.* Hillsdale, NJ: The Analytic Press, 367–406.

Crittenden, P.M., Partridge, M.F. and Clausen, A.H. (1991) Family patterns of relationship in normative and dysfunctional families. *Development and Psychopathology* **3**, 491–512.

Crockenberg, S.B. (1981) Infant irritability, maternal support and social support influences on the security of infant–mother attachment. *Child Development* **52**, 857–69.

Crowell, J. (1990) *Current Relationship Interview.* Unpublished manuscript, State University of New York, Stony Brook, NY.

Crowell, J. and Treboux, D. (1995) A review of adult attachment measures: implications for theory and research. *Social Development* 4, 294–327.

Crowell, J., Waters, E., Treboux, D. *et al.* (1996) Discriminant validity of the Adult Attachment Interview. *Child Development* 67, 2584–90.

Cummings, E.M. and Cicchetti, D. (1990) Toward a transactional model of relations between attachment and depression. In Greenberg, M.T., Cicchetti, D. and Cummings, E.M. (Eds), *Attachment in the preschool years.* Chicago: University of Chicago Press, 339–72.

Cummings, E.M. and Davies, P. (1994) *Children and marital conflict.* New York: Guilford Press.

Davis, K., Kirkpatrick, L., Levy, M. and O'Hearn, R. (1994) Stalking the elusive love style: attachment styles, love styles, and relational development. In Erber, R. and Gilmour, R. (Eds), *Theoretical frameworks for personal relationships.* Hillsdale, NJ: Erlbaum, 179–210.

Del Carmen, R., Pederson, F.A., Huffman, L.C. and Bryan, Y.E. (1993) Dyadic distress management predicts subsequent security of attachment. *Infant Behavior and Development* 16, 131–47.

Demos, V. (1986) Crying in early infancy: an illustration of the motivational function of affect. In Brazelton, T.B. and Yogman, M. (Eds), *Affect and early infancy.* New York: Ablex, 39–73.

DeMulder, E.K. and Radke-Yarrow, M. (1991) Attachment with affectively ill and well mothers: concurrent behavioral correlates. *Developmental and Psychopathology* 3, 227–42.

De Wolff, M.S. and van IJzendoorn, M.H. (1997) Sensitivity and attachment: a meta-analysis on parental antecedents of infant attachment. *Child Development* 68, 571–91.

Dodge, K.A. (1989) Coordinating responses to aversive stimuli: introduction to special section on development of emotion regulation. *Developmental Psychology* 25, 339–42.

Dollard, J. and Miller, N.E. (1950) *Personality and psychotherapy.* New York: McGraw-Hill.

Donovan, W. and Leavitt, L. (1985) Physiologic assessment of mother–infant attachment. *Journal of the American Academy of Child Psychiatry* 24, 65–70.

Dozier, M., Cue, K. and Barnett, L. (1994). Clinicians as caregivers: the role of attachment organization in treatment. *Journal of Consulting and Clinical Psychology* 62, 793–800.

Dozier, M. and Kobak, R.R. (1992) Psychophysiology in attachment interviews: converging evidence for deactivating strategies. *Child Development* 63, 1473–80.

Dozier, M. and Lee, S.W. (1995) Discrepancies between self- and other-report of psychiatric symptomatology: effects of dismissing attachment strategies. *Development and Psychopathology* 7, 217–26.

Dozier, M., Stevenson, A., Lee, S.W. and Velligan, D. (1991) Attachment organization and familial overinvolvement for adults with serious psychopathological disorders. *Development and Psychopathology* 3, 475–89.

Dozier, M., Stovall, K.C. and Albus, K. (1999) Attachment and psychopathology in adulthood. In Cassidy, J. and Shaver, P.R. (Eds), *Handbook of attachment theory and research.* New York: Guilford Press, 497–519.

Dunn, J. and Kendrick, C. (1982) Siblings and their mothers: developing relationships within the family. In Lamb, M.E. and Sutton-Smith, B. (Eds), *Sibling relationships: their nature and significance across the lifespan.* Hillsdale, NJ: Erlbaum, 39–60.

Durrett, M.E., Otaki, M. and Richards, P. (1984) Attachment and the mother's perception of support from the father. *International Journal of Behavioral Develop ment* 7, 167–76.

Easterbrooks, M.A. and Goldberg, W.A. (1990) Security of toddler–parent attachment: relation to children's sociopersonality functioning in kindergarten. In Greenberg, M.T., Cicchetti, D. and Cummings, E.M. (Eds), *Attachment in the preschool years.* Chicago: University of Chicago Press, 221–44.

Egeland, B. and Farber, A.E. (1984) Infant–mother attachment: factors related to its development and changes over time. *Child Development* 55, 753–71.

Egeland, B. and Sroufe, L.A. (1981) Attachment and early maltreatment. *Child Development* 52, 44–52.

Emde, R.N. (1991) The wonder of our complex enterprise: steps enabled by attachment and the effects of relationships on relationships. *Infant Mental Health Journal* 12, 164–73.

Emde, R.N., Katz, E.L. and Thorpe, J.K. (1978) Emotional expression in infancy: early deviations in Down syndrome. In Lewis, M. and Rosenblum, L.A. (Eds), *The development of affect.* London: Plenum, 351–60.

Emde, R.N., Osofsky, J.D. and Butterfield, P.M. (1993) The IFEEL Pictures: a new instrument for interpreting emotions. *Clinical Infant Reports. No. 5.* Madison, CT: International Universities Press.

Entwhistle, D. and Doering, S. (1981) *The first birth: a family turning point.* Baltimore, MD: Johns Hopkins University Press.

Erickson, M.F., Sroufe, L.A. and Egeland, B. (1985) The relationship between quality of attachment and behavior problems in preschool in a high-risk sample. In Bretherton, I. and Waters, E. (Eds), Growing points of attachment theory and research. *Monographs of the Society for Research in Child Development* 50, 147–66.

Escher-Graeub, D. and Grossmann, K.E. (1983) *Attachment security in the second year of life.* Unpublished report, University of Regensburg.

Ewart, C.K. (1991) Social action theory for a public health psychology. *American Psychologist* 46, 931–46.

Fahrenfort, J. (1993) *Attachment and early hospitalization.* Amsterdam: Thesis Publishers.

Feeney, J.A. and Noller, P. (1990) Attachment style as a predictor of adult romantic relationships. *Journal of Personality and Social Psychology* 58, 281–91.

Feeney, J.A. and Noller, P. (1992) Attachment style and romantic love: relationship dissolution. *Australian Journal of Psychology* 44, 69–74.

Feeney, J.A., Noller, P. and Hanrahan, M. (1994) Assessing adult attachment. In Sperling, M.B. and Berman, W.H. (Eds), *Attachment in adults: clinical and developmental perspectives.* New York: Guilford Press, 128–54.

Feldman, R., Greenbaum, C.W. and Yirmiya, N. (1999) Mother–infant affect synchrony as an antecedent of the emergence of self-control. *Developmental Psychology* 35, 223–31.

Field, T.M. (1977) The effects of early separation, interactive deficits and experimental manipulations on infant–mother face-to-face interaction. *Child Development* 48, 763–71.

Field, T.M. (1978) Interaction behaviors of primary versus secondary caretaker fathers. *Developmental Psychology* 14, 183–5.

Field, T.M. (1992) Infants of depressed mothers. *Development and Psychopathology* 4, 49–66.

Finkel, D., Wille, D.E. and Matheny, A.P. (1998) Preliminary results from a twin study of infant–caregiver attachment. *Behavior Genetics* **28**, 1–8.

Fischer-Fay, A., Goldberg, S., Simmons, R.J. and Levison, H. (1988) Chronic illness and infant–mother attachment: cystic fibrosis. *Journal of Developmental and Behavioral Pediatrics* **9**, 266–70.

Flavell, J.H. (1979) Meta-cognition and cognitive monitoring: a new area of cognitive-developmental inquiry? *American Psychologist* **34**, 906–11.

Fonagy, P., Leigh, T., Steele, M. *et al.* (1996) The relation of attachment status, psychiatric classification and response to therapy. *Journal of Consulting and Clinical Psychology* **64**, 22–31.

Fonagy, P., Steele, H. and Steele, M. (1991) Maternal representations of attachment during pregnancy predict the organization of infant–mother attachment at one year of age. *Child Development* **62**, 891–905.

Fonagy, P., Steele, M., Steele, H. *et al.* (1995) Attachment, the reflective self, and borderline states. In Goldberg, S., Muir, R. and Kerr, J. (Eds), *Attachment theory: social, developmental and clinical perspectives*. Hillsdale, NJ: The Analytic Press, 233–78.

Fonagy, P., Steele, M., Steele, H., Moran, G.S. and Higgett, A.C. (1991) The capacity for understanding mental states: the reflective self in parent and child and its significance for security of attachment. *Infant Mental Health Journal* **12**, 201–18.

Fonagy, P., Target, M., Steele, M. *et al.* (1997) Morality, disruptive behaviour, borderline personality disorder, crime and their relationship to security of attachment. In Atkinson, L. and Zucker, K. (Eds), *Attachment and psychopathology*. New York: Guilford Press, 223–76.

Fox, N.A. (1977) Attachment of kibbutz infants to mothers and metapelet. *Child Development* **48**, 1228–39.

Fox, N.A. (1994) Dynamic cerebral processes underlying emotion regulation. In Fox, N.A. (Ed.), The development of emotion regulation: biological and behavioral considerations. *Monographs of the Society for Research in Child Development* **59**, 152–66.

Fox, N.A. (1995) Of the way we were: adult memories about attachment experiences and their role in determining infant–parent relationships: a commentary on van IJzendoorn (1995). *Psychological Bulletin* **117**, 404–10.

Fox, N.A. and Fein, G. (1990) *Infant day care: the current debate*. Norwood, NJ: Ablex.

Fox, N.A., Kimmerly, N.L. and Schafer, W.D. (1991a) Attachment to mother, attachment to father: a meta-analysis. *Child Development* **62**, 210–25.

Fox, N.A., Kimmerly, N.L. and Schafer, W.D. (1991b) Erratum to 'Attachment to mother/attachment to father: a meta-analysis.' *Child Development* **62**, 424.

Frodi, A. (1983) Attachment behaviour and sociability with strangers in premature and full-term infants. *Infant Mental Health Journal* **4**, 14–22.

Fury, G., Carlson, E. and Sroufe, L.A. (1997) Children's representations of attachment relationships in family drawings. *Child Development* **68**, 1154–64.

Gaensbauer, T.J., Harmon, R.J., Culp, A.M., Schultz, L.A., van Doornick, W.J. and Dawson, P. (1985) Relationships between attachment behavior in the laboratory and the caretaking environment. *Infant Behavior and Development* **8**, 355–69.

George, C., Kaplan, N. and Main, M. (1984) (revised in 1985 and 1996) *Adult Attachment Interview*. Unpublished manuscript, Department of Psychology, University of California, Berkeley, CA.

George, C. and Solomon, J. (1999) Attachment and caregiving: the caregiving behavioral system. In Cassidy, J. and Shaver, P.R. (Eds), *Handbook of attachment*. New York: Guildford Press, 649–70.

George, C., West, M. and Pettem, O. (1999) Adult attachment projective. Training announcement. Oakland, CA: Mills College.

Gewirtz, J. (1969) Mechanisms of social learning: some roles of stimulation and behaviour in early development. In Goslin, D.A. (Ed.), *Handbook of socialization theory and research.* Chicago: Rand McNally, 57–212.

Gewirtz, J. and Boyd, E.F. (1977a) Does maternal responding imply reduced infant crying? A critique of the 1972 Bell and Ainsworth report. *Child Development* **48**, 1200–7.

Gewirtz, J. and Boyd, E.F. (1977b) In reply to the rejoinder to our critique of the 1972 Bell and Ainsworth report. *Child Development* **48**, 1217–18.

Goldberg, S. (1982) Some biological aspects of early parent–infant interaction. In Moore, S.G. and Cooper, C.R. (Eds), *The young child: reviews of research.* Washington, DC: National Association for the Education of Young Children.

Goldberg, S. (1997) Attachment and childhood behavior problems in normal, at-risk and clinical samples. In Atkinson, L. and Zucker, K. (Eds), *Attachment and psychopathology.* New York: Guilford Press, 171–95.

Goldberg, S., Blokland, K. and Myhal, N. (in press) A tale of two stories: temperament, attachment and emotion regulation. In Tarabulsy, G. Larose, S., Pederson, D. and Moran, G. (Eds), *Attachment et developpement. I. Petite et jeune enfance.* Quebec: Les Presses de l'Université du Quebec.

Goldberg, S. and DiVitto, B. (1995) Parenting children born preterm. In Bornstein, M.H. (Ed.), *Handbook of parenting. Vol. 1. Children and parenting.* Mahwah, NJ: Erlbaum, 209–32.

Goldberg, S., Gotowiec, A. and Simmons, R. J. (1995) Infant–mother attachment and behavior problems in healthy and chronically ill preschoolers. *Development and Psychopathology* **7**, 267–82.

Goldberg, S., Grusec, J. and Jenkins, J. (1999) Confidence in protection: arguments for a narrow definition of attachment. *Journal of Family Psychology* **13**, 475–83.

Goldberg, S., Lojkasek, M., Minde, K. and Corter, C. (1990) Prediction of behavior problems in 4-year-olds born prematurely. *Development and Psychopathology* **2**, 15–30.

Goldberg, S., MacKay-Soroka, S. and Rochester, M. (1994) Affect, attachment and maternal responsiveness. *Infant Behavior and Development* **17**, 335–40.

Goldberg, S., Perrotta, M., Minde, K.M. and Corter, C. (1986) Maternal behaviour and attachment in low birthweight twins and singletons. *Child Development* **57**, 34–46.

Goldberg, S., Simmons, R.J., Neuman, J., Campbell, K. and Fowler, R. (1991) Congenital heart disease, parent stress, and infant–mother attachment. *Journal of Pediatrics* **119**, 661–6.

Goldberg, S., Washington, J., Myhal, N. *et al.* (1998) *Stability and change in attachment from infancy to preschool.* Unpublished paper, Hospital for Sick Children, Toronto, ON.

Goldberg, W.A. and Easterbrooks, M.A. (1984) The role of marital quality in toddler development. *Developmental Psychology* **20**, 504–14.

Goldfarb, W. (1943a) Infant rearing and problem behaviour. *American Journal of Orthopsychiatry* **13**, 249–65.

Goldfarb, W. (1943b) The effects of early institutional care on adolescent personality. *Journal of Experimental Education* **12**, 106–29.

Goldfarb, W. (1945) Effects of psychological deprivation in infancy and subsequent adjustment. *American Journal of Psychiatry* **102**, 18–33.

Goldfarb, W. (1955) Emotional and intellectual consequences of psychological deprivation in infancy: a re-evaluation. In Hoch, P.H. and Zubin, J. (Eds), *Psychopathology of childhood*. New York: Grune & Stratton, 101–99.

Goldsmith, H.H. and Alansky, J. (1987) Maternal and infant temperamental predictors of attachment: a meta-analytic review. *Journal of Clinical and Consulting Psychology* 55, 805–16.

Goldsmith, H.H. and Rothbart, M. (1996) *Laboratory Temperament Assessment Battery. Unpublished manual*. Madison, WI: Department of Psychology, University of Wisconsin.

Goossens, F.A. and van IJzendoorn, M.H. (1990) Quality of infants' attachments to professional caregivers: relation to infant–parent attachment and day-care characteristics. *Child Development* 61, 832–7.

Gordon, A.N. and Jameson, J. (1979) Infant–mother attachment in patients with non-organic failure to thrive syndrome. *Journal of the American Academy of Child Psychiatry* 18, 251–9.

Gottlieb, L.N. and Mendelson, M.J. (1990) Parental support and firstborn girls' adaptation to the birth of a sibling. *Journal of Applied Developmental Psychology* 11, 29–48.

Greenberg, M.T., Speltz, M.L. and DeKlyen, M. (1993) The role of attachment in the early development of disruptive behavior problems. *Development and Psychopathology* 5, 191–213.

Greenberg, M.T., Speltz, M.L. and DeKlyen, M. and Endriga, M.C. (1991) Attachment security in preschoolers with and without externalizing problems: a replication. *Development and Psychopathology* 3, 413–30.

Greenough, W.T., Black, J.E. and Wallace, C.S. (1987) Experience and brain development. *Child Development* 58, 539–59.

Grice, H.P. (1975) Logic and conversation. In Cole, P. and Moran, J.L. (Eds), *Syntax and semantics. Vol. 3*. New York: Academic Press, 41–58.

Grossmann, K.E. (1995) The evolution and history of attachment research and theory. In Goldberg, S., Muir, R. and Kerr, J. (Eds), *Attachment theory: social, developmental and clinical perspectives*. Hillsdale, NJ: The Analytic Press, 85–122.

Grossmann, K.E. and Grossmann, K. (1984) The development of conversational styles in the first year of life and its relationship to sensitivity and attachment quality between mother and child. Paper presented at the Congress of the German Society for Psychology, Vienna, September 1984.

Grossmann, K.E. and Grossmann, K. (1990) The wider concept of attachment in cross-cultural research. *Human Development* 33, 31–47.

Grossmann, K.E. and Grossmann, K. (1991) Attachment quality as an organizer of emotional and behavioral responses in a longitudinal perspective. In Parkes, C.M., Stevenson-Hinde, J. and Marris, P. (Eds), *Attachment across the life cycle*. London: Tavistock/Routledge, 93–114.

Grossman K., Grossman, K.E., Spangler, G., Suess, G. and Unzer, L. (1985) Maternal sensitivity and newborn orientation responses as related to quality of attachment in Northern Germany. In Bretherton, I. and Waters, E. (Eds), Growing points of attachment theory and research. *Monographs of the Society for Research in Child Development* 50, 233–56.

Gunnar, M.R. (1986) Human development psychoendocrinology: a review of research on neuroendocrine responses to challenge and threat in infancy and childhood. In Lewis, M. and Worobey, J. (Eds), *Infant stress and coping*. San Francisco, CA: Jossey-Bass, 3–18.

Gunnar, M.R. (1990) The psychobiology of infant temperament. In Columbo, J. and Fagan, J. (Eds), *Individual differences in infancy*. Hillsdale, NJ: Erlbaum, 387–410.

Gunnar, M.R. (1992) Reactivity of the hypothalamic-pituitary-adrenocortical system to stressors in normal infants and children. *Pediatrics* **90**, 491–7.

Gunnar, M.R. (1999) Early adversity and the development of stress reactivity and regulation. In Nelson, C.A. (Ed.), *Minnesota Sympsium on Child Psychology. Vol. 31 The effects of adversity on neurobehavioral development.* Mahwah, NJ: Erlbaum.

Gunnar, M.R., Broderson, L., Nachmias, M., Buss, K. and Rigatuso, J. (1996a) Stress reactivity and attachment security. *Developmental Psychobiology* **29**, 191–204.

Gunnar, M.R., Broderson, L., Krueger, K. and Rigatuso, J. (1996) Dampening of adrenocortical responses during infancy: normative changes and individual differences. *Child Development* **67**, 877–89.

Gunnar, M.R., Mangelsdorf, S., Larson, M. and Hertsgaard, L. (1993) Attachment, temperament and adrenocortical activity in infancy: a study of psychoendocrine regulation. *Developmental Psychology* **25**, 355–63.

Haft, W.L. and Slade, A. (1989) Affect attunement and maternal attachment: a pilot study. *Infant Mental Health Journal* **10**, 157–72.

Hamilton, C.E. (1994) *Continuity and discontinuity in attachment from infancy through adolescence.* Unpublished doctoral dissertation, University of California, Los Angeles, CA.

Hansburg, H.G. (1972) *Adolescent separation anxiety.* Springfield, IL: Charles Thomas.

Harlow, H.F. and Harlow, M.K. (1962) Social deprivation in monkeys. *Scientific American* **207**, 136.

Harlow, H.F. and Harlow, M.K. (1965) The affectional systems. In Schrier, A.M., Harlow, H.F. and Stollnitz, F. (Eds), *Behavior of nonhuman primates.* New York: Academic Press, 287–334.

Harlow, H.F., Harlow, M.K. and Suomi, S.J. (1971) From thought to therapy: lessons from a primate laboratory. *American Scientist* **59**, 538–49.

Harris, J.R. (1998) *The nurture assumption: why children turn out the way they do.* New York: Free Press.

Harris, T. and Bifulco, A. (1991) Loss of parent in childhood, attachment style, and depression in adulthood. In Parkes, C.M., Stevenson-Hinde, J. and Marris, P. (Eds), *Attachment across the life cycle.* London: Routledge, 234–67.

Harris, T., Brown, G.W. and Bifulco, A. (1986) Loss of parent in childhood and adult psychiatric disorder: the role of lack of adequate parental care. *Psychological Medicine* **16**, 641–59.

Harwood, R.L. (1992) The influence of culturally derived values on Anglo and Puerto Rican mothers' perceptions of attachment behaviour. *Child Development* **63**, 822–39.

Harwood, R.L., Miller, J.G. and Irizarry, N.L. (1995) *Culture and attachment.* New York: Guilford Press.

Hazan, C. and Shaver, P.R. (1987) Romantic love conceptualized as an attachment process. *Journal of Personality and Social Psychology* **52**, 511–24.

Hazan, C. and Shaver, P.R. (1990) Love and work: an attachment theoretical perspective. *Journal of Personality and Social Psychology* **59**, 270–80.

Hersher, L., Moore, A.U. and Richmond, J.B. (1958) Effect of post-partum separation of mother and kid on maternal care in the domestic goat. *Science* **128**, 1342–3.

Hertsgaard, L., Gunnar, M., Erickson, M.F. and Nachmias, M. (1995) Adrenocortical responses to the strange situation in infants with disorganized/disoriented attachment relationships. *Child Development* **66**, 1100–6.

Hesse, E. (1996) Discourse, memory and the Adult Attachment Interview: a brief note with emphasis on the emerging Cannot Classify category. *Infant Mental Health Journal* **17**, 4–11.

Hillburn-Cobb, C. (1993) *Adolescent–parent attachments and family problem-solving styles.* Unpublished doctoral dissertation, York University, Toronto, ON.

Hillburn-Cobb, C. (1996) Adolescent–parent attachments and family problem-solving styles. *Family Process* **35**, 57–82.

Hillburn-Cobb, C. (1998) Controlling versus frankly disorganized behaviour in adolescent psychopathology. Paper presented at the Second International Conference on Attachment and Psychopathology. Toronto, ON, October 1998.

Hodapp. R.M. (1995) Parenting children with Down syndrome and other types of mental retardation. In Bornstein, M.H. (Ed.), *Handbook of parenting. Vol. 1. Children and parenting.* Mahwah, NJ: Erlbaum, 233–53.

Hodges, J. and Tizard, B. (1989a) IQ and behavioral adjustment of ex-institutional adolescents. *Journal of Child Psychology and Psychiatry* **30**, 53–75.

Hodges, J. and Tizard, B. (1989b) Social and family relationships of ex-institutional adolescents. *Journal of Child Psychology and Psychiatry* **30**, 77–97.

Hofer, M.A. (1973a) The effects of brief maternal separations on behavior and heart rate of two-week-old rat pups. *Physiology and Behaviour* **10**, 423–7.

Hofer, M.A. (1973b) The role of nutrition in the physiological and behavioral effects of early maternal separation on infant rats. *Psychosomatic Medicine* **35**, 350–9.

Hofer, M.A. (1975) Studies on how early maternal separation produces behavioral change in young rats. *Psychosomatic Medicine* **37**, 245–64.

Hofer, M.A. (1995) Hidden regulators in attachment and loss. In Goldberg, S., Muir, R. and Kerr, J. (Eds), *Attachment theory: social, developmental, and clinical perspectives.* Hillsdale, NJ: The Analytic Press, 203–30.

Hofer, M.A. and Shair, H.N. (1978) Ultrasonic vocalizations during social interaction and isolation in 2-week-old rats. *Developmental Psychobiology* **11**, 495–504.

Hoffman, L.W. (1979) Maternal employment. *American Psychologist* **34**, 859–65.

Hoffman, L.W. (1989) Effects of maternal employment in the two-parent family. *American Psychologist* **44**, 283–92.

Holahan, C.J. and Moos, R.H. (1987) Personal and contextual determinants of coping strategies. *Journal of Personality and Social Psychology* **52**, 946–55.

Holmes, D., Ruble, N., Kowalski, J. and Lavesen, B. (1984) Predicting quality of attachment at one year from neonatal characteristics. Paper presented at the International Conference on Infant Studies, New York, NY, April 1984.

Holmes, J. (1993) *John Bowlby and attachment theory.* London: Routledge.

Holmes, J. (1995) 'Something there is that doesn't love a wall': John Bowlby, attachment theory and psychoanalysis. In Goldberg, S., Muir, R. and Kerr, J. (Eds), *Attachment theory: social, developmental and clinical perspectives.* Hillsdale, NJ: The Analytic Press, 19–44.

Holtzworth-Munroe, A., Hutchinson, G. and Stuart, G.I. (1992) Attachment patterns of maritally violent vs. nonviolent men: data from the Adult Attachment Interview. Paper presented at the Meeting of the Association for the Advancement of Behavior Therapy, Boston, MA.

Howes, C. and Hamilton, C.E. (1992a) Children's relationships with caregivers: mothers and child care teachers. *Child Development* **63**, 856–9.

Howes, C. and Hamilton, C.E. (1992b) Children's relationships with child care teachers: stability and concordance with parental attachments. *Child Development* **63**, 867–78.

Howes, C., Matheson, C.C. and Hamilton, C.E. (1994) Maternal, teacher and child care history correlates of children's relationships with peers. *Child Development* **65**, 264–73.

Howes, P. and Markman, H.J. (1989) Marital quality and child functioning: a longitudinal investigation. *Child Development* **60**, 1044–51.

Hubel, D.H. and Wiesel, T.N. (1965) Receptive fields and functional architecture in two nonstriate visual areas (18 and 19) of the cat. *Journal of Neurophysiology* **28**, 228–89.

Izard, C.E. and Malatesta, C.Z. (1987) Perspectives on emotional development. 1. Differential emotions theory of early emotional development. In Osofsky, J.D. (Ed.), Handbook of infant development, 2nd edn. New York: John Wiley, 494–554.

Jacobsen, T., Edelstein, W. and Hofmann, V. (1994) A longitudinal study of the relation between representations of attachment in childhood and cognitive functioning in childhood and adolescence. *Developmental Psychology* **30**, 112–24.

Jacobson, J.L. and Wille, D.E. (1986) The influence of attachment pattern on developmental changes in peer interaction from the toddler to the preschool period. *Child Development* **57**, 338–47.

Jacobvitz, D., Hazen, N. and Riggs, S. (1997) Disorganized mental processes in mothers, frightening/frightened caregiving, and disoriented/disorganized behavior in infancy. Symposium paper presented at the Meeting of the Society for Research in Child Development, Washington, DC, April 1997.

Janus, M. and Goldberg, S. (1997) Securely attached infants are healthier: attachment and health in the first three years of life. Presented at the Meeting of the Society for Research in Child Development, Washington, DC, April 1997.

Kagan, J. (1994) *Galen's prophecy*. New York: Basic Books.

Kagan, J. (1998) *Three seductive ideas*. Cambridge, MA: Harvard University Press.

Kagan, J., Kearsley, R. and Zelazo, P. (1978) *Infancy: its place in human development.* Cambridge, MA: Harvard University Press.

Kaplan, N. and Main, M. (1986) *Instructions for the classification of children's family drawings in terms of representation of attachment.* Unpublished manuscript, University of California, Berkeley, CA.

Karen, R. (1994) *Becoming attached.* New York: Warner Books.

Kerns, K.A. (1994) A longitudinal examination of links between mother–child attachment and children's friendships in early childhood. *Journal of Social and Personal Relationships* **11**, 379–81.

Kirkpatrick, L. and Hazan, C. (1994) Attachment styles and close relationships: a four-year prospective study. *Personal Relationships* **1**, 123–42.

Kirsch, S.J. and Cassidy, J. (1997) Preschoolers' attention to and memory for attachment-relevant information. *Child Development* **68**, 1143–54.

Kirschbaum, C. and Hellhammer, D.H. (1989) Salivary cortisol in psychobiological research: an overview. *Neuropsychobiology* **22**, 150–69.

Klagsbrun, M. and Bowlby, J. (1976) Responses to separation from parents: a clinical test for young children. *British Journal of Professional Psychology* **21**, 7–21.

Klaus, M.H. and Kennell, J.H. (1976) *Mother–infant bonding.* Baltimore, MD: C.V. Mosby.

Kobak, R.R. (1989) *The Attachment Interview Q-set.* Unpublished manuscript, University of Delaware, Newark.

Kobak, R.R., Cole, H.E., Ferenz-Gillies, R. and Fleming, W.S. (1987) Attachment in late adolescence: working models, affect regulation, and representation of self and others. *Child Development* **64**, 231–45.

Kobak, R.R., Cole, H.E., Ferenz-Gillies, R., Fleming, W.S. and Gamble, W. (1993)

Attachment and emotion regulation during mother–teen problem-solving: a control theory analysis. *Child Development* **64**, 231–45.

Kobak, R.R. and Hazan, C. (1991) Attachment in marriage: effects of security and accuracy of working models. *Journal of Personality and Social Psychology* **60**, 861–9.

Kobak, R.R. and Sceery, A. (1988) Attachment in late adolescence: working models, affect regulation and representations of self and others. *Child Development* **59**, 135–46.

Kobak, R.R., Sudler, N. and Gamble, W. (1991) Attachment and depressive symptoms during adolescence: a developmental pathways analysis. *Development and Psychopathology* **3**, 461–74.

Kochanska, G. (1998) Mother–child relationship, child fearfulness and emerging attachment: a short-term longitudinal study. *Developmental Psychology* **34**, 480–90.

Kogan, K.L. and Taylor, N. (1973) Mother–child interaction in young physically handicapped children. *American Journal of Mental Deficiency* **77**, 492–7.

Kopp, C. (1989) Regulation of distress and negative emotions: a developmental view. *Developmental Psychology* **25**, 343–54.

Kotelchuck, M. (1976) The infant's relationship to the father: Experimental evidence. In Lamb, M.E. (Ed.), *The role of the father in child development*. New York: John Wiley, 329–44.

Kotler, T., Buzwell, S., Romeo, Y. and Bowland, J. (1994) Avoidant attachment as a risk factor for health. *British Journal of Medical Psychology* **67**, 237–45.

Kraemer, G.W. (1992) A psychobiological theory of attachment. *Behavioral and Brain Sciences* **15**, 493–541.

Kraemer, G.W., Ebert, M.H., Schmidt, D.E. and McKinney, W.T. (1989) A longitudinal study of the effects of different rearing environments on cerebrospinal fluid norepinephrine and biogenic amine metabolites in rhesus monkeys. *Neuropsychopharmacology* **2**, 175–89.

Kuczynski, L., Kochanska, G., Radke-Yarrow, M. and Girnius-Brown, O. (1987) A developmental interpretation of young children's non-compliance. *Developmental Psychology* **23**, 799–806.

Laible, D.L. and Thompson, R.A. (1998) Attachment and emotional understanding in preschool children. *Developmental Psychology* **34**, 1038–45.

Lamb, M.E. (1977) Father–infant and mother–infant interaction in the first year of life. *Child Development* **48**, 167–81.

Lamb, M.E. and Fracasso, M.P. (1998) Dimensions du tempérament: physiologie, comportements et perceptions maternelles (Dimensions of temperament: physiology, behaviour and maternal perceptions). In Tarabulsy, G.M., Tessier, R. and Kappas, A. (Eds), *Le tempérament de l'enfant: cinq etudes (Child temperament: five studies)*. Québec: Presses de l'Université du Québec, 77–92.

Lamb, M.E., Hwang, C.P., Frodi, A. and Frodi, M. (1982) Security of mother- and father–infant attachment and its relation to sociability with strangers in traditional and non-traditional Swedish families. *Infant Behavior and Development* **5**, 355–67.

Lamb, M.E. and Sternberg, K. (1990) Do we really know how day care affects children? *Journal of Applied Developmental Psychology* **11**, 351–79.

Lamb, M.E., Sternberg, K. and Prodrimidis, M. (1992) Nonmaternal care and the security of attachment: a reanalysis of the data. *Infant Behavior and Development* **15**, 71–83.

Lamb, M.E., Thompson, R.A., Gardner, W.P. and Charnov, E.L. (1985) *Infant–mother attachment*. Hillsdale, NJ: Erlbaum.

Lamb, M.E., Thompson, R.A., Gardner, W.P. and Charnov, E.L. and Estes, D. (1984) Security of infantile attachment as assessed in the 'strange situation': its study and biological interpretation. *Behavioral and Brain Sciences* 7, 127–72.

Larson, M.C., Gunnar, M.R. and Hertsgaard, L. (1991) The effects of morning naps, car trips and maternal separation on adrenocortical activity in human infants. *Child Development* 62, 362–72.

Laudenslager, M.L., Boccia, M.L. and Reite, M.L. (1993) Biobehavioral consequences of loss in nonhuman primates: individual differences. In Stroebe, M.S., Stroebe, W. and Hanssen, R.O. (Eds), *The handbook of bereavement*. Cambridge: Cambridge University Press, 129–42.

Lay, K.L., Waters, E., Posada, G. and Ridgeway, D. (1995) Attachment security, affect regulation and defensive responses to mood induction. In Waters, E., Vaughn, B.E., Posada, G. and Kondo-Ikemura, K. (Eds), Caregiving, cultural, and cognitive perspectives on secure base behavior and working models: new growing points of attachment theory and research. *Monographs of the Society for Research in Child Development* 60, 179–96.

Lazarus, R.S. and Folkman, S. (1984) *Stress, appraisal, and coping*. New York: Springer.

Levine, S., Haltmeyer, G.C., Karas, G.G. and Denenberg, V.H. (1967) Physiological and behavioral effects of infantile stimulation. *Physiology and Behavior* 2, 55–63.

Levitt, M.J., Weber, R.A. and Clark, M.C. (1986) Social networks as sources of maternal support and well-being. *Developmental Psychology* 22, 310–16.

Levy, K.N., Blatt, S.J. and Shaver, P.R. (1998) Attachment styles and parent representations. *Journal of Personality and Social Psychology* 74, 407–19.

Lewis, J.M., Owen, M.T. and Cox, M.J. (1988) The transition to parenthood. III. Incorporation of the child into the family. *Family Process* 27, 411–21.

Lewis, M. (1997) *Altering fate: why the past does not predict the future*. New York: Guilford Press.

Lewis, M. and Feiring, C. (1989a) Infant, mother, and mother–infant interaction behavior and subsequent attachment. *Child Development* 60, 831–7.

Lewis, M. and Feiring, C. (1989b) Early predictors of childhood friendship. In Berndt, T.J. and Ladd, G.W. (Eds), *Peer relationships in child development*. New York: John Wiley, 247–73.

Lewis, M., Feiring, C., McGuffog, C. and Jaskir, J. (1984) Predicting psychopathology in 6-year-olds from early social relations. *Child Development* 55, 123–36.

Lewis, M. and Michalson, L. (1983) *Children's emotions and moods*. New York: Plenum.

Lewis, M., Ramsay, D. and Kawakami, K. (1993) Differences between Japanese and Caucasian American infants in behavioral and cortisol responses to inoculation. *Child Development* 64, 1772–81.

Lewis, M. and Thomas, D. (1990) Cortisol release in infants in response to inoculation. *Child Development* 61, 50–59.

Lieberman, A.F. (1977) Preschooler's competence with a peer: relations with attachment and peer experience. *Child Development* 48, 1277–87.

Lieberman, A.F. (1997) Toddlers' internalization of maternal attributions as a factor in quality of attachment. In Atkinson, L. and Zucker, K. (Eds), *Attachment and psychopathology*. New York: Guilford Press, 277–91.

Lieberman, A.F. and Pawl, J.H. (1988) Clinical applications of attachment theory. In Belsky, J. and Nezworski, T. (Eds), *Clinical implications of attachment*. Hillsdale, NJ: Erlbaum, 327–47.

Lieberman, A.F., Weston, D. and Pawl, J.H. (1991) Preventive intervention and outcome with anxiously attached dyads. *Child Development* **62**, 199–209.

Liotti, G. (1995) Disorganized/disoriented attachment in the psychotherapy of the dissociative disorders. In Goldberg, S., Muir, R. and Kerr, J. (Eds), *Attachment theory: social, developmental and clinical perspectives*. Hillsdale, NJ: The Analytic Press, 343–66.

Liu, D., Diorio, J., Tannenbaum, B. *et al.* (1997) Maternal care, hippocampal glucocorticoid receptors and hypothalamic-pituitary-adrenal responses to stress. *Science* **277**, 1659–61.

Londerville, S. and Main, M. (1981) Security, compliance and maternal training methods in the second year of life. *Developmental Psychology* **17**, 289–99.

Lorenz, K.Z. (1935) Der Kumpan in der Umwelt des Vogels: die Aartgenosse als ausloseudes Moment sozialer Verhaltungwiesen. *Journal of Orintuology* **83**, 137–213, 289–413.

Luecken, L.J. (1998) Childhood attachment and loss experiences affect adult cardiovascular and cortisol function. *Psychosomatic Medicine* **60**, 765–72.

Lutkenhaus, P., Grossmann, K.E. and Grossmann, K. (1985) Infant–mother attachment at 12 months and style of interaction with a stranger at 3 years. *Child Development* **56**, 1538–72.

Lynch, M. and Cicchetti, D. (1991) Patterns of relatedness in maltreated and non-maltreated children: connections among multiple representational models. *Development and Psychopathology* **3**, 207–26.

Lyons-Ruth, K. (1996) Attachment relationships among children with aggressive behavior problems: the role of disorganized early attachment patterns. *Journal of Consulting and Clinical Psychology* **64**, 64–73.

Lyons-Ruth, K., Alpern, L. and Repacholi, B. (1993) Disorganized attachment classification and maternal psychological problems as predictors of hostile-aggressive behavior in the preschool classroom. *Child Development* **64**, 572–85.

Lyons-Ruth, K. and Block, D. (1996) The disturbed caregiving system: relations among childhood trauma, maternal caregiving and infant affect and attachment. *Infant Mental Health Journal* **17**, 257–75.

Lyons-Ruth, K. Bronfman, E. and Atwood, G. (1999) A relational diathesis model of hostile–helpless states of mind: expressions in mother–infant interaction. In Solomon, J. and George, C. (Eds), *Attachment disorganization*. New York: Guilford Press, 33–70.

Lyons-Ruth, K., Bronfman, E. and Parsons, E. (1997) Maternal frightened, frightening or atypical behaviour and disorganized infant attachment patterns. In Vondra, J. and Barnett, D. (Eds), *Atypical attachment in infancy and early childhood. Monographs of the Society for Research in Child Development*.

Lyons-Ruth, K., Connell, D. and Zoll, D. (1987) Infants at social risk: relations among infant maltreatment, maternal behaviour and infant attachment. *Developmental Psychology* **23**, 223–32.

McCartney, K. and Phillips, D. (1988) Motherhood and child care. In Birns, B. and Hay, D. (Eds), *The different faces of motherhood*. New York: Plenum Press, 157–83.

McCrone, E.R., Egeland, B., Kalkoske, M. and Carlson, E.A. (1994) Relations between early maltreatment and mental representations of relationships assessed with projective storytelling in middle childhood. *Development and Psychopathology* **6**, 99–120.

MacDonald, K. (1992) Warmth as a developmental construct: an evolutionary analysis. *Child Development* **63**, 753–73.

McFarlane, J.A. (1975) Olfaction in the development of social preferences in the human neonate. In *Parent–infant interaction. CIBA Foundation Symposium 33.* Amsterdam: Elsevier, 103–13.

McKim, M.K., Cramer, K.M., Stuart, B. and O'Connor, D. L. (1999) Infant care decisions and attachment security: the Canadian 'Transition to Child Care' study. *Canadian Journal of Behavioural Science* **31**, 92–106.

Maccoby, E. and Feldman, S. (1972) Mother attachment and stranger reactions in the third year of life. *Monographs of the Society for Research in Child Development* **37**.

Maier, S.F., Watkins, L.R. and Fleshner, M. (1994) Psychoneuroimmunology: the interface between behavior, brain and immunity. *American Psychologist* **49**, 1004–17.

Main, M. (1983) Exploration, play, and cognitive functioning as related to infant–mother attachment. *Infant Behavior and Development* **6**, 167–74.

Main, M. (1990) Cross-cultural studies of attachment organization: recent studies of changing methodologies, and the concept of conditional strategies. *Human Development* **33**, 48–61.

Main, M. (1991) Metacognitive knowledge, metacognitive monitoring, and singular (coherent) vs. multiple (incoherent) model of attachment: findings and directions for future work. In Parkes, C.M., Stevenson-Hinde, J. and Marris, P. (Eds), *Attachment across the life cycle.* London: Routledge, 127–59.

Main, M. (1995) Recent studies in attachment. In Goldberg, S., Muir, R. and Kerr, J. (Eds), *Attachment theory: social, developmental and clinical perspectives.* Hillsdale, NJ: The Analytic Press, 407–74.

Main, M. (1999) Attachment theory: eighteen points with suggestions for future studies. In Cassidy, J. and Shaver, P.R. (Eds), *Handbook of attachment.* New York: Guilford Press, 845–88.

Main, M. and Cassidy, J. (1988) Categories of response to reunion with parents at age 6: predictable from infant attachment and stable over a 1-month period. *Developmental Psychology* **24**, 415–26.

Main, M. and Hesse, E. (1990) Parents' unresolved traumatic experiences are related to infant disorganized attachment status: is frightened and/or frightening behavior the linking mechanism? In Greenberg, M.T., Cicchetti, D. and Cummings, E.M. (Eds), *Attachment in the preschool years.* Chicago: University of Chicago Press, 161–82.

Main, M. and Hesse, E. (1992) Disorganized/disoriented infant behavior in the strange situation, lapses in the monitoring of reasoning and discourse during the parent's Adult Attachment Interview and dissociative states. In Ammaniti, M. and Stern, D. (Eds), *Attachment and psychoanalysis.* Rome: Guis, Laterza & Figli, 161–84 (in Italian).

Main, M., Kaplan, N. and Cassidy, J. (1985) Security in infancy, childhood and adulthood: a move to the level of representation. In Bretherton, I. and Waters, E. (Eds), Growing points of attachment theory and research. *Monographs of the Society for Research in Child Development* **50**, 66–104.

Main, M. and Solomon, J. (1986) Discovery of a new, insecure-disorganized/disoriented attachment pattern. In Brazelton, T.B. and Yogman, M. (Eds), *Affective development in infancy.* Norwood, NJ: Ablex, 95–124.

Main, M. and Solomon, J. (1990) Procedures for identifying infants as disorganized/disoriented during the Ainsworth Strange Situation. In Greenberg, M.T., Cicchetti, D. and Cummings, E.M. (Eds), *Attachment in the preschool years.* Chicago: University of Chicago Press, 121–60.

Main, M., Tomasini, L. and Tolan, W. (1979) Differences among mothers of infants judged to differ in security. *Developmental Psychology* **15**, 472–3.

Malatesta, C.Z., Culver, C., Tesman, J.R. and Shepard, B. (1989) The development of emotion expression in the first two years of life. *Monographs of the Society for Research in Child Development* **54**.

Manassis, K., Bradley, S., Goldberg, S., Hood, J. and Swinson, R.P. (1994) Attachment in mothers with anxiety disorders and their children. *Journal of the Academy of Child and Adolescent Psychiatry* **33**, 1106–13.

Mangelsdorf, S., Gunnar, M., Kestenbaum, R., Lang, S. and Andreas, D. (1990) Infant proneness-to-distress, temperament, maternal personality and mother–infant attachment. *Child Development* **61**, 820–31.

Marcovitch, S., Goldberg, S., Gold, A. *et al.* (1997) Determinants of behavioural problems in Romanian children adopted in Ontario. *International Journal of Behavioral Development* **20**, 17–31.

Marvin, R.S. (1977) An ethological-cognitive model for the attenuation of mother–child attachment behavior. In Alloway, T., Krames, L. and Pliner, P. (Eds), *Attachment behavior*. New York: Plenum Press, 189–216.

Marvin, R.S. and Britner, P.A. (1999) Normative development: the otogeny of attachment. In Cassidy, J. and Shaver, P.R. (Eds), *Handbook of attachment theory and research*. New York: Guildford Press, 44–67.

Marvin, R.S. and Greenberg, M.T. (1982) Preschoolers' changing conception of their mothers: a social-cognitive study of mother–child attachment. In Forbes, D. and Greenberg, M.T. (Eds), *Children's planning strategies. No. 18. New directions in child development*. San Francisco, CA: Jossey-Bass, 47–60.

Marvin, R.S. and O'Connor, T.G. (1999) The formation of parent–child attachment following privation. Paper presented at the Society for Research in Child Development, Albuquerque, NM, April 1999.

Marvin, R.S. and Stewart, R.B. (1990) A family systems framework for the study of attachment. In Greenberg, M.T., Ciccetti, D. and Cummings, E.M. (Eds), *Attachment in the preschool years*. Chicago: University of Chicago Press, 51–86.

Marvin, R.S., Van Devender, T.L., Iwanga, M.I., LeVine, S. and LeVine, R.A. (1977) Infant–caregiver attachment among the Hausa of Nigeria. In McGurk, H.M. (Ed.), *Ecological factors in human development*. Amsterdam: North Holland Publishing, 247–60.

Mason, W.A. and Capitano, J.P. (1988) Formation and expression of filial attachment in rhesus monkeys raised with living and inanimate mother substitutes. *Developmental Psychobiology* **21**, 401–30.

Matas, L., Arend, R.A. and Sroufe, L.A. (1978) Continuity and adaptation in the second year. The relationship between quality of attachment and later competence. *Child Development* **49**, 549–56.

Maunder, R.G., Lancee, W.J., Greenberg, G.R. and Hunter, J.J. (1999) Insecure attachment in a subgroup of ulcerative colitis defined by ANCA status. Presented at the Meeting of the American Psychosomatic Society, Vancouver, BC, March 1999.

Melhuish, E.C., Mooney, A., Martin, S. and Lloyd, E. (1990) Type of childcare at 18 months. I. Differences in interactional experience. *Journal of Child Psychology and Psychiatry* **31**, 849–59.

Mikulincer, M., Florian, V. and Weller, A. (1993) Attachment styles, coping strategies, and post-traumatic psychological distress: the impact of the Gulf War on Israel. *Journal of Personality and Social Psychology* **64**, 817–26.

Minuchin, S. (1974) *Families and family therapy*. Cambridge, MA: Harvard University Press.

Miyake, K., Chen, S. and Campos, J.J. (1985) Infant temperament, mother's mode of interaction, and attachment in Japan: an interim report. In Bretherton, I. and

Waters, E. (Eds), Growing points of attachment theory and research. *Monographs of the Society for Research in Child Development* 50, 276–97.

Morelli, G.A. and Tronick, E.Z. (1991) Multiple caretaking and attachment. In Gewirtz, J.L. and Kurtines, W.M. (Eds), *Intersections with attachment*. Hillsdale, NJ: Erlbaum, 41–51.

Moss, E., Parent, S., Gosselin, C. and Dumont, M. (1993) Attachment and the development of metacognitive and collaborative strategies. *International Journal of Educational Research* 19, 555–71.

Moss, E., St Laurent, D. and Parent, S. (1999) Disorganized attachment and developmental risk at school age. In George, C. and Solomon, J. (Eds), *Attachment disorganization*. New York: Guilford, 160–88.

Mrazek, D.A., Casey, B. and Anderson, I. (1987) Insecure attachment in severely asthmatic preschool children: is it a risk factor? *Journal of the American Academy of Child and Adolescent Psychiatry* 26, 516–20.

Nachmias, M., Gunnar, M., Mangelsdorf, S., Parritz, R.H. and Buss, K. (1996) Behavioral inhibition and stress reactivity: the moderating role of attachment security. *Child Development* 67, 508–22.

Neuman, J. and Goldberg, S. (1990) Temperament and attachment: health and illness. Paper presented at the International Conference on Infant Studies, Montreal, PQ, April 1990.

NICHD Early Child Care Research Network (1997) The effects of infant child care on infant–mother attachment security: results of the NICHD study of early child care. *Child Development* 68, 860–79.

Ninio, A. and Rinott, N. (1988) Fathers' involvement in the care of their infants and their attributions of cognitive competence to infants. *Child Development* 59, 652–63.

Oppenheim, D., Sagi, A. and Lamb, M.E. (1988) Infant–adult attachments on the kibbutz and their relation to socioemotional development four years later. *Developmental Psychology* 24, 427–33.

Oppenheim, D. and Waters, H.S. (1995) Narrative processes and attachment representations: issues of development and assessment. In Waters, E., Vaughn, B., Posada, G. and Kondo-Ikemura, K. (Eds), Caregiving, cultural and cognitive perspectives on secure-base behavior and working models. *Monographs of the Society for Research in Child Development* 60, 197–215.

Osofsky, J. and Osofsky, H. (1984) Psychological and developmental perspectives on expectant and new parenthood. In Parke, R.D. (Ed.), *Review of child development research. Vol. 7. The family*. Chicago: University of Chicago Press, 372–97.

Owens, G. and Crowell, J.A. (1992) *Scoring manual for the Current Relationship Interview*. Unpublished document. Stony Brook, NY: State University of New York.

Owens, G. and Crowell, J.A. (1993) *Current relationship scoring system*. Unpublished manuscript. Stony Brook, NY: State University of New York.

Owens, G. and Crowell, J.A., Pan, H., Treboux, D., O'Connor, E. and Waters, E. (1995) The prototype hypothesis and origins of attachment working models: adult relationships with parents and romantic partners. In Waters, E., Vaughn, B., Posada, G. and Kondo-Ikemura, K. (Eds), Caregiving, cultural and cognitive perspectives on secure-base behavior and working models. *Monographs of the Society for Research in Child Development* 60, 216–33.

Park, K.A. and Waters, E. (1989) Security of attachment and preschool friendships. *Child Development* 60, 1076–81.

Parke, R.D. and Sawin, D.B. (1975) Infant characteristics and behavior as elicitors of maternal and paternal responsibility in the newborn period. Paper presented at the Meeting of the Society for Research in Child Development. Denver, CO, April 1975.

Patrick, M., Hobson, R.P., Castle, D., Howard, R. and Maughan, B. (1994) Personality disorder and the representation of early social experience. *Development and Psychopathology* 6, 375–88.

Pearson, J.L., Cohn, D.A., Cowan, P.A. and Cowan, C.P. (1994) Earned and continuous-security in adult attachment: relation to depressive symptomatology and parenting style. *Development and Psychopathology* 6, 359–73.

Pearson, J.L., Cowan, P.A., Cowan, C.P. and Cohn, D.A. (1993) Adult attachment and adult–child–older parent relationships. *American Journal of Orthopsychiatry* 63, 606–13.

Pedersen, F.A. and Robson, K.S. (1969) Father participation in infancy. *American Journal of Orthopsychiatry* 39, 466–72.

Pederson, D.R., Gleason, K.E., Moran, G. and Bento, S. (1998) Maternal attachment representations, maternal sensitivity and the infant–mother attachment relationship. *Developmental Psychology* 34, 925–33.

Pederson, D.R. and Moran, G. (1995) A categorical description of infant–mother relationships in the home and its relation to Q-sort measures of infant–mother interaction. In Waters, E., Vaughn, B., Posada, G. and Kondo-Ikemura, K. (Eds), Caregiving, cultural and cognitive perspectives on secure-base behavior and working models. *Monographs of the Society for Research in Child Development* 60, 111–33.

Pederson, D.R. and Moran, G. (1996) Expressions of the attachment relationship outside of the strange situation. *Child Development* 67, 915–27.

Pederson, D.R. and Moran, G. (1998) Describing mother–infant interactions in the home: the Pederson–Moran Maternal Behaviour Q-sort. Presented at the International Conference on Infant Studies, Atlanta, GA, April 1998.

Phelps, J.L., Belsky, J. and Crnic, K. (1998) Earned security, daily stress, and parenting: a comparison of five alternative models. *Development and Psychopathology* 10, 21–38.

Phillips, D.A., McCartney, K., Scarr, S. and Howes, C. (1987) Selective review of day care research: a cause for concern. *Zero to Three* 7, 18–21.

Phipps, S., Fairclough, D. and Mulhern, R.K. (1995). Avoidant coping in children with cancer. *Journal of Pediatric Psychology* 20, 217–32.

Piaget, J. (1952) *The origins of intelligence in children.* New York: International Universities Press.

Pianta, R.C., Longmaid, K. and Ferguson, J.E. (1999) Attachment-based classifications of children's family drawings: psychometric properties and relations with children's adjustment in kindergarten. *Journal of Clinical Child Psychology* 28, 244–55.

Plotsky, P.M. and Meany, M.J. (1993) Early postnatal experience alters corticotropin-releasing factor (CRF) mRNA, median eminence CRF content and stress-induced release in adult rats. *Molecular Brain Research* 18, 195–200.

Plunkett, J.W., Klein, T. and Meisels, S.J. (1988) The relationship of preterm infant–mother to stranger sociability at 3 years. *Infant Behavior and Development* 11, 83–96.

Plunkett, J.W., Meisels, S.J., Steifel, G.S., Pasick, P.L. and Roloff, D.W. (1986) Patterns of attachment among preterm infants of varying biological risk. *Journal of the American Academy of Child Psychiatry* 25, 794–800.

Porter, R.H., Makin, J.W., Davis, L.B. and Christensen, K.M. (1992) Breast-fed infants respond to olfactory cues from their own mother and unfamiliar lactating females. *Infant Behavior and Development* 15, 85–93.

Posada, G., Gao, Y., Wu, F. *et al.* (1995) The secure-base phenomenon across cultures: children's behavior, mothers' preferences, and experts' concept. In Waters, E., Vaughn, B.E., Posada, G. and Kondo-Ikemura, K. (Eds), Caregiving, cultural and cognitive perspectives on secure-base behavior and working models: new growing points of attachment theory and research. *Monographs of the Society for Research in Child Development* **60**, 27–48.

Posada, G. and Jacobs, A.E. (1999) Maternal caregiving behavior and attachment security in emergency and everyday situations. Paper presented at the Meeting of the Society for Research in Child Development, Albuquerque, NM, April 1999.

Power, T.C. and Parke, R.D. (1983) Patterns of early socialization: mother and father–infant interaction in the home. *International Journal of Behavioral Development* **9**, 331–41.

Price, D.A., Close, C.C. and Fielding, B.A. (1983) Age of appearance of circadian rhythm in salivary cortisol values in infancy. *Archives of Diseases of Childhood* **58**, 454–6.

Provence, S. and Lipton, R.C. (1962) *Infants in institutions.* New York: International Universities Press.

Radke-Yarrow, M., Cummings, E.M., Kuczynski, L. and Chapman, M. (1985) Patterns of attachment in two- and three-year-olds in normal families and families with parental depression. *Child Development* **56**, 591–615.

Ramey, C.T. and Mills, P. (1977) Social and intellectual consequences of day care for high-risk infants. In Webb, R. (Ed.), *Social development in childhood: day-care programs and research.* Baltimore, MD: Johns Hopkins University Press, 79–110.

Reiss, D. (1981) *The family's construction of reality.* Cambridge, MA: Harvard University Press.

Renken, B., Egeland, B., Marvinney, D., Mangelsdorf, S. and Sroufe, L.A. (1989) Early childhood antecedents of aggression and passive-withdrawal in early elementary school. *Journal of Personality* **57**, 591–615.

Resnick, G. (1997) Correspondence between the strange situation at 12 months and the Separation Anxiety Test at 11 years in an Israeli kibbutz sample. Presented at the Meeting of the Society for Research in Child Development, Indianapolis, IN, April 1997.

Ricciuti, A.E. (1992) *Child–mother attachment: a twin study.* Unpublished doctoral dissertation. Virginia, VA: University of Virginia.

Richards, M.P.M., Dunn, J.F. and Antonis, B. (1977) Caretaking in the first year of life: the role of fathers' and mothers' social isolation. *Child: Care, Health and Development* **3**, 23–6.

Richters, J. and Waters, E. (1990) Attachment and socialization. The positive side of social influence. In Feinman, S. and Lewis, M. (Eds), *Social influences and behavior.* New York: Plenum, 185–213.

Richters, J. and Waters, E. and Vaughn, B. (1988) An empirical classification system for the strange situation. *Child Development* **59**, 512–22.

Robertson, J. (1953) *A two-year-old goes to hospital* (Film). University Park, PA: Pennsylvania State Audio Visual Services.

Roggmann, L.A., Langlois, J.H., Hubbs-Tait, L. and Reiser-Danner, L.A. (1994) Infant day-care, attachment and the 'file-drawer problem.' *Child Development* **65**, 1429–43.

Rosen, K.S. and Burke, P. (1999) Multiple attachment relationships within families with two young children. *Developmental Psychology* **35**, 436–44.

Rosenstein, D.S. and Horowitz, H.A. (1996) Adolescent attachment and psychopathology. *Journal of Consulting and Clinical Psychology* **64**, 244–53.

Rothbart, M. and Derryberry, D. (1981) Development of individual differences in temperament. In Lamb, M.E. and Brown, A.L. (Eds), *Advances in developmental psychology.Vol. 1.* Hillsdale, NJ: Erlbaum, 37–86.

Russell, G. (1982) Shared caregiving families: an Australian study. In Lamb, M.E. (Ed.), *Non-traditional families.* Hillsdale, NJ: Erlbaum, 139–72.

Rutter, M. (1997) Clinical implications of attachment concepts: retrospect and prospect. In Atkinson, L. and Zucker, K. (Eds), *Attachment and psychopathology.* NewYork: Guilford Press, 17–46.

Saarni, C. (1979) Children's understanding of display rules for expressive behaviour. *Developmental Psychology* 15, 424–9.

Sabbagh, R. (1995) *Attachment and behaviour toward strangers in Romanian preschoolers adopted into Canadian families.* Unpublished Masters Thesis. Toronto, ON: University of Toronto.

Sagi, A., Lamb, M.E., Lewkowicz, K.S., Shoham, R., Dvir, R. and Estes, D. (1985) Security of infant–mother, father and metapelet attachments among kibbutz-reared Israeli children. In Bretherton, I. and Waters, E. (Eds), Growing points of attachment theory and research. *Monographs of the Society for Research in Child Development* 50, 257–75.

Sagi, A., Lamb, M.E., Shoham, R., Dvir, R. and Lewkowicz, K.S. (1985) Parent–infant interaction in families on Israeli kibbutzim. *International Journal of Behavioral Development* 8, 273–84.

Sagi, A., van IJzendoorn, M.H., Aviezer, A. *et al.* (1995) Attachments in a multiple-caregiver and multiple-infant environment: the case of the Israeli kibbutzim. In Waters, E.,Vaughn, B.E., Posada, G. and Kondo-Ikemura, K. (Eds), Caregiving, cultural, and cognitive perspectives on secure-base behavior and working models: new growing points of attachment theory and research. *Monographs of the Society for Research in Child Development* 60, 71–94.

Sagi, A., van IJzendoorn, M.H., Aviezer, A., Donnell, F. and Mayseless, O. (1994a) Sleeping away from home in a kibbutz communal arrangement: it makes a difference for infant–mother attachment. *Child Development* 65, 992–1004.

Sagi, A., van IJzendoorn, M.H., Scharf, M.H., Korne-Karie, N., Joels, T. and Mayseless, O. (1994b) Stability and discriminant validity of the Adult Attachment Interview: a psychometric study in young Israeli adults. *Developmental Psychology* 30, 771–7.

Salter, M. (1940) *An evaluation of adjustment based on the concept of security.* Toronto: University of Toronto Press.

Sander, L. (1975) Infant and caretaking environment: investigation and conceptualization of adaptive behavior in a system of increasing complexity. In Anthony, E. (Ed.), *Explorations in child psychiatry.* NewYork: Plenum, 129–66.

Sapolsky, R.M. (1992) Stress: the aging brain and the mechanisms of neuron death. Cambridge, MA: MIT Press.

Schaffer, H.R. and Emerson, P.E. (1964) The development of social attachments in infancy. *Monographs of the Society for Research in Child Development* 29.

Schank, R.C. (1982) *Dynamic memory: a theory of reminding and learning in computers and people.* Cambridge: Cambridge University Press.

Schneider-Rosen, K. (1990) The developmental reorganization of attachment relationships: guidelines for classification beyond infancy. In Greenberg, M.T., Cicchetti, D. and Cummings, E.M. (Eds), *Attachment in the preschool years.* Chicago: University of Chicago Press, 161–82.

Schore, A.N. (1996) The experience-dependent maturation of a regulatory system in the orbital prefrontal cortex and the origin of developmental psychopathology. *Development and Psychopathology* 8, 59–87.

Schuengel, C., Bakermans-Kranenburg, M.J. and van IJzendoorn, M.H. (1999)

Frightening maternal behavior linking unresolved loss and disorganized infant attachment. *Journal of Consulting and Clinical Psychology* **67**, 54–63.

Sears, R.R. (1963) Dependency motivation. In Jones, M.R. (Ed.), *The Nebraska Symposium on Motivation*. Lincoln, NB: University of Nebraska Press, 25–64.

Seifer, R. and Schiller, M. (1995) The role of parenting sensitivity, infant temperament, and dyadic interaction in attachment theory and assessment. In Waters, E., Vaughn, B.E., Posada, G. and Kondo-Ikemura, K. (Eds), Caregiving, cultural and cognitive perspectives on secure-base behavior and working models: new growing points of attachment theory and research. *Monographs of the Society for Research in Child Development* **60**, 146–76.

Seifer, R. and Schiller, M., Sameroff, A.J., Resnick, S. and Riordan, K. (1996) Attachment, maternal sensitivity and temperament during the first year of life. *Developmental Psychology* **32**, 12–25.

Selye, H. (1946) The general adaptation syndrome and the diseases of adaptation. *Journal of Clinical Endocrinology* **6**, 117–73.

Serafica, F. and Cicchetti, D. (1976) Down's syndrome children in the strange situation: attachment and exploratory behaviors. *Merrill-Palmer Quarterly* **21**, 137–50.

Shouldice, A. and Stevenson-Hinde, J. (1992) Coping with security distress: the Separation Anxiety Test and attachment classification at 4.5 years. *Journal of Child Psychology and Psychiatry* **33**, 331–48.

Silven, M. and Laine, P. (1996) Can attachment predict children's developing theory of others' emotions? Presented at the Fourteenth Biennial Conference of the International Society for the Study of Behavioural Development, Quebec City, August 1996.

Simmons, R.J., Goldberg, S., Washington, J. Fischer-Fay, A. and MacLusky, I. (1995) Infant–mother attachment and nutrition in children with cystic fibrosis. *Journal of Developmental and Behavioral Pediatrics* **16**, 183–6.

Simpson, J. (1990) Influence of attachment styles on romantic relationships. *Journal of Personality and Social Psychology* **59**, 971–80.

Simpson, J., Rholes, W. and Nelligan, J. (1992) Support-seeking and support-giving within couples in an anxiety-provoking situation: the role of attachment styles. *Journal of Personality and Social Psychology* **62**, 434–46.

Skeels, H.M. (1996) Adult status of children with contrasting life experiences: a longitudinal study. *Monographs of the Society for Research in Child Development* **31**, No. 105.

Skodak, M. and Skeels, H.M. (1949) A final follow-up study of one hundred adopted children. *Journal of Genetic Psychology* **75**, 85–125.

Skolnick, A. (1986) Early attachment and personal relationships across the life span. In Balthes, T., Featherman, D. and Lerner, R. (Eds), *Life span development and behavior*. Hillsdale, NJ: Erlbaum, 173–206.

Slade, A. (1999) Individual psychotherapy: an attachment perspective. In Cassidy, J. and Shaver, P.R. (Eds), *Handbook of attachment theory and research*. New York: Guilford Press, 575–94.

Slough, N.M., Goyette, M. and Greenberg, M.T. (1988) *Scoring indices for the Seattle version of the Separation Anxiety Test*. Unpublished manuscript. University of Washington, Seattle, WA.

Sluckin, W. (1965) *Imprinting and early learning*. London: Methuen.

Solomon, J. and George, C. (1994) Disorganization of maternal caregiving strategies: an attachment approach to role reversal. Paper presented at the Meeting of the American Psychological Association, Los Angeles, CA, August 1994.

Spangler, G. (1991) The emergence of adrenocortical circadian function in newborns and infants and its relationship to sleep, feeding and maternal adreno-cortical activity. *Early Human Development* 25, 197–208.

Spangler, G. and Grossmann, K.E. (1993) Biobehavioral organization in securely and insecurely attached infants. *Child Development* 64, 1439–50.

Spangler, G. and Schieche, M. (1998) Emotional and adrenocortical responses of infants to the strange situation: the differential function of emotional expression. *International Journal of Behavioural Development* 22, 681–706.

Speltz, M.L., Endriga, M.C., Fisher, P.A. and Mason, C.A. (1997) Early predictors of attachment in infants with cleft lip and/or palate. *Child Development* 68, 12–25.

Speltz, M.L., Greenberg, M.T. and DeKlyen, M. (1990) Attachment in pre-schoolers with disruptive behavior. *Development and Psychopathology* 2, 31–46.

Sperling, M.B. and Berman, W.H. (1991) An attachment classification of desperate love. *Journal of Personality Research* 56, 45–55.

Spieker, S.J. and Booth, C.L. (1988) Maternal antecedents of attachment quality. In Belsky, J. and Nezworski, T. (Eds), *Clinical implications of attachment*. Hillsdale, NJ: Erlbaum, 95–135.

Spitz, R.A. (1945) Hospitalism. An inquiry into the genesis of psychiatric conditions in early childhood. *Psychoanalytic Study of the Child* 1, 53–74.

Spitz, R.A. (1946) Hospitalism. An inquiry into the genesis of psychiatric conditions in early childhood. A follow-up report. *Psychoanalytic Study of the Child* 2, 113–17.

Spitz, R.A. (1956) The influence of the mother–child relationship and its disturbances. In Soddy, K. (Ed.), *Mental health and infant development. Vol. 1*. Papers and discussion. New York: Basic Books, 103–8.

Sroufe, L.A. (1983) Infant–caregiver attachment and patterns of adaptation in preschool: the roots of maladaptation and competence. In Perlmutter, M. (Ed.), *Minnesota Symposium in Child Psychology. Vol. 16*. Hillsdale, NJ: Erlbaum, 41–81.

Sroufe, L.A. (1985) Attachment classification from the perspective of infant–caregiver relationships and infant temperament. *Child Development* 56, 1–14.

Sroufe, L.A. (1997) Psychopathology as outcome of development. *Development and Psychopathology* 9, 251–68.

Sroufe, L.A., Egeland, B. and Carlson, E.A. (in press) One social world: the integrated development of parent–child and peer relationships. In Collins, W.A. and Laursen, B. (Eds), *Relationships as developmental contexts: Minnesota Symposium on Child Psychology. Vol. 30*. Hillsdale, NJ: Erlbaum, 241–61.

Sroufe, L.A. and Fleeson, J. (1986) Attachment and the construction of relationships. In Hartup, W. and Rubin, Z. (Eds), *The nature and development of relationships*. Hillsdale, NJ: Erlbaum, 51–71.

Sroufe, L.A. and Waters, E. (1977a) Heart rate as a convergent measure in clinical and developmental research. *Merrill-Palmer Quarterly* 23, 3–27.

Sroufe, L.A. and Waters, E. (1977b) Attachment as an organizational construct. *Child Development* 48, 1184–99.

Stansbury, K. and Gunnar, M. (1994) Adrenocortical activity and emotion regulation. In Fox, N. (Ed.), The development of emotion regulation: biological and behavioral considerations. *Monographs of the Society for Research in Child Development* 59, 108–43.

Statistics Canada (1996) *Labour force annual averages*. Ottawa, Ontario: Statistics Canada.

Steele, H., Steele, M. and Fonagy, P. (1996) Associations among attachment classifications of mothers, fathers and their infants. *Child Development* 67, 541–55.

Stein, H., Jacobs, N.J., Ferguson, K.S., Allen, J.G. and Fonagy, P. (1998) What do adult attachment scales measure? *Bulletin of the Menninger Clinic* 62, 33–82.

Stevenson-Hinde, J. (1990) Attachment within family systems: an overview. *Infant Mental Health Journal* **11**, 218–27.

Stovall, K. C. and Dozier, M. (1998). Infants in foster care: an attachment theory perspective. *Adoption Quarterly* **2**, 55–88.

Stovall, K. C. and Dozier, M. (in press) The evolution of attachment in new relationships: single subject analyses for ten foster infants. *Development and Psychopathology*.

Stroebe, M.S., Stroebe, W. and Hanssen, R.O. (1993) *The handbook of bereavement.* Cambridge: Cambridge University Press.

Suomi, S.J. (1991) Early stress and emotional reactivity in the rhesus monkey. In Barker, D. (Ed.), *The childhood environment and adult disease.* Chichester: John Wiley, 171–88.

Suomi, S.J. (1995) Attachment theory and non-human primates. In Goldberg, S., Muir, R. and Kerr, J. (Eds), *Attachment theory: social, developmental, and clinical perspectives.* Hillsdale, NJ: The Analytic Press, 203–30.

Suomi, S.J. (1997) Early determinants of behaviour: evidence from primate studies. *British Medical Bulletin* **53**, 170–84.

Susman-Stillman, A., Kalkoske, M., Egeland, B. and Waldman, I. (1996) Infant temperament and maternal sensitivity as predictors of attachment security. *Infant Behavior and Development* **19**, 33–47.

Sutton, D.B. (1994) Attachment, emotion socialization and emotion regulation: relationships between 14, 24 and 58 months. Unpublished doctoral dissertation, University of Maryland.

Szajnberg, N.M., Skrinjaric, J. and Moore, A. (1989) Affect attunement, attachment, temperament and zygosity: a twin study. *Journal of the American Academy of Child and Adolescent Psychiatry* **28**, 249–53.

Takahashi, K. (1990) Are the key assumptions of the 'strange situation' procedure universal? A view from Japanese research. *Human Development* **33**, 23–30.

Tarabulsy, G.M., Tessier, R., Gagnon, J. and Piche, C. (1996) Attachment classification and infant responsiveness during interactions. *Infant Behavior and Development* **19**, 131–43.

Taylor, S.E. (1990) Health psychology: the science and the field. *American Psychologist* **45**, 40–50.

Teti, D.M. and Ablard, K.E. (1989) Security of attachment and infant–sibling relationships: a laboratory study. *Child Development* **60**, 1519–28.

Teti, D.M., Sakin, J.W., Kucera, E.M. and Corns, K.M. (1996) And baby makes four: predictors of attachment security among preschool-age firstborns during the transition to siblinghood. *Child Development* **67**, 579–96.

Thomas, A., Chess, S. and Birch, H.G. (1968) *Temperament and behavior disorders in children.* New York: New York University Press.

Thompson, R.A. (1988) The effects of infant day care through the prism of attachment theory. *Early Childhood Research Quarterly* **3**, 273–82.

Thompson, R.A. (1994) Emotion regulation: a theme in search of a definition. In Fox, N.A. (Ed.), The development of emotion regulation: biological and behavioral considerations. *Monographs of the Society for Research in Child Development* **59**, 25–52.

Thompson, R.A. (1997) Sensitivity and security: questions to ponder. *Child Development* **68**, 595–7.

Thompson, R.A. (1998) Early sociopersonality development. In Damon, W. (Ed.), *Handbook of child psychology, 5th edn. Vol. 3. Social, emotional, and personality development.* New York: John Wiley, 25–104.

Thompson, R.A. (1999) Early attachment and later development. In Cassidy, J. and Shaver, P. (Eds), *The handbook of attachment*. New York: Guilford Press, 265–86.

Thompson, R.A., Cicchetti, D., Lamb, M. and Malkin, K. (1985) The emotional responses of Down syndrome and normal infants in the strange situation: the organization of affective behavior in infants. *Developmental Psychology* 21, 828–41.

Thompson, R.A. and Lamb, M.E. (1983) Security of attachment and stranger sociability in infancy. *Developmental Psychology* 19, 184–91.

Tizard, B. (1977) *Adoption: a second chance*. London: Open Books.

Tizard, B. and Hodges, J. (1978) The effect of early institutional rearing on the development of eight-year-old children. *Journal of Child Psychology and Psychiatry* 19, 99–118.

Tizard, B. and Rees, J. (1974) A comparison of the effects of adoption, restoration to the natural mother, and continued institutionalization on the cognitive development of four-year-old children. *Child Development* 45, 92–9.

Treboux, D., Crowell, J. and Colon-Downs, C. (1992) Attachment histories and working models: relations to best friendships and romantic relationships. Presented at the Society for Research on Adolescence, Washington, DC, March 1992.

Tronick, E.Z. (1989) Emotions and emotion communcation in infants. *American Psychologist* 44, 112–19.

Tronick, E.Z., Morelli, G.A. and Ivey, P.K. (1992) The Efe forager infant and toddler's pattern of social relationships: multiple and simultaneous. *Developmental Psychology* 28, 568–77.

Troy, M. and Sroufe, L.A. (1987) Victimization among preschoolers: the role of attachment relationship theory. *Journal of the American Academy of Child and Adolescent Psychiatry* 26, 166–72.

Tulving, E. (1972) Episodic and semantic memory. In Tulving, E. and Donaldson, W. (Eds), *Organization of memory*. New York: Academic Press, 381–403.

Tulving, E. (1985) How many memory systems are there? *American Psychologist* 40, 385–98.

Turner, P. (1991) Relations between attachment, gender and behaviour problems with peers in preschool. *Child Development* 62, 1475–88.

Tyrrell, C. and Dozier, M. (1999) Alienating behavioral strategies of late-placed foster infants. *Adoption Quarterly* 2, 49–64.

Tyrrell, C. and Dozier, M., Teague, G.B. and Fallot, R.D. (1999) Effective treatment relationships for persons with serious psychiatric disorders: the importance of attachment states of mind. *Journal of Consulting and Clinical Psychology* 67, 725–33.

Uchino, B.N., Cacioppo, J.T. and Kiecolt-Glaser, J.K. (1996) The relationship between social support and physiological processes: a review with emphasis on underlying mechanisms and implications for health. *Psychological Bulletin* 119, 488–531.

Valenzuela, M. (1990) Attachment in clinically underweight young children. *Child Development* 61, 1984–96.

van Dam, M. and van IJzendoorn, M.H. (1988) Measuring attachment security. *Journal of Genetic Psychology* 149, 447–57.

Vandell, D.L., Owen, M.T., Wilson, K.S. and Henderson, V.K. (1988) Social development in infant twins: peer and mother–child relationships. *Child Development* 59, 168–77.

van den Boom, D. (1990) Preventive intervention and the quality of mother–infant interaction and infant exploration in irritable infants. In Koops, W. (Ed.), *Developmental psychology behind the dikes*. Amsterdam: Eburon, 249–70.

van den Boom, D. (1995) The influence of temperament and mothering on attachment and exploration. *Child Development* 65, 1449–69.

van Emmichoven, I.A.Z. (1998) Attachment and perceptual defense: a tachisto scopic study in a non-clinical and anxiety-disordered sample. Presented at the Second International Conference on Attachment and Psychopathology, Toronto, October 1998.

van IJzendoorn, M.H. (1995) Adult attachment representations, parental responsiveness and infant attachment: a meta-analysis on the predictive validity of the Adult Attachment Interview. *Psychological Bulletin* 117, 387–403.

van IJzendoorn, M.H. and Bakermans-Kranenburg, M.J. (1996) Attachment representations in mothers, fathers, adolescents and clinical groups: a meta-analytic search for normative data. *Journal of Consulting and Clinical Psychology* 64, 8–21.

van IJzendoorn, M.H. and De Wolff, M.S. (1997) In search of the absent father – meta-analyses of infant–father attachment: a rejoinder to our discussants. *Child Development* 68, 609–14.

van IJzendoorn, M.H., Dijkstra, J. and Bus, A.G. (1995) Attachment, intelligence, and language: a meta-analysis. *Social Development* 4, 115–28.

van IJzendoorn, M.H., Feldbrugge, J.T.M., Derks, F. *et al.* (1997a) Attachment representations of personality-disordered criminal offenders. *American Journal of Orthopsychiatry* 67, 449–59.

van IJzendoorn, M.H., Goldberg, S., Kroonenberg, P.M. and Frenkel, O.J. (1992) The relative effects of maternal and child problems on the quality of attachment: a meta-analysis of attachment in clinical samples. *Child Development* 63, 840–58.

van IJzendoorn, M.H., Juffer, F. and Duyvesteyn, M.G.C. (1995) Breaking the intergenerational cycle of insecure attachment: a review of the effects of attachment-based interventions on maternal sensitivity and infant security. *Journal of Child Psychology and Psychiatry* 36, 225–48.

van IJzendoorn, M.H. and Kroonenberg, P.M. (1988) Cross-cultural patterns of attachment: a meta-analysis of the strange situation. *Child Development* 58, 147–56.

van IJzendoorn, M.H. and Riksen-Walraven, M.J.M.A. (in press) Is the Attachment Q-sort a valid measure of attachment security in young children? In Vaughn, B.E. and Waters, E. (Eds), *Patterns of secure base behavior: Q-sort perspectives on attachment and caregiving.* Hillsdale, NJ: Erlbaum.

van IJzendoorn, M.H. and Sagi, A. (1999) Cross-cultural patterns of attachment: universal and contextual dimensions. In Cassidy, J. and Shaver, P.R. (Eds), *Handbook of attachment.* New York: Guilford Press, 713–34.

van IJzendoorn, M.H., Schuengel, C. and Bakermans-Kranenburg, M.J. (1997b) *Disorganized attachment in early childhood: meta-analysis of precursors, concomitants and sequelae.* Unpublished manuscript.

Vaughn, B.E., Deane, K.E. and Waters, E. (1985) The impact of out-of-home-care on child–mother attachment quality: another look at some enduring questions. In Bretherton, I. and Waters, E. (Eds), Growing points of attachment theory and research. *Monographs of the Society for Research in Child Development* 50, 110–35.

Vaughn, B.E., Goldberg, S., Atkinson, L., Marcovitch, S., MacGregor, D. and Seifer, R. (1994) Quality of toddler–mother attachments in children with Down syndrome: limits to interpretation of strange situation behaviour. *Child Development* 65, 95–108.

Vaughn, B.E., Leftover, G.B., Seifer, R. and Barglow, P. (1989) Attachment behavior, attachment security and temperament during infancy. *Child Development* 60, 728–37.

Vaughn, B.E. and Seifer, R. (1989) Classifying attachment for Down syndrome children. Paper presented at the Gatlinburg Conference on Mental Retardation, Gatlinburg, TN.

Vaughn, B.E., Stevenson-Hinde, J., Waters, E. *et al.* (1992) Attachment security and temperament in infancy and childhood: some conceptual clarifications. *Developmental Psychology* **28**, 463–73.

Vaughn, B.E. and Waters, E. (1990) Attachment behavior at home and in the laboratory: Q-sort observations and strange-situation classifications of one-year-olds. *Child Development* **61**, 1965–73.

Verscheurren, K., Marcoen, A. and Schoefs, V. (1996) The internal working model of the self, attachment and competence in five-year-olds. *Child Development* **67**, 2493–511.

Volling, B. and Belsky, J. (1992) Infant, father, and marital antecedents of infant–father attachment security in dual-earner and single-earner families. *International Journal of Behavioral Development* **15**, 83–100.

Ward, M.J. and Carlson, E.A. (1995) Associations among adult attachment representations, maternal sensitivity, and infant–mother attachment in a sample of adolescent mothers. *Child Development* **66**, 69–79.

Ward, M.J., Kessler, D.B. and Altman, S.C. (1993) Infant–mother attachment in children with failure to thrive. *Infant Mental Health Journal* **14**, 208–20.

Ward, M.J., Vaughn, B.E. and Robb, M.D. (1988) Socioemotional adaptation and infant–mother attachment in siblings: role of the mother in cross-sibling consistency. *Child Development* **59**, 643–51.

Warren, S.L., Huston, L., Egeland, B. and Sroufe, L.A. (1997) Child and adolescent anxiety disorders and early attachment. *Journal of the American Academy of Child and Adolescent Psychiatry* **36**, 637–44.

Wartner, U.W., Grossmann, K., Fremmer-Bombik, E. and Suess, G. (1994) Attachment patterns at age 6 in South Germany: predictability from infancy and implications for preschool behavior. *Child Development* **66**, 69–79.

Waters, E. (1978) The reliability and stability of individual differences in infant–mother attachment. *Child Development* **39**, 483–94.

Waters, E. and Deane, K.E. (1985) Defining and assessing individual differences in attachment relationships: Q-methodology and the organization of behavior in infancy and early childhood. In Bretherton, I. and Waters, E. (Eds), Growing points of attachment theory and research. *Monographs of the Society for Research in Child Development* **50**, 41–64.

Waters, E., Kondo-Ikemura, K., Posada, G. and Richters, J.E. (1991) Learning to love: mechanisms and milestones. In Gunnar, M. and Sroufe, L.A. (Eds), *Minnesota Symposium on Child Psychology. Vol. 23.* Hillsdale, NJ: Erlbaum, 217–55.

Waters, E., Merrick, S.K., Albersheim, L.J. and Treboux, D. (1995) Attachment security from infancy to early adulthood: a 20-year longitudinal study. Presented at the Meeting of the Society for Research in Child Development, Indianapolis, IN, March 1995.

Waters, E., Vaughn, B.E. and Egeland, B.R. (1980) Individual differences in infant–mother attachment relationships at age one: antecedents in neonatal behavior in an urban, economically disadvantaged sample. *Child Development* **51**, 208–16.

Waters, E., Vaughn, B.E., Posada, G. and Kondo-Ikemura, K. (Eds) (1995) Caregiving, cultural and cognitive perspectives on secure-base behavior and working models. *Monographs of the Society for Research in Child Development*, **60**.

Waters, E., Wippman, J. and Sroufe, L.A. (1979) Attachment, positive affect and competence in the peer group: two studies in construct validation. *Child Development* 50, 821–9.

Waters, H.S. and Hou, F. (1987) Children's production and recall of narrative passages. *Journal of Experimental Child Psychology* 55, 348–63.

Wedell-Monnig, J. and Lumley, J.M. (1980) Child deafness and mother–child interaction. *Child Development* 49, 580–89.

West, M. and Sheldon-Keller, A.E. (1994) *Patterns of relating: an adult attachment perspective*. New York: Guilford Press.

West, M., Sheldon-Keller, A.E. and Reiffer, L. (1987) An approach to delineation of adult attachment: scale development and reliability. *Journal of Nervous and Mental Disease* 175, 738–41.

Winnicott, D.W. (1964) *The child, the family and the outside world*. Harmondsworth: Penguin.

Wright, J.C., Binney, V. and Smith, P.K. (1995) Security of attachment in 8 to 12-year-olds: a revised version of the Separation Anxiety Test, its psychometric properties and clinical interpretation. *Journal of Child Psychology and Psychology* 36, 757–74.

Yogman, M.W. (1983) Development of the father–infant relationship. In Fitzgerald, H.E., Lester, B.M. and Yogman, M.W. (Eds), *Theory and research in behavioral pediatrics. Vol. 1*. New York: Plenum, 221–80.

Youngblade, L.M. and Belsky, J. (1992) Parent–child antecedents of 5-year-olds' close friendships: a longitudinal analysis. *Developmental Psychology* 28, 700–13.

Zeanah, C.H. (1996) Beyond insecurity: a reconceptualization of attachment disorders in infancy. *Journal of Consulting and Clinical Psychology* 64, 42–52.

Zeanah, C.H., Benoit, D., Barton, M., Regan, C., Hirschberg, L. and Lipsett, L. (1993) Representations of attachment in mothers and their one-year-old infants. *Journal of the Academy of Child and Adolescent Psychiatry* 32, 278–86.

Zeanah, C.H., Benoit, D., Hirshberg, L., Barton, M.L. and Regan, C. (1994) Mothers' representations of their infants are concordant with infant attachment classifications. *Developmental Issues in Psychiatry and Psychology* 1, 1–14.

Zeanah, C.H., Finley-Belgrad, E. and Benoit, D. (1997) Intergenerational transmission of relationship psychopathology: a mother–infant case study. In Atkinson, L. and Zucker, K. (Eds), *Attachment and psychopathology*. New York: Guilford Press, 292–318.

Zimmerman, P. (1994) *Bindung im judendalter: Entwicklung und umgang mit aktuellen anforderungen (Attachment in adolescence: development while coping with actual challenges)*. Unpublished doctoral dissertation. University of Regensburg, Regensburg, Germany.

Author index

Subject index